Chemotherapy for Leukemia

Takanori Ueda
Editor

Chemotherapy for Leukemia

Novel Drugs and Treatment

Springer

Editor
Takanori Ueda
Vice-President, University of Fukui
Fukui, Japan

ISBN 978-981-10-3330-8 ISBN 978-981-10-3332-2 (eBook)
DOI 10.1007/978-981-10-3332-2

Library of Congress Control Number: 2017939138

Printed on acid-free paper

This Springer imprint is published by Springer Nature
The registered company is Springer Nature Singapore Pte Ltd.
The registered company address is: 152 Beach Road, #21-01/04 Gateway East, Singapore 189721, Singapore

Preface

Chemotherapy for Leukemia: Novel Drugs and Treatment covers the most recent progress in chemotherapy for leukemia and related diseases, including promising studies that are still in progress.

The book consists of three parts:

1. Molecular targeted therapy
2. Novel chemotherapeutic agents, including antimetabolite analogues
3. Therapy targeting leukemic stem cells

Every drug presented will be of great interest to hemato-oncologists. The focus is on the drug and not treatment protocols. The book is designed to be a practical guide for drug selection decisions, and drugs are described basically, pharmacokinetically, and clinically by leading experts in each field.

I will be very happy if this book helps hemato-oncologists to cure, or improve the outcomes of, leukemia patients.

I would like to thank very much the contributing authors from many countries for providing their input despite their busy schedules and Dr. Takahiro Yamauchi for his excellent scientific advice. Thanks are also due to Ms. Yoko Arai for the proposal to publish this book and her editorial advice, Ms. Tamaki Yamamoto and Ms. Makie Kambara for the editorial assistance, and Ms. Juri Hashimoto, Ms. Rie Yamagishi, and Ms. Hitomi Takeuchi for the excellent secretarial assistance.

Finally, I owe much to my wife, children, and grandchildren, who have provided invaluable support.

Fukui, Japan
November 2016

Takanori Ueda

Contents

An Overview

1

Takanori Ueda

Abstract

There has been remarkable progress in chemotherapy for leukemia and related diseases, including promising studies that are still in progress. The contents consist of three parts:

1. Molecular targeted therapy
2. Novel chemotherapeutic agents, including antimetabolite analogs
3. Therapy targeting leukemic stem cells

In this chapter, an overview of these drugs presented in this book is briefly described.

Keywords

Molecular targeted therapy • Leukemic stem cells • Oncogenic addiction • Bcr-Abl tyrosine kinase inhibitors

In the last 20 years, there has been remarkable progress in leukemia chemotherapy (Table 1.1), and the factors listed below are the main reasons for the significant improvements in patient outcomes (Fig. 1.1):

1. The development of effective and less toxic molecular targeted drugs
2. The development of other highly effective anticancer chemotherapeutic agents
3. The introduction of immunotherapy

T. Ueda (✉)
Vice-President, University of Fukui, 3-9-1 Bunkyo, Fukui 910-8507, Japan
e-mail: tueda@u-fukui.ac.jp

T. Ueda (ed.), *Chemotherapy for Leukemia*, DOI 10.1007/978-981-10-3332-2_1

Table 1.1 Novel agents for leukemia chemotherapy

1. *Bcr-Abl tyrosine kinase inhibitors (TKIs)*
Imatinib
Nilotinib, dasatinib, ponatinib, and other TKIs
2. *New antibodies for leukemia*
Rituximab for chronic lymphocytic leukemia
Alemtuzumab for chronic lymphocytic leukemia
Inotuzumab ozogamicin for acute lymphoblastic leukemia
Blinatumomab for acute lymphoblastic leukemia
Mogamulizumab, anti-chemokine receptor 4 (anti CCR4) for adult T-cell leukemia/lymphoma
3. *Signaling inhibitors*
Aurora-kinase inhibitors[a]
FLT3 inhibitors
4. *Differentiating agents*
Retinoic acid: all-trans-retinoic acid (ATRA) and tamibarotene
Arsenic trioxide
5. *New chemotherapeutic agents, including antimetabolites*
Nelarabine, specifically active in T-cell neoplasms
Forodesine, specifically active in lymphoid neoplasms
Clofarabine, active for lymphoid and myeloid neoplasms
Epigenetic regulators
Isocitrate dehydrogenase (IDH) 1 and 2 inhibitor[a]
6. *Therapy targeting leukemic stem cells*

[a]Not described in this book

4. The identification of leukemic stem cells [1], the realization that these cells are crucial players in leukemia drug resistance, and the development of strategies to target this cell population
5. Progress in stem cell transplantation for refractory and chemotherapy-resistant leukemia
6. Outstanding progress in supportive care for anticancer chemotherapy

Recently, about 80% of patients suffering from adult acute myeloid leukemia achieved complete remission [2]. However, even among low-risk patients with core-binding factor leukemias, there was a high mortality rate of 40% at 5 years from the start of chemotherapy [3], suggesting that more than 50% of the patients in complete remission had relapsed.

Many molecular targeted drugs have been introduced to leukemia chemotherapy in an attempt to improve cure rates, and previously we proposed three categories for clinical use [4].

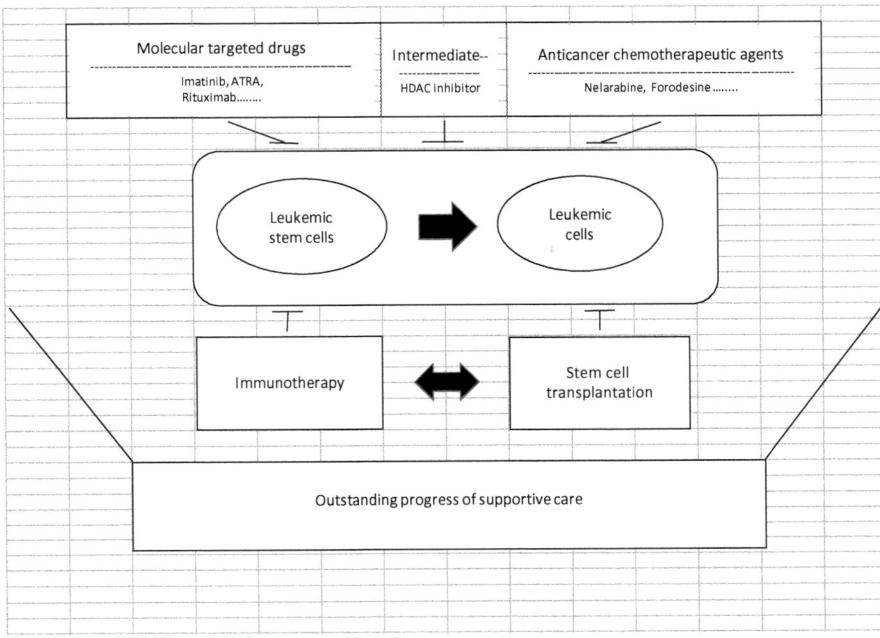

Fig. 1.1 Recent progress of chemotherapy for leukemia

1.1 Category 1 Drugs

This category includes drugs targeting abnormal small molecules that are specific to neoplastic cells that show typical oncogenic addiction [5]. However, only two kinds of drugs have been shown to be effective, including imatinib and the related Bcr-Abl tyrosine kinase inhibitors (TKIs) for chronic myeloid leukemia (CML) [6] and retinoids (all-trans-retinoic acid) [7], tamibarotene [8]), and arsenic trioxide [7] for acute promyelocytic leukemia (APL).

It is important to understand not only why the drugs mentioned above are so effective for the treatment of CML and APL but also why so many drugs are ineffective.

In this regard, it is curious that other cancers with specific driver genes do not necessarily show marked oncogenic addiction. Is the effectiveness of the targeted CML and APL drugs based on the pharmacodynamic action of the drugs on the specific target molecules of the disease, or might there also be other reasons why imatinib and ATRA are so effective?

CML is relatively resistant to standard antileukemic chemotherapy, and almost all patients who do not receive allogeneic stem cell transplantation die within 10 years from onset. However, even before the imatinib era, CML was known to be relatively sensitive to interferon-α [9]. Donor leukocyte infusion (DLI) [10] after allogeneic stem cell transplantation is also effective for CML. Although both treatment modalities were originally expected to be highly effective for the treatment of a broad spectrum of malignancies, this was not actually the case. The effectiveness of interferon-α and DLI suggests that CML is a somewhat unique disease entity compared with other leukemias, although the reasons for the interferon-α and DLI sensitivity have not been determined.

The pathogenesis of APL is shown to be linked to the inhibition of granulocyte differentiation. Inhibition of differentiation is involved in the pathogenesis of leukemia and even some solid cancers. However, like CML, APL is unique because of the dramatic success of new treatment modalities, namely, differentiation induction therapy, to overcome the PML-RARA fusion gene-mediated inhibition of differentiation of myeloid cells. Moreover, although arsenic trioxide is remarkably effective for the treatment of APL [7], the differentiation inducer does not have a prominent effect on other leukemias.

The success of these pioneering drugs for the treatment of CML and APL appears to be disease specific and based on the unique molecular targets present in these cancers, although other unique biological and/or genetic characteristics of CML and APL are likely to be important. Interestingly, although several fascinating molecular targeted drugs, such as aurora-kinase inhibitors, have been assessed experimentally and clinically for the treatment of non-CML/APL leukemias, these drugs have not had the spectacular success seen with imatinib/CML and ATRA/APL.

Thus, the strategy for the introduction of new molecular targeted drugs requires a detailed understanding of the biological characteristics, as well as the principal molecular aberrations of the leukemia cells in question.

As described above, CML (as a Bcr-Abl disease) and APL were thought to be typical rare cases of oncogenic addiction [5], in which inactivation of a single critical oncogene can induce cancer cells to differentiate into cells with a normal phenotype or to undergo apoptosis. To comprehensively understand CML and APL pathogenesis and ultimately develop more effective targeted treatments, it is crucial to clarify the mechanisms that drive and maintain oncogene addiction.

1.2 Category 2 Drugs

This category includes drugs that target proteins that are selectively overexpressed, or are more active, in neoplastic cells compared with normal cells. Most molecular targeted drugs belong to this category. For example, erlotinib [11] is a specific inhibitor of epidermal growth factor receptor tyrosine kinase, which is abundantly expressed in various types of neoplastic cells compared with normal cells. Similarly, cytarabine (ara-C) is an inhibitor of DNA polymerase α and β (in high concentration), which is more active in neoplastic cells compared with normal cells. As these drugs target normal cells as well as cancer cells, there may not be significant qualitative differences between category 2 drugs and some classical anticancer drugs. Indeed, although classical anticancer agents are usually more toxic than molecular targeted drugs, the latter sometimes induce specific severe side effects, such as interstitial lung disease [12] and cytokine storm [13]. Thus, classical anticancer agents might be a good match for at least some category 2 molecular targeted drugs in total clinical benefit.

Among recently developed molecular targeted drugs, FLT3 inhibitors show promise [14], with effects similar to category 1 drugs.

1.3 Category 3 Drugs

This category of molecular targeted drugs includes monoclonal antibodies effective for the treatment of patients with leukemia. Typical therapeutic monoclonal antibodies [15, 16] cause the death of neoplastic cells by direct induction of apoptosis, antibody-dependent cell-mediated cytotoxicity (ADCC), or complement-dependent cytotoxicity (CDC). Monoclonal antibodies coupled to radioactive agents (ibritumomab tiuxetan Y-90) [17] or cytotoxic agents (inotuzumab ozogamicin) [18] are also available. Among them, rituximab [15], alemtuzumab [16], inotuzumab ozogamicin [18], blinatumomab [19], and mogamulizumab [20] are key, or promising, agents for the treatment of patients with leukemia.

The recent progress in cancer chemotherapy is not only limited to molecular targeted drugs; classical chemotherapeutic agents still play important roles. Examples include the newly available antimetabolites, nelarabine [21], forodesine [22], and clofarabine [23], which are antipurinergic agents mainly effective for lymphoid malignancies. The remarkable progress in supportive care, including infection control, suggests that these drugs could be safely introduced into the clinic.

As alluded to above, the borderline between molecular targeted drugs and anticancer chemotherapeutic drugs is sometimes blurred. Good examples are the antimetabolites, azacitidine [24, 25], and decitabine [26]. Although both are cytidine derivatives that have antineoplastic activity similar to ara-C analogs, at low doses these drugs were recently shown to act as epigenetic regulators [27] such as HDAC inhibitors, azacytidine, and decitabine.

1.4 Leukemic Stem Cells

It is clear that the elimination of leukemic stem cells is a key to improve outcomes [1]. All leukemias contain leukemic stem cells, with specific characteristics depending on the type of leukemia [28]. Clinically, the most crucial characteristics of leukemic stem cells are deregulated self-renewal and proliferation and a range of chemoresistance characteristics, including a high population of dormant cells in the niche [29, 30], multidrug resistance mechanisms [31, 32], and a high level of reactive oxygen species (ROS) [33].

At present, the targets of leukemia chemotherapy are leukemic clones, and the strategy is to prevent the emergence of resistant clones by prompt and intensive combination chemotherapy. In leukemic relapse, the disease is usually refractory to multiple drugs by multifactorial mechanisms of resistance [34]. The mechanisms may be specific for the particular multidrug combination chemotherapy and different from the summation of the resistance mechanisms associated with single drug administration

[35]. It is possible that this phenomenon could be overcome by high-dose chemotherapy or novel drugs with different modes of action and/or new targets.

If the real target is leukemic stem cells, we might not need to be as concerned about the leukemic cells at different maturation stages. It is interesting that about 40% of low-risk leukemia patients are cured, suggesting that current treatment protocols effectively kill both leukemic cells and leukemic stem cells. On the other hand, for relapse patients, combination chemotherapy is clearly ineffective, suggesting that current high-intensity protocols do not eliminate leukemic stem cells. Ongoing detailed analyses of the differences in pharmacokinetics/pharmacodynamics between leukemic cells and leukemic stem cells will provide invaluable clues for the design of new drugs capable of targeting and eliminating leukemic stem cell populations.

References

1. Bonnet D, Dick JE. Human acute myeloid leukemia is organized as a hierarchy that originates from a primitive hematopoietic cell. Nat Med. 1997;3:730–7.
2. Ohtake S, Miyawaki S, Fujita H, Kiyoi H, Shinagawa K, Usui N, et al. Randomized study of induction therapy comparing standard-dose idarubicin with high-dose daunorubicin in adult patients with previously untreated acute myeloid leukemia: the JALSG AML201 Study. Blood. 2011;117:2358–65.
3. Burnett A, Wetzler M, Löwenberg B. Therapeutic advances in acute myeloid leukemia. J Clin Oncol. 2011;29:487–94.
4. Ueda T. Update on molecular-targeted therapy in hematologic malignancies. Int J Clin Oncol. 2007;12:311–2.
5. Weinstein IB. Addiction to oncogenes – the Achilles heal of cancer. Science. 2002;297:63–4.
6. Apperley JF. Chronic myeloid leukaemia. Lancet. 2015;385:1447–59.
7. Lo-Coco F, Avvisati G, Vignetti M, Thiede C, Orlando SM, Iacobelli S, et al. Retinoic acid and arsenic trioxide for acute promyelocytic leukemia. N Engl J Med. 2013;369:111–21.
8. Shinagawa K, Yanada M, Sakura T, Ueda Y, Sawa M, Miyatake J, et al. Tamibarotene as maintenance therapy for acute promyelocytic leukemia: results from a randomized controlled trial. J Clin Oncol. 2014;32:3692–6.
9. Talpaz M, Kantarjian HM, McCredie K, Trujillo JM, Keating MJ, Gutterman JU. Hematologic remission and cytogenetic improvement induced by recombinant human interferon alpha A in chronic myelogenous leukemia. N Engl J Med. 1986;314:1065–9.
10. Kolb HJ, Schattenberg A, Goldman JM, Hertenstein B, Jacobsen N, Arcese W, et al. Graft-versus-leukemia effect of donor lymphocyte transfusions in marrow grafted patients. Blood. 1995;86:2041–50.
11. Shepherd FA, Rodriques Pereira J, Ciuleanu T, Tan EH, Hirsh V, Thonqprasert S, et al. Erlotinib in previously treated non-small-cell lung cancer. N Engl J Med. 2005;353:123–32.
12. Ando M, Okamoto I, Yamamoto N, Takeda K, Tamura K, Seto T, et al. Predictive factors for interstitial lung disease, antitumor response, and survival in non-small-cell lung cancer patients treated with gefitinib. J Clin Oncol. 2006;24:2549–56.
13. Suntharalingam G, Perry MR, Ward S, Brett SJ, Castello-Cortes A, Brunner MD, et al. Cytokine storm in a phase 1 trial of the anti-CD28 monoclonal antibody TGN1412. N Engl J Med. 2006;355:1018–28.
14. Galanis A, Ma H, Rajkhowa T, Ramachandran A, Small D, Cortes J, et al. Crenolanib is a potent inhibitor of FLT3 with activity against resistance-conferring point mutants. Blood. 2014;123:94–100. doi:10.1182/blood-2013-10-529313.
15. Reff ME, Carner K, Chambers KS, Chinn PC, Leonard JE, Raab R, et al. Depletion of B cells in vivo by a chimeric mouse human monoclonal antibody to CD20. Blood. 1994;83:435–45.

16. Keating ML, Flinn I, Jain V, Binet JL, Hillmen P, Byrd J, et al. Therapeutic role of alemtuzumab (Campath-1H) in patients who have failed fludarabine: results of a large international study. Blood. 2002;99:3554–61.
17. Matesan M, Rajendran J, Press OW, Maloney DG, Storb RF, Cassaday JM, et al. 90Y-ibritumomab tiuxetan therapy in allogeneic transplantation in B-cell lymphoma with extensive marrow involvement and chronic lymphocytic leukemia: utility of pretransplantation biodistribution. Nucl Med Commun. 2014;35:1132–42.
18. Kantarjian HM, DeAngelo DJ, Stelljes M, Martinelli G, Liedtke M, Stock W, et al. Inotuzumab Ozogamicin versus standard therapy for acute lymphoblastic leukemia. N Engl J Med. 2016; doi:10.1056/NEJMoa1509277.
19. Topp MS, Gökbuget N, Stein AS, Zugmaier G, O'Brien S, Bargou RC, et al. Safety and activity of blinatumomab for adult patients with relapsed or refractory B-precursor acute lymphoblastic leukaemia: a multicentre, single-arm, phase 2 study. Lancet Oncol. 2014;15:57–66.
20. Ishida T, Joh T, Uike N, Yamamoto K, Utsunomiya A, Yoshida S. Defucosylated anti-CCR4 monoclonal antibody (KW-0761) for relapsed adult T-cell leukemia-lymphoma: a multicenter phase II study. J Clin Oncol. 2012;30:837–42.
21. Cohen MH, Johnson JR, Massie T, Sridhara R, McGuinn Jr WD, Abraham S, et al. Approval summary: nelarabine for the treatment of T-cell lymphoblastic leukemia/lymphoma. Clin Cancer Res. 2006;12:5329–35.
22. Gandhi V, Kilpatrick JM, Plunkett W, Ayres M, Harman L, Du M, et al. A proof-of-principle pharmacokinetic, pharmacodynamic, and clinical study with purine nucleoside phosphorylase inhibitor immucillin-H (BCX-1777, forodesine). Blood. 2005;106:4253–60.
23. Kantarjian H, Gandhi V, Cortes J, Verstovsek S, Du M, Garcia-Manero G, et al. Phase 2 clinical and pharmacologic study of clofarabine in patients with refractory or relapsed acute leukemia. Blood. 2003;102:2379–86.
24. Cihak A. Biological effects of 5-azacytidine in eukaryotes. Oncology. 1974;30:405–22.
25. Issa JP, Kantarjian HM, Kirkpatrick P. Azacitidine. Nat Rev Drug Discov. 2005;4:275–6.
26. Kantarijian H, Issa JP, Rosenfeld CS, Bennett JM, DiPersio J, Klimek V, et al. Decitabine improves patient outcomes in myelodysplastic syndromes. Cancer. 2006;106:1794–803.
27. Merlevede J, Droin N, Qin T, Meldi K, Yoshida K, Morabito M, et al. Mutation allele burden remains unchanged in chronic myelomonocytic leukaemia responding to hypomethylating agents. Nat Commun. 2016; doi:10.1038/ncomms10767.
28. Anderson K, Lutz C, van Delft FW, Bateman CM, Guo Y, Colman SM, et al. Genetic variegation of clonal architecture and propagating cells in leukaemia. Nature. 2011;469:356–61.
29. Aguirre-Ghiso JA. Models, mechanisms and clinical evidence for cancer dormancy. Nat Rev Cancer. 2007;7:834–46.
30. Ishikawa F, Yoshida S, Saito Y, Hijikata H, Kitamura H, Tanaka S, et al. Chemotherapy-resistant human AML stem cells home to and engraft within the bone-marrow endosteal region. Nat Biotechnol. 2007;25:1315–21.
31. Chen CJ, Chin JE, Ueda K, Clark DP, Pastan I, Gottesman MM, et al. Internal duplication and homology with bacterial transport proteins in the mdr1 (P-glycoprotein) gene from multidrug-resistant human cells. Cell. 1986;47:381–9.
32. Dean M, Fojo T, Bates S. Tumour stem cells and drug resistance. Nat Rev Cancer. 2005;5:275–84.
33. Takubo K, Goda N, Yamada W, Iriuchishima H, Ikeda E, Kubota Y, et al. Regulation of the HIF-1alpha level is essential for hematopoietic stem cells. Cell Stem Cell. 2010;7:391–402.
34. Urasaki Y, Ueda T, Nakamura T. Circumvention of daunorubicin resistance by a new tamoxifen derivative, toremifene, in multidrug-resistant cell line. Jpn J Cancer Res. 1994;85:659–64.
35. Takemura H, Urasaki Y, Yoshida A, Fukushima T, Ueda T. Simultaneous treatment with 1-beta-D-arabinofuranosylcytosine and daunorubicin induces cross-resistance to both drugs due to a combination-specific mechanism in HL60 cells. Cancer Res. 2001;61:172–7.

Part I

Bcr-Abl Tyrosine Kinase Inhibitors (TKIs)

Imatinib: Basic Results

2

Fujiko Tsukahara and Yoshiro Maru

Abstract

Chronic myeloid leukemia (CML) is a clonal hematopoietic stem cell disorder characterized by the reciprocal translocation t(9;22), which leads to the production of the Philadelphia (Ph) chromosome, encoding BCR-ABL tyrosine kinase. BCR-ABL is constitutively activated and induces malignant transformation of primitive hematopoietic cells. Imatinib mesylate (also known as STI571, GLEEVEC, or GLIVEC) is a 2-phenylaminopyrimidine derivative that received FDA approval as the first mechanism-based targeted small-molecule protein kinase inhibitor in 2001. Imatinib acts as an ATP-competitive inhibitor via interaction with the ABL kinase domain that results in the formation of six hydrogen bonds and through direct inhibition of BCR-ABL kinase activity. It inhibits BCR-ABL's ability to transfer phosphate groups to tyrosine residues on the substrate, which blocks the subsequent activation of the proliferative signals. Although imatinib is an effective frontline therapy that has provided a remarkable success in the treatment of CML, the resistance to the inhibitor is still an obstacle. Quiescent leukemic stem cells are unresponsive to imatinib. BCR-ABL-dependent and BCR-ABL-independent mechanisms of drug resistance have been reported. To overcome imatinib resistance, the pharmacological targeting of key pathways alone or in combination with tyrosine kinase inhibitor (TKI) is being investigated.

Keywords

Imatinib • Chronic myeloid leukemia • BCR-ABL

F. Tsukahara • Y. Maru (✉)
Department of Pharmacology, Tokyo Women's Medical University School of Medicine,
8-1 Kawada-cho, Shinjuku-ku, Tokyo 162-8666, Japan
e-mail: maru.yoshiro@twmu.ac.jp

T. Ueda (ed.), *Chemotherapy for Leukemia*, DOI 10.1007/978-981-10-3332-2_2

2.1 Development of Imatinib

In 1845, Bennet, Craigie, and Virchow independently recognized and described a distinct entity of white blood [1]. Virchow first used the term "leukemia" in 1857. In 1960, two Philadelphia researchers, Nowell and Hungerford, discovered a consistent chromosomal abnormality characteristic of chronic myelogenous leukemia (CML), and this chromosome was subsequently named the Philadelphia (Ph) chromosome [2]. This was the first demonstration of a chromosomal rearrangement being consistently linked to a malignant disease. In 1967, the presence of the Ph chromosome in the hematopoietic stem cell of CML patients was confirmed by cell surface markers [3]. In 1973, Rowley et al. discovered that the Ph chromosome was the product of a reciprocal translocation between the long arms of chromosomes 9 and 22 t(9;22)-(q34;q11) [4]. In 1984, the ABL gene on chromosome 9, a human homolog of v-ABL [5, 6], and the translocation partner breakpoint cluster region (BCR) gene on chromosome 22 were identified in the Ph chromosome [7, 8]. The chimeric BCR-ABL gene product was found to have deregulated tyrosine kinase activity [9]. Mice-administered transplants of the bone marrow cells infected with a retrovirus-mediated expression of p210 BCR-ABL developed CML-like diseases [10], and p185/p190 BCR-ABL transgenic mice developed acute leukemia [11]. Thus, BCR-ABL was found to be not only a marker but also the cause of the hematopoietic malignancy of CML and acute lymphocytic leukemia (ALL). Thus, targeting the BCR-ABL kinase was thought important in the treatment of the hematopoietic malignancy.

In the late 1980s, investigators at Ciba-Geigy, now Novartis, originally initiated a random screening of archived inhibitors for the protein kinase Cα and identified a 2-phenylaminopyrimidine derivative as a lead compound [12]. From this compound, a series of derivatives were further synthesized, and their specificity for several serine/threonine and tyrosine kinases was profiled. In 1996, Druker and colleagues found that CGP57148 selectively inhibited both the growth of BCR-ABL-expressing cells and BCR-ABL-induced tumor in mice. Colony formation of peripheral blood or bone marrow from CML patients was also selectively inhibited [13]. This compound was first named STI571 and then imatinib. In 1998, phase 1 study of imatinib mesylate treatment in chronic CML patients started, and the drug received FDA approval as the first mechanism-based targeted small-molecule protein kinase inhibitor in 2001 [14, 15] (Fig. 2.1).

2.2 Molecular Biology of CML

2.2.1 Ph Chromosome

The Ph chromosome results from a reciprocal translocation, which involves the BCR gene on chromosome 22 at band q11 and the ABL proto-oncogene on chromosome 9 at band q34, t(9; 22)(q34; q11) [4] (Fig. 2.2a). Depending on the breakpoints in the BCR gene, there are three different forms of the BCR-ABL

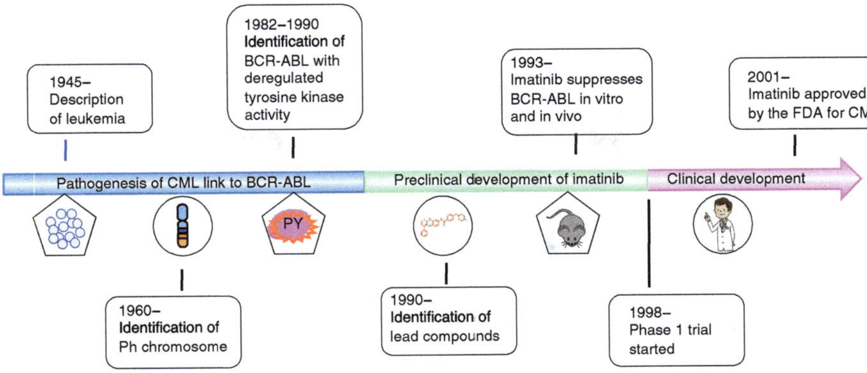

Fig. 2.1 Timeline of BCR-ABL findings and development of imatinib

oncogene: p185/p190 (m-bcr breakpoint), p210 (M-bcr breakpoint), and p230 (μ-bcr breakpoint) (Fig. 2.2b, c). p210 BCR-ABL is observed in 90% of CML, p185/190 BCR-ABL in 20–30% of ALL, and p230 BCR-ABL in a subset of patients with chronic neutrophilic leukemia (CNL) patients [16].

2.2.2 Structure and Intramolecular Interaction of BCR-ABL

The structure of p210 BCR-ABL is shown in Fig. 2.3a. The tyrosine kinase c-ABL is negatively regulated by interactions between its SH3 and SH2 domains and the distal surface of the kinase domain. The myristoyl group of c-ABL is inserted into the hydrophobic pocket of the kinase domain to dock of the SH2 and SH3 domains onto the kinase domain [17]. The interface between the SH3 domain and the linker segment connecting the SH2 and the kinase domains also provides negative regulation [18]. In contrast, BCR-ABL exists primarily as a dimmer or tetramer to facilitate trans-autophosphorylation. The N-terminal coiled-coil oligomerization domain in the BCR sequence plays an essential role in the activation of BCR-ABL, which is similar to ligand-induced dimerization and subsequent activation of receptor tyrosine kinases [19, 20]. In an activated state of BCR-ABL, the inhibition through the SH3 domain and the linker region is released, and the SH2 domain not only binds the N-lobe via tight interactions between I145 and T272/Y312 but also the SH2-binding domain in the BCR sequence as well as SH2 ligands [21] (Fig. 2.3b).

2.2.3 Signaling Pathways Downstream of BCR-ABL

The deregulated BCR-ABL activates a large number of signal transduction pathways including Ras, signal transducer and activator of transcription-5 (STAT5), phosphatidylinositol 3-kinase (PI3), Myc, RhoA-Rac, and cyclin D1, which lead to uncontrolled proliferation and differentiation, resistance to apoptosis,

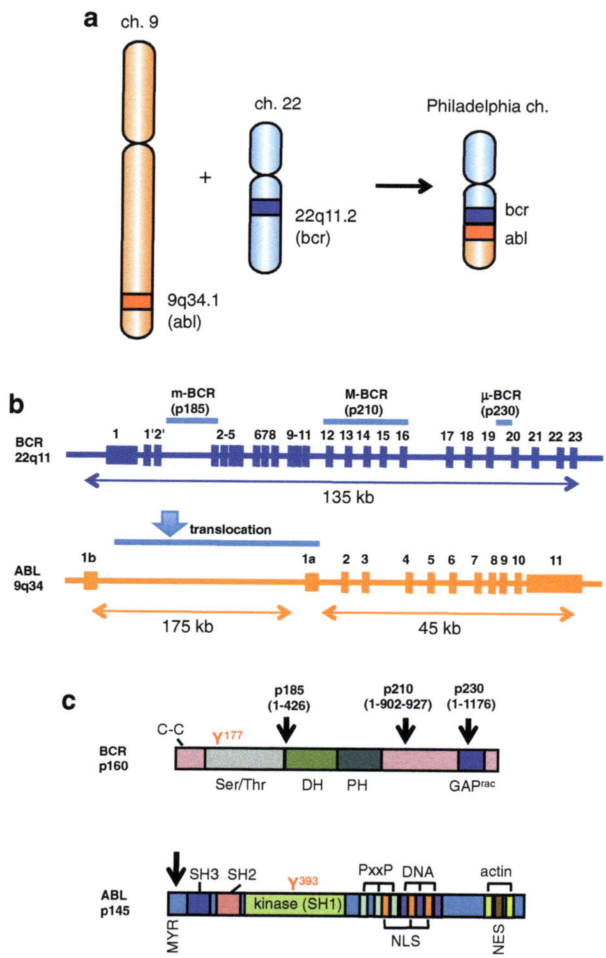

Fig. 2.2 Philadelphia chromosome (**a**) and localization of the breakpoints in the ABL and BCR genes (**b**) and proteins (**c**). **a** The fusion BCR-ABL gene is formed within Ph chromosome as a result of a reciprocal translocation between chromosomes 22 and 9. **b** BCR has three breakpoint cluster regions indicated as m-BCR, M-BCR, and µ-BCR, for p185/190, p210, and p230 BCR-ABL genes, respectively. The ABL gene has alternately spliced first exons Ib and Ia. An *arrowhead* indicates the region of the translocation. **c** BCR consists of the coiled-coil (C–C) domain and a region exhibiting serine/threonine kinase activity in the N-terminus region. Y177 is the autophosphorylation site crucial for binding to growth factor receptor-bound protein 2 (Grb2). The center region contains a dbl-like domain (DH) and pleckstrin homology (PH) domains. Toward the C-terminus is a domain with an activating function for Rac-GTPase (Rac-GAP). ABL consists of a myristoylation (MYR) site and SH3 and SH2 domains in the N-terminus region. Y393 is the major site of autophosphorylation within the kinase (SH1) domain. The middle region consists of proline-rich regions (PxxP), nuclear localization signal (NLS), nuclear export signal (NES), and DNA-binding region (DNA). The C-terminus contains G- and F-actin-binding domain (actin). *Arrowheads* indicate the position of the breakpoints in the p185/190, 210, and 230 BCR-ABL proteins, respectively

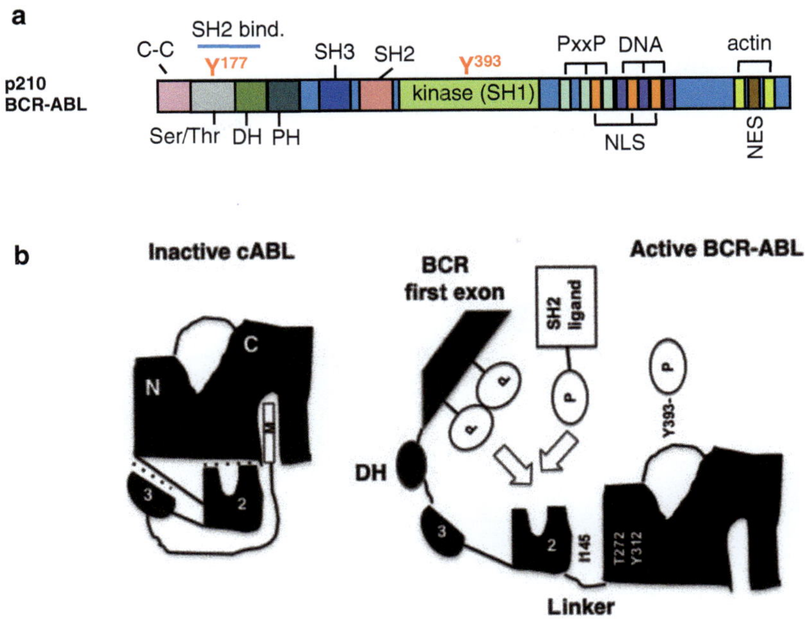

Fig. 2.3 Structure and intramolecular interaction of BCR-ABL. **a** The p210 BCR-ABL protein contains the coiled-coil (C–C) domain, Ser/Thr kinase domain, dbl-like domain (DH), and pleckstrin homology (PH) domains from BCR, as well as the SH domains, proline-rich (PxxP), nuclear localization signal (NLS), nuclear export signal (NES), DNA-binding (DNA), and actin-binding domains (actin) from ABL. The tyrosine residues in the Ser/Thr (Y177) and SH1 kinase (Y393) domains have been highlighted. **b** Intramolecular inhibitory folding through the interactions between domains is shown with *dotted lines*, including binding between (1) the SH3 domain and the SH2 linker, (2) the SH2 and the tyrosine kinase domains, and (3) the myristoyl group in N-terminal ABL and the tyrosine kinase domain. The inhibitory folding in the inactive state in c-ABL is released in BCR-ABL, allowing autophosphorylation in the activation loop at Y393 and the interaction between (1) the SH2 domain and the N-lobe and (2) the SH2 ligands and the SH2 domain (see details in the text; Maru [22])

cell migration, and unique metabolism and defect in DNA repair in progenitor cells [22] (Fig. 2.4).

2.3 Mechanism of BCR-ABL Inhibition by Imatinib

Imatinib acts as an ATP-competitive tyrosine kinase inhibitor (TKI) via interaction with the ABL kinase domain. Binding of imatinib prevents BCR-ABL's ability to transfer a phosphate group onto tyrosine on the substrate and its subsequent activation, which blocks the transmission of proliferative signals to the nucleus, thus inducing apoptosis in the leukemic cell [23] (Fig. 2.5).

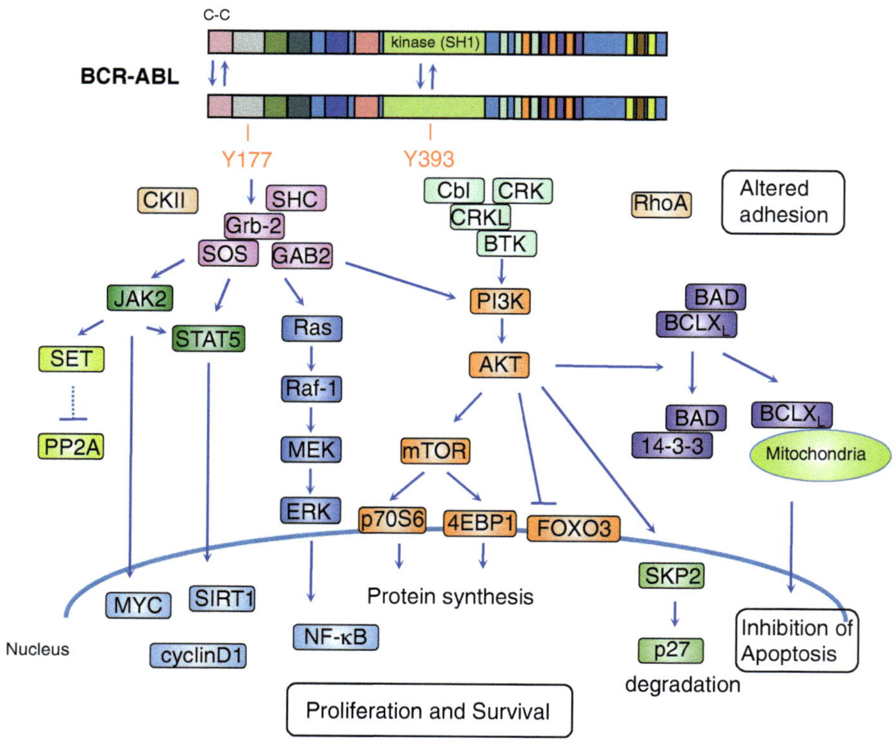

Fig. 2.4 Schematic representation of the downstream molecular pathways of BCR-ABL. Dimerization of BCR-ABL via the N-terminal coiled-coil domain activates BCR-ABL kinase leading to autophosphorylation of Y393 in ABL followed by Y177 in BCR. The phosphorylation of Y177 recruits Grb2, SOS (a guanine nucleotide exchanger of RAS), and Grb2-associated-binding protein 2 (GAB2) complex. This complex activates Ras/MAPK/ERK, phosphatidylinositol 3-kinase (PI3K)/AKT, and JAK/STAT signaling pathways. The activated AKT induces mTOR activation, suppression of forkhead O (FOXO) transcription factor, and proteosomal degradation of p27. PI3K-AKT also promotes phosphorylation of the proapoptotic protein Bad, leading to its interaction with chaperone protein 14-3-3, which in turn results in the restriction of Bad to the cytoplasm. This attenuates Bad opposing BCL2 and BCL-XL inhibition of apoptosis in the mitochondria. Both, through activation of JAK2, directly and indirectly, activate STAT5. JAK2 also activates the PP2A inhibitor, SET, leading to PP2A inhibition. These downstream signaling pathways of BCR-ABL promote proliferation and survival and inhibit apoptosis

2.3.1 Imatinib: Chemical Structure

Imatinib is a 4-[(4-methyl-1-piperazinyl)methyl]-n-[4-methyl-3-[[4-(3-pyridinyl)-2-pyrimidinyl]amino]phenyl]-benzamide monomethanesulfonate. N-methylpiperazine, as a polar side chain, is associated with good water solubility and oral bioavailability. The introduction of a flag-methyl group at the 6-position of the anilino phenyl ring increases the selectivity for ABL kinase. Cellular activity is enhanced by the addition of a 3′-pyridyl group at the 3′-position of the pyrimidine [15, 23] (Fig. 2.6).

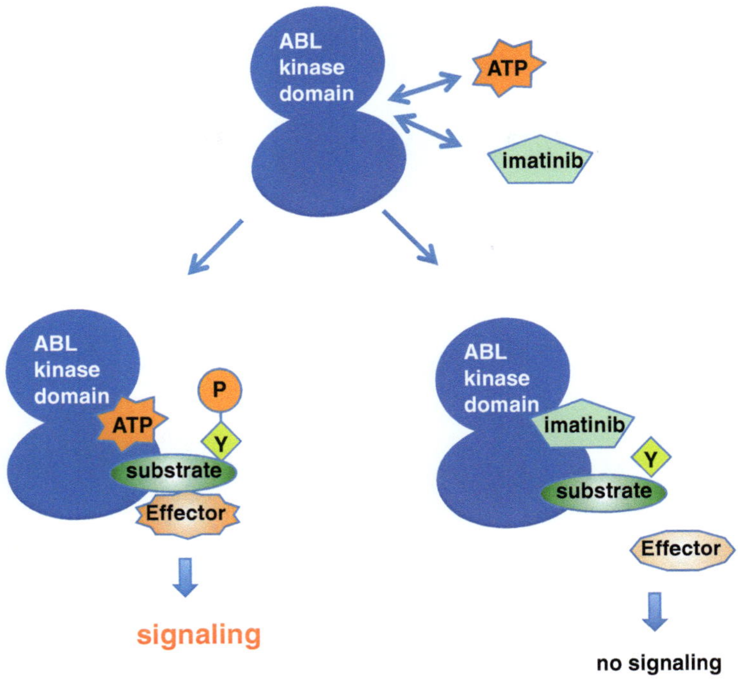

Fig. 2.5 Imatinib acts as an ATP-competitive inhibitor. The deregulated tyrosine kinase, BCR-ABL, functions by transferring phosphate from ATP to tyrosine residues on the substrates, which promotes downstream signaling pathways that lead to the stimulation of proliferation and inhibition of apoptosis. Imatinib competes with ATP at the BCR-ABL kinase domain and specifically inhibits the downstream signaling cascade

2.3.2 Imatinib and ABL Kinase Domain Interactions

The catalytic domain of protein kinase is well-conserved and consists of the N-lobe and the C-lobe. Imatinib functions through competitive inhibition of ATP at the ATP-binding site of the BCR-ABL kinase domain. The Asp-Phe-Gly (DFG) motif in the activation loop of the N-lobe, adjacent to the ATP-binding site, is very important for the kinase's inhibitors. The αC-helix in the C-lobe contributes to an on-off switch related to the conformational status of "ready-to-phosphorylate substrates." Type I and II inhibitors are the predominant groups of targeted protein kinase inhibitors [24]. The type I inhibitors recognize the active conformation of the kinase, while imatinib, which belongs to the type II protein kinase inhibitors, recognizes the inactive conformation of the enzyme [25]. The binding to a specific "DFG-out" conformation of BCR-ABL contributes to the selectivity of type II inhibitors. Imatinib interacts with 21 amino acid residues in the ABL kinase domain, forming six hydrogen bonds (Fig. 2.6). The aromatic ring of the inhibitor also interacts with the protein through van der Waals interactions [26].

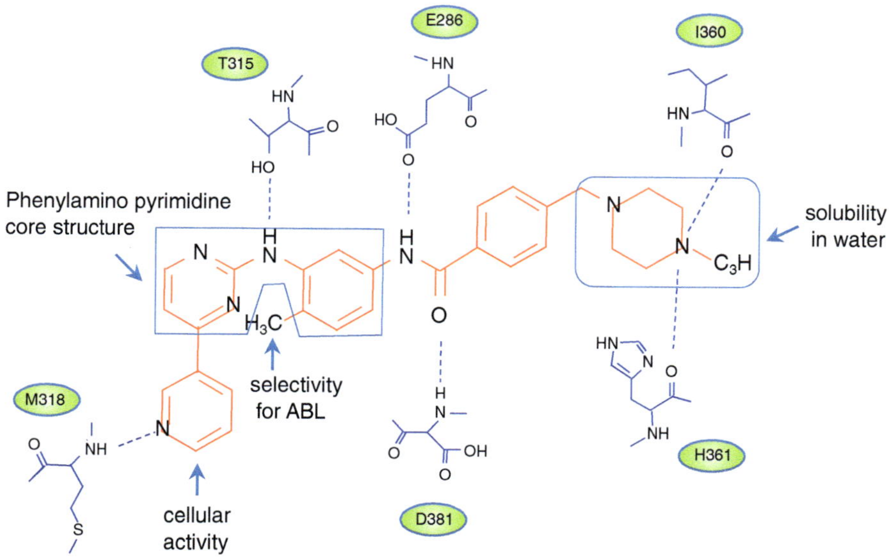

Fig. 2.6 Imatinib and ABL kinase domain interactions. Chemical structures of imatinib and schematic diagram showing the six hydrogen bonds between imatinib and the BCR-ABL kinase domain (see details in the text)

2.3.3 Imatinib: Pharmacodynamic Properties

In vitro kinase assay showed that imatinib potently inhibits ABL kinase and its active derivatives, BCR-ABL and v-ABL with IC_{50} values in the range of 0.025 μM for autophosphorylation. Imatinib also inhibits the platelet-derived growth factor receptor (PDGFR) and Steel factor receptor (c-KIT) kinases at a similar concentration. On the contrary, a large number of other kinases including Src family kinases such as c-Src, c-Lyn, and c-Lck and the epidermal growth factor receptor (EGFR) exhibited at least 100-fold higher IC_{50} values [13, 23] (Table 2.1). According to the substrate specificity, imatinib is not only approved for the treatment of Ph+ CML and ALL but also for the treatment of KIT-mutant-positive gastrointestinal stromal tumor (GIST) and myelodysplastic diseases with PDGFR gene rearrangements and hypereosinophilic syndrome with Fip1-like-1 (FIP1L1)-PDGFRα fusion proteins [27].

2.3.4 Effects of Imatinib on CML Mouse

Imatinib inhibits tumor growth in mice injected with BCR-ABL-transformed 32D cells and in nude mice injected with human BCR-ABL-positive KU812 cells [13, 28]. Imatinib significantly prolonged the survival of the murine bone marrow transduction-transplantation model of CML. Although all the animals exhibited prolonged survival after imatinib treatment, approximately 20% died of leukemia [29].

Table 2.1 Selectivity profile of imatinib

	IC_{50} (μM)
p210 BCR-ABL	0.025*
p185 BCR-ABL	0.025*
c-ABL	0.025*
v-ABL	0.038
PDGF receptor	0.038
c-Kit	0.41
FLT3	> 10
EGF receptor	> 100
Insulin receptor	> 10
IGF-1 receptor	> 10
c-Src	> 100
c-Lyn	> 100
c-Lck	9.0
JAK2	> 100*

Imatinib concentrations that cause 50% inhibition (IC_{50}) of autophosphorylation are given
PDGF platelet-derived growth factor, *FLT3* fms-related tyrosine kinase 3, *EGF* epidermal growth factor, *IGF-1* insulin-like growth factor-1
*IC_{50} was determined in immunocomplex assays (Deininger [23])

2.3.5 Mechanism of Imatinib-Induced Apoptosis

Imatinib induces apoptosis in BCR-ABL leukemic cells through upregulation of the proapoptotic proteins Bim and Bad. Suppression of Bim expression is sufficient to confer imatinib resistance [30–32].

2.4 Imatinib Resistance and Targeting Strategies to Overcome the Resistance

Although 80% of patients quickly achieved a complete cytogenetic response, a small proportion of patients in the chronic phase (CP) and a substantial proportion in the accelerated phase (AP) and the blast phase (BP) failed to respond to imatinib. The precise mechanism of disease progression is still uncertain, but the additional genetic changes involving activation of the oncogenic factor and/or inactivation of the tumor suppressor appear to cause more advanced CML-AP or CML-BP [33] (Fig. 2.7). As CML stem cells are not addicted to BCR-ABL, imatinib failed to kill BCR-ABL-expressing CML stem cells [34, 35]. Several mechanisms of imatinib resistance have been reported, including BCR-ABL-dependent mechanisms (i.e., mutations in specific amino acids within ABL kinase or overexpression of the

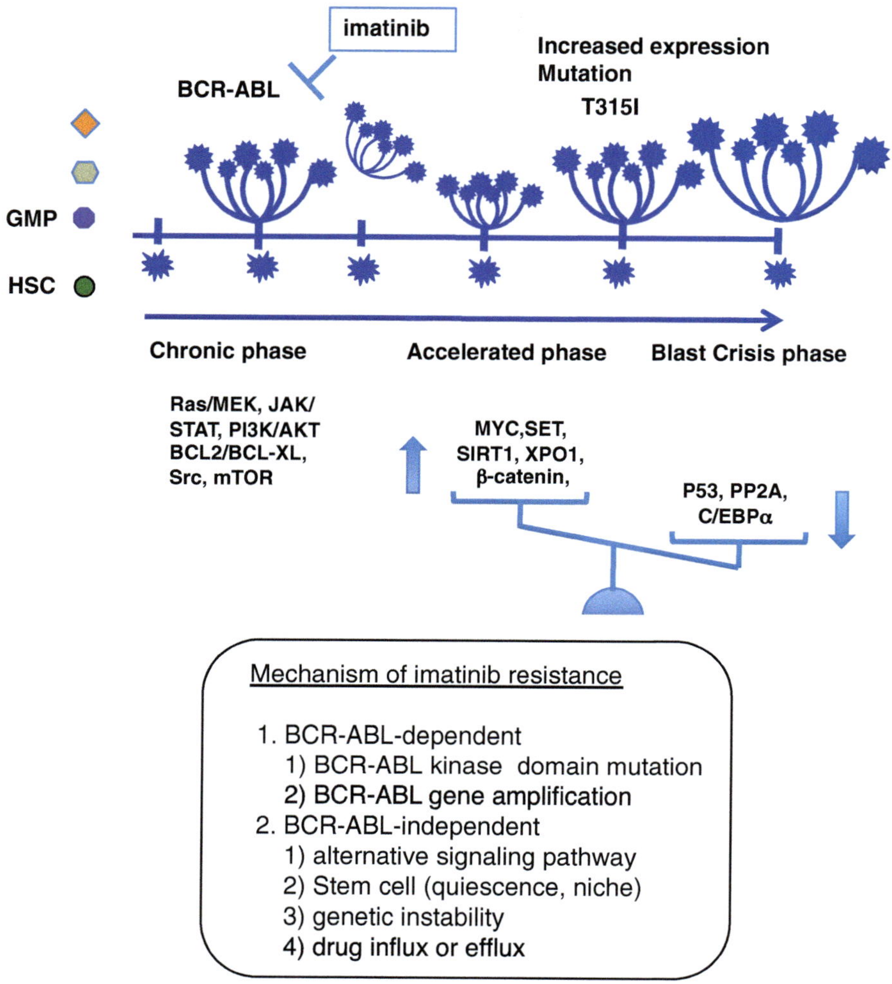

Fig. 2.7 Mechanism of imatinib resistance. Imatinib fails to kill BCR-ABL-expressing CML stem cells. During treatment with imatinib, accumulation of genetic changes involving activation of the oncogenic factor and/or inactivation of the tumor suppressor appears to induce more advanced CML-AP or CML-BP (Maru [22])

BCR-ABL protein) and BCR-ABL-independent mechanisms (i.e., drug import or export, additional genetic abnormalities, and the activation of alternative signaling pathways, such as Ras/Raf/MEK kinase, STAT or Src family kinases) [36, 37]. To overcome imatinib/TKIs resistance, several strategies are being investigated (Fig. 2.8, Table 2.2).

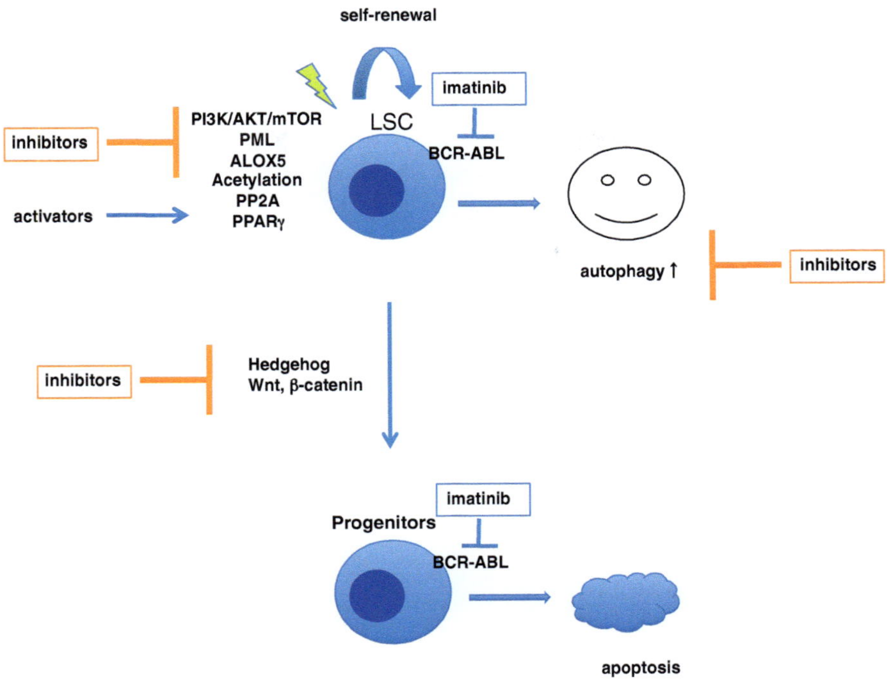

Fig. 2.8 Pharmacological targeting CML stem cells to overcome imatinib resistance. Imatinib effectively inhibits BCR-ABL kinase activity leading to apoptosis in the more mature progenitor cells. In contrast, the quiescent CML stem cells are less sensitive to imatinib, and furthermore imatinib-induced autophagy eliminates defective mitochondria, a source of reactive oxygen species, to promote cell survival. Autophagy inhibitors are under investigation alone and in combination with imatinib/TKI. Several inhibitors and activators targeting CML stem cells and bone marrow niche are also being investigated

2.4.1 BCR-ABL-Dependent Imatinib Resistance

2.4.1.1 BCR-ABL Kinase Domain Mutations

The presence or acquisition of mutations in the BCR-ABL kinase domain has been shown to confer variable degrees of resistance to imatinib [38]. The mutations responsible for imatinib resistance mainly occur at seven sites: G250, Y253, E255 (in the phosphate-binding region or P-loop), T315I (in the imatinib-binding site), M351, F359 (near the catalytic domain), and H396 (in the activation loop) [39]. The substitution of the "gatekeeper" residue T315 with the bulkier and more hydrophobic isoleucine results in the loss of an important hydrogen bond between imatinib and the kinase domain. Second-generation TKIs, dasatinib and nilotinib, are more effective than imatinib in preventing the progression to accelerated phase and blast crisis. These drugs are highly potent against imatinib-resistant ABL kinase mutations, except T315I mutation. The third-generation TKI, ponatinib, can inhibit BCR-ABL with a T315I mutation [40].

Table 2.2 Target signaling pathways and compounds to overcome imatinib resistance

Signaling pathway	Target	Compound	Reference
Autophagy	autophagy	Chloroquine, Hydroxychloroquine, Bafilomycin A1	[73] [74] [75]
Wnt/β-catenin	COX , Wnt/ β-catenin, GSK3,	Indomethacin, Av65, SB216763	[63] [70] [91]
Hedgehog	Smoothened	Cyclopamine, LDE 225	[67] [68] [69]
CXCR4/CXCL12	CXCR4	BKT140, AMD3465	[71] [72]
P13K/AKT/ mTOR	mTORC1/2, PI3K	Rapamycin, KU-0063794, BEZ235, PP242, OSI027, GDC0941	[76] [77] [92] [93] [94]
FOXO/TGF-β	TGF-β	Ly364947, SB431542	[95] [96]
JAK-STAT	JAK2	AG490, TG101209, CYT387, ONO44580, Ruxolitinib	[50] [97] [98] [99] [100]
PP2A	SET, SIP, PP2A	FTY20, OP449	[101] [102] [103]
PML	PML	Arsenic trioxide	[45] [78]
Acetylation	Pan-HDAC, SIRT1	SAHA, LAQ824, LBH589, Valproic acid, tenovin-6	[57] [56] [58] [59] [61]
Eicosanoid metabolism	ALOX5, prostaglandin (PG)	Zileuton, 15d-PGJ$_2$/Δ12-PGJ$_3$	[79] [104]
Nuclear export	CRM1	KPT-330	[105]
Interferon (IFN)	immunomodulator	IFN-α	[106] [107] [108] [109]
Hsp90 inhibitor	Hsp90	Geldanamycin analog Non-ansamycin synthetic molecules	[42] [43]
BCL2 family	BCL2	Sabutoclax	[110]
PPARγ	PPARγ	Pioglitazone	[80]

2.4.1.2 Gene Amplification and Upregulation of BCR-ABL Protein

Gene amplification results in the overexpression of the BCR-ABL protein. Moreover, the binding of imatinib to the ABL kinase domain appears to stabilize the BCR-ABL protein [41]. Newly synthesized BCR-ABL proteins are initially stabilized by Hsc70 and then passed on to Hsp90 and cochaperone Cdc37 to achieve maturation or kinase activation. Hsp90 inhibitors can ubiquitinate and degrade BCR-ABL proteins with or without mutations (e.g., T315I and E255K) via an E3 ligase CHIP and a c-Cbl-mediated proteasome machinery [41, 42]. The second generation of Hsp90 inhibitors has entered clinical trials [43]. Protein phosphatase 2A (PP2A) agonists can inhibit BCR-ABL kinase, also leading to degradation of the BCR-ABL protein [44]. Arsenic trioxide (As_2O_3) downregulates BCR-ABL protein via an autophagic or a proteasomal degradation mechanism [45].

2.4.2 BCR-ABL-Independent Imatinib Resistance

2.4.2.1 Alternative Signaling Pathways

The ABL kinase domain-independent scaffolding function of BCR-ABL appears to activate pro-survival signaling pathways, leading to imatinib resistance. The Src family kinase, Hck, is activated by BCR-ABL in a kinase-independent manner, and the activated Hck can phosphorylate Y177 in BCR, leading to an activation of the STAT5 signaling pathway [46, 47]. Y177 phosphorylation is also induced by the reciprocal activation between JAK2 and BCR-ABL, which results in BCR-ABL protein stability and activation of STAT5, Ras, and Lyn-mediated stimulation of the PI3K-AKT pathway [48]. Highly activated Lyn has been observed in TKI-resistant patients [49]. Inhibition of both BCR-ABL and the Src family kinases by the second- and third-generation TKIs is expected to overcome the Src family kinase-dependent imatinib resistance. A non-ATP-competitive dual inhibitor for JAK2 and BCR-ABL is effective in T315I BCR-ABL [50].

2.4.2.2 Genetic Instability

BCR-ABL appears to induce genomic instability in CML-CP stem cells during imatinib treatment, which may result from an aberrant cellular response to enhanced DNA damage caused by higher levels of reactive oxygen species (ROS) [51]. The inefficient repair generates not only TKI-resistant point mutations in BCR-ABL kinase but also point mutations in other genes (e.g., p53 and Ras). BCR-ABL-induced deregulated mechanisms of DNA repair appear to involve downregulation of the catalytic subunit of DNA-PK, disruption of the Fanconi anemia/BRCA DNA repair pathway, activation of Rad51 and the Werner syndrome helicase (WRN), and inhibition of uracil DNA glycosylase UNG [52–55]. In addition, the genetic mutations may tend to occur through BCR-ABL-induced alterations of epigenetic regulators involving histone acetyltransferases and deacetylases (HDAC). HDAC inhibitors enhance imatinib-induced apoptosis of CML cells [56–60]. Inhibition of SIRT1, an NAD-dependent histone deacetylase, enhances p53 acetylation leading to its transcriptional activity, which promotes elimination of CML stem cells following imatinib treatment [61].

2.4.2.3 Stem Cells and Bone Marrow Niche

As mentioned above, imatinib is unable to eradicate quiescent $CD34^+$ CML stem cells [34, 35]. In the hypoxic microenvironment of the hematopoietic stem cell (HSC) niche, HIF1-α signaling supports CML stem cells persistence independent of BCR-ABL kinase activity [62]. Wnt-β-catenin signaling leads to self-renewal in stem cells by activating the expression of Myc and cyclin D1 [63]. Aberrant activation of Wnt signaling endows granulocyte-macrophage progenitor cells (GMPs) with self-renewal capacity in CML-BC [64]. A close interplay between the Wnt-β-catenin pathway and N-cadherin in the bone marrow mesenchymal stromal cell also protects CML stem and progenitor cells during TKI treatment [65]. The Hedgehog pathway is a developmental signaling pathway that also plays a role in primitive and adult hematopoiesis [66]. BCR-ABL-induced upregulation of Smo activates the Hedgehog pathway in CML stem cells via the Gli family of transcriptional effectors. The inhibitors for the Wnt and the Hedgehog signaling pathways in combination with imatinib are expected to eradicate CML stem cells [63, 67–70].

The bone marrow microenvironment has been implicated in the protection of CML stem cells from imatinib-induced apoptosis. CXCL12, also called stromal cell-derived factor-1 (SDF-1), a chemokine produced by bone marrow stromal cells, and its receptor CXCR4 regulate HSC migration to and from the bone marrow. BCR-ABL downregulates CXCR4 expression, leading to a defective adhesion of CML cells to bone marrow stroma. Imatinib-induced upregulation of CXCR4 promotes migration of CML cells to bone marrow stroma, which results in the survival of quiescent CML progenitor cells [71]. CXCR4 inhibitor-induced disruption of stroma-mediated protection enhances imatinib sensitivity [72].

Autophagy appears to act as a double-edged sword for tumor cells. Autophagy selectively removes damaged organelles, especially dysfunctional mitochondria that are the source of reactive oxygen species. BCR-ABL-induced activation of the PI3K-AKT-mTOR signaling pathway inhibits autophagy, which results in high ROS levels that induce genome instability [73, 74]. On the contrary, treatment with imatinib induces autophagy that is associated with endoplasmic reticulum stress, which results in stem cell survival. The combination of TKI and an autophagy inhibitor resulted in a dramatic growth inhibition of $CD34^+$ cells from CML patients [75]. The mTOR inhibitor, rapamycin, also decreased the viability of K562 cells and can block cell proliferation in imatinib-resistant CML patients [76, 77].

The promyelocytic leukemia protein (PML) tumor suppressor, which acts as a negative regulator of mTOR, plays a critical role in HSCs. As_2O_3 induces PML degradation and thereby inhibits maintenance of CML stem cells [78]. BCR-ABL induced upregulation of arachidonate 5-lipoxygenase (ALOX5), which is not inhibited by imatinib, suggesting that kinase independence is essential for the induction of CML in mice. The ALOX5 inhibitor-induced depletion of CML, but not normal, stem cells, and imatinib-induced elimination of differentiated leukemia cells could be a good combination [79]. Glitazone-induced activation of peroxisome proliferator-activated receptor-γ (PPARγ) has recently been shown to decrease STAT5 expression and that of its downstream key molecules such as HIF2α and CITED2 in quiescent stem cells. The combination of imatinib and pioglitazone can synergistically decrease CML stem cells [80].

2.4.2.4 Imatinib Influx or Efflux

Imatinib is a substrate of the influx transporter, organic cation transporter 1 (OCT1) and the efflux transporters, P-glycoprotein (P-gP, ABCB1, or MDR1), and breast cancer-related protein (BCRP or ABCG2) [81–83]. Increased efflux and decreased influx of imatinib may be associated with the imatinib resistance. Several studies have shown a clinical determinant of intracellular drug levels and resistance to imatinib [81]. An ABCB1 inhibitor, cyclosporine, resensitized imatinib-resistant K562 cells to imatinib in vitro [84]. Statins also inhibited ABCB1 and ABCG2 efflux pump activity, which resulted in potentiation of antileukemic activity of imatinib in primary CD34+ CML-CP and CML-BP cells [85].

2.5 Effects of Imatinib on Other Tyrosine Kinases

Imatinib has been shown to be able to inhibit other tyrosine kinases including c-ABL, PDGFR, and c-Kit. Thus, imatinib may be used to treat various other tumors caused by imatinib-specific abnormalities of PDGFR and c-Kit [86]. Imatinib also affects energy metabolism, bone metabolism, or endocrine pathways [87]. Imatinib appears to cause dysregulation of bone remodeling through attenuation of osteoclasts via inhibition of c-Kit, c-fms, and PDGFR and activation of osteoblast activity via inhibition of PDGFR [88]. c-ABL participates in the regulation of the endothelial barrier. Inhibition of c-ABL by imatinib causes a reduction of endothelial permeability in response to VEGF and the inflammatory mediators, thrombin, and histamine [89]. PDGF is involved in cardiovascular diseases, such as atherosclerosis, pulmonary arterial hypertension, angiogenesis, and diabetes. Inhibition of PDGFR by imatinib may improve the cardio-metabolic dysfunctions [90].

References

1. Piller G. Historical review LEUKAEMIA – a brief historical review from ancient times to 1950. Br J Haematol. 2001;112:282–92.
2. Nowell P, Hungerford D. A minute chromosome in human chronic granulocytic leukemia. Science. 1960;132:1497.
3. Fialkow PJ, Gartler SM, Yoshida A. Clonal origin of chronic myelocytic leukemia in man. Proc Natl Acad Sci U S A. 1967;58(4):1468–71.
4. Rowley JD. A new consistent chromosomal abnormality in chronic myelogenous leukaemia identified by quinacrine fluorescence and giemsa staining. Nature. 1973;243(5405):290–3. doi:10.1038/243290a0.
5. Abelson HT, Rabstein LS. Lymphosarcoma: virus-induced thymic-independent disease in mice. Cancer Res. 1970;30:2213–22.
6. Bartram CR, de Klein A, Hagemeijer A, van Agthoven T, Geurts van Kessel A, Bootsma D, et al. Translocation of c-abl oncogene correlates with the presence of a Philadelphia chromosome in chronic myelocytic leukaemia. Nature. 1983;306:277–80.
7. Canaani E, Gale RP, Steiner-Saltz D, Berrebi A, Aghai E, Januszewicz E. Altered transcription of an oncogene in chronic myeloid leukaemia. Lancet. 1984;1:593–5.
8. Groffen J, Stephenson JR, Heisterkamp N, de Klein A, Bartram CR, Grosveld G. Philadelphia chromosomal breakpoints are clustered within a limited region, bcr, on chromosome 22. Cell. 1984;36(1):93–9. doi:10.1016/0092-8674(84)90077-1.
9. Lugo TG, Pendergast A-M, Muller AJ, Witte ON. Tyrosine kinase activity and transformation potency of bcr-abl oncogene products. Science. 1990;247:1079–82.

10. Daley GQ, Van Etten RA, Baltimore D. Induction of chronic myelogenous leukemia in mice by the P210bcr/abl gene of the Philadelphia chromosome. Science. 1990;247:824–30.
11. Heisterkamp N, Jenster G, ten Hoeve J, Zovich D, Pattengale PK, Groffen J. Acute leukaemia in bcr/abl transgenic mice. Nature. 1990;344(6263):251–3.
12. Zimmermann J, Buchdunger E, Mett H, Meyer T, Lydon NB. Potent and selective inhibitors of the Abl-kinase: phenylamino-pyrimidine (PAP) derivatives. Bioorg Med Chem Lett. 1997;7(2):187–92.
13. Druker BJ, Tamura S, Buchdunger E, Ohno S, Segal GM, Fanning S, et al. Effects of a selective inhibitor of the Abl tyrosine kinase on the growth of Bcr-Abl positive cells. Nat Med. 1996;2:561–6.
14. Wu P, Nielsen TE, Clausen MH. FDA-approved small-molecule kinase inhibitors. Trends Pharmacol Sci. 2015;36(7):422–39. doi:10.1016/j.tips.2015.04.005.
15. Capdeville R, Buchdunger E, Zimmermann J, Matter A. Glivec (STI571, imatinib), a rationally developed, targeted anticancer drug. Nat Rev Drug Discov. 2002;1(7):493–502. doi:10.1038/nrd839.
16. Melo JV. The diversity of BCR-ABL fusion proteins and their relationship to leukemia phenotype. Blood. 1996;88(7):2375–84.
17. Nagar B, Hantschel O, Young MA, Scheffzek K, Veach D, Bornmann W, et al. Structural basis for the autoinhibition of c-Abl tyrosine kinase. Cell. 2003;112:859–71.
18. Smith KM, Yacobi R, Van Etten RA. Autoinhibition of Bcr-Abl through its SH3 domain. Mol Cell. 2003;12(1):27–37. doi:10.1016/s1097-2765(03)00274-0.
19. McWhirter JR, Galasso DL, Wang JY. A coiled-coil oligomerization domain of Bcr is essential for the transforming function of Bcr-Abl oncoproteins. Mol Cell Biol. 1993;13(12):7587–95.
20. Heldin CH. Dimerization of cell surface receptors in signal transduction. Cell. 1995;80:213–23.
21. Nagar B, Hantschel O, Seeliger M, Davies JM, Weis WI, Superti-Furga G, et al. Organization of the SH3-SH2 unit in active and inactive forms of the c-Abl tyrosine kinase. Mol Cell. 2006;21(6):787–98. doi:10.1016/j.molcel.2006.01.035.
22. Maru Y. Molecular biology of chronic myeloid leukemia. Cancer Sci. 2012;103(9):1601–10. doi:10.1111/j.1349-7006.2012.02346.x.
23. Deininger MWN. Imatinib – an overview. Haematol Rep. 2005;1(8):20–7.
24. Roskoski Jr R. Classification of small molecule protein kinase inhibitors based upon the structures of their drug-enzyme complexes. Pharmacol Res. 2016;103:26–48. doi:10.1016/j.phrs.2015.10.021.
25. Schindler T, Bornmann TW, Pellicena P, Miller T, Clarkson B, Kuriyan J. Structural mechanism for STI-571 inhibition of abelson tyrosine kinase. Science. 2000;289(5486):1938–42. doi:10.1126/science.289.5486.1938.
26. Nagar B, Bornmann WG, Pellicena P, Schindler T, Veach DR, Miller WT, et al. Crystal structures of the kinase domain of c-Abl in complex with the small molecule inhibitors PD173955 and imatinib (STI-571). Cancer Res. 2002;62:4236–43.
27. USFDA approved protein kinase inhibitors compiled by Robert Roskoski Jr. www.brimrorg/PKI/PKIshtm. Accessed 23 Mar 2016.
28. Coutre P, Mologni L, Cleris L, Marchesi E, Buchdunger E, Giardini R, et al. In vivo eradication of human BCR/ABL-positive leukemia cells with an ABL kinase inhibitor. J Natl Cancer Inst. 1999;91(2):163–8.
29. Wolff NC, Ilaria Jr RL. Establishment of a murine model for therapy-treated chronic myelogenous leukemia using the tyrosine kinase inhibitor STI571. Blood. 2001;98:2808–16.
30. Kuribara R, Honda H, Matsui H, Shinjyo T, Inukai T, Sugita K, et al. Roles of Bim in apoptosis of normal and Bcr-Abl-expressing hematopoietic progenitors. Mol Cell Biol. 2004;24(14):6172–83. doi:10.1128/MCB.24.14.6172-6183.2004.
31. Kuroda J, Puthalakath H, Cragg MS, Kelly PN, Bouillet P, Huang DCS, et al. Bim and Bad mediate imatinib-induced killing of Bcr/Abl+ leukemic cells, and resistance due to their loss

is overcome by a BH3 mimetic. Proc Natl Acad Sci. 2006;103(40):14907–12. doi:10.1073/pnas.0608505103.
32. Ng KP, Hillmer AM, Chuah CT, Juan WC, Ko TK, Teo AS, et al. A common BIM deletion polymorphism mediates intrinsic resistance and inferior responses to tyrosine kinase inhibitors in cancer. Nat Med. 2012;18(4):521–8. doi:10.1038/nm.2713.
33. Perrotti D, Jamieson C, Goldman J, Skorski T. Chronic myeloid leukemia: mechanisms of blastic transformation. J Clin Invest. 2010;120(7):2254–64. doi:10.1172/JCI41246.
34. Corbin AS, Agarwal A, Loriaux M, Cortes J, Deininger MW, Druker BJ. Human chronic myeloid leukemia stem cells are insensitive to imatinib despite inhibition of BCR-ABL activity. J Clin Invest. 2011;121(1):396–409. doi:10.1172/JCI35721.
35. Graham SM, Jørgensen HG, Allan E, Pearson C, Alcorn MJ, Richmond L, et al. Primitive, quiescent, Philadelphia-positive stem cells from patients with chronic myeloid leukemia are insensitive to STI571 in vitro. Blood. 2002;99:319–25.
36. Barnes DJ, Palaiologou D, Panousopoulou E, Schultheis B, Yong AS, Wong A, et al. Bcr-Abl expression levels determine the rate of development of resistance to imatinib mesylate in chronic myeloid leukemia. Cancer Res. 2005;65(19):8912–9. doi:10.1158/0008-5472.CAN-05-0076.
37. Bixby D, Talpaz M. Seeking the causes and solutions to imatinib-resistance in chronic myeloid leukemia. Leukemia. 2011;25(1):7–22. doi:10.1038/leu.2010.238.
38. Soverini S, Hochhaus A, Nicolini FE, Gruber F, Lange T, Saglio G, et al. BCR-ABL kinase domain mutation analysis in chronic myeloid leukemia patients treated with tyrosine kinase inhibitors: recommendations from an expert panel on behalf of European LeukemiaNet. Blood. 2011;118(5):1208–15. doi:10.1182/blood-2010-12-326405.
39. Apperley JF. Part I: mechanisms of resistance to imatinib in chronic myeloid leukaemia. Lancet Oncol. 2007;8(11):1018–29. doi:10.1016/s1470-2045(07)70342-x.
40. Mathisen MS, Kantarjian HM, Cortes J, Jabbour EJ. Practical issues surrounding the explosion of tyrosine kinase inhibitors for the management of chronic myeloid leukemia. Blood Rev. 2014;28(5):179–87. doi:10.1016/j.blre.2014.06.001.
41. Tsukahara F, Maru Y. Bag1 directly routes immature BCR-ABL for proteasomal degradation. Blood. 2010;116(18):3582–92. doi:10.1182/blood-2009-10-249623.
42. Peng C, Brain J, Hu Y, Goodrich A, Kong L, Grayzel D, et al. Inhibition of heat shock protein 90 prolongs survival of mice with BCR-ABL-T315I-induced leukemia and suppresses leukemic stem cells. Blood. 2007;110(2):678–85. doi:10.1182/blood-2006-10-054098.
43. Soga S, Akinaga S, Shiotsu Y. Hsp90 inhibitors as anti-cancer agents, from basic discoveries to clinical development. Curr Pharm Des. 2013;19:366–76.
44. Neviani P, Santhanam R, Trotta R, Notari M, Blaser BW, Liu S, et al. The tumor suppressor PP2A is functionally inactivated in blast crisis CML through the inhibitory activity of the BCR/ABL-regulated SET protein. Cancer Cell. 2005;8(5):355–68. doi:10.1016/j.ccr.2005.10.015.
45. Goussetis DJ, Gounaris E, Wu EJ, Vakana E, Sharma B, Bogyo M, et al. Autophagic degradation of the BCR-ABL oncoprotein and generation of antileukemic responses by arsenic trioxide. Blood. 2012;120(17):3555–62. doi:10.1182/blood-2012-01-402578.
46. Warmuth M, Bergmann M, Priess A, Hauslmann K, Emmerich B, Hallek M. The Src family kinase Hck interacts with Bcr-Abl by a kinase-independent mechanism and phosphorylates the Grb2-binding site of Bcr. J Biol Chem. 1997;272(52):33260–70. doi:10.1074/jbc.272.52.33260.
47. Klejman A, Schreiner SJ, Nieborowska-Skorska M, Slupianek A, Wilson M, Smithgall TE, et al. The Src family kinase Hck couples BCR/ABL to STAT5 activation in myeloid leukemia cells. EMBO J. 2001;21:5766–74.
48. Samanta A, Perazzona B, Chakraborty S, Sun X, Modi H, Bhatia R, et al. Janus kinase 2 regulates Bcr-Abl signaling in chronic myeloid leukemia. Leukemia. 2011;25(3):463–72. doi:10.1038/leu.2010.287.

49. Wu J, Meng F, Kong LY, Peng Z, Ying Y, Bornmann WG, et al. Association between imatinib-resistant BCR-ABL mutation-negative leukemia and persistent activation of LYN kinase. J Natl Cancer Inst. 2008;100(13):926–39. doi:10.1093/jnci/djn188.
50. Jatiani SS, Cosenza SC, Reddy MV, Ha JH, Baker SJ, Samanta AK, et al. A non-ATP-competitive dual inhibitor of JAK2V617F and BCR-ABLT315I kinases: elucidation of a novel therapeutic spectrum based on substrate competitive inhibition. Genes Cancer. 2010;1(4):331–45. doi:10.1177/1947601910371337.
51. Bolton-Gillespie E, Schemionek M, Klein H-U, Flis S, Hoser G, Lange T, et al. Genomic instability may originate from imatinib-refractory chronic myeloid leukemia stem cells. Blood. 2013;121:4175–83. doi:10.1182/blood-2012-11-.
52. Deutsch E, Dugray A, AbdulKarim B, Marangoni E, Maggiorella L, Vaganay S, et al. BCR-ABL down-regulates the DNA repair protein DNA-PKcs. Blood. 2001;97:2084–90.
53. Valeri A, Alonso-Ferrero ME, Rio P, Pujol MR, Casado JA, Perez L, et al. Bcr/Abl interferes with the Fanconi anemia/BRCA pathway: implications in the chromosomal instability of chronic myeloid leukemia cells. PLoS ONE. 2010;5(12):e15525. doi:10.1371/journal.pone.0015525.
54. Slupianek A, Poplawski T, Jozwiakowski SK, Cramer K, Pytel D, Stoczynska E, et al. BCR/ABL stimulates WRN to promote survival and genomic instability. Cancer Res. 2011;71(3):842–51. doi:10.1158/0008-5472.CAN-10-1066.
55. Slupianek A, Falinski R, Znojek P, Stoklosa T, Flis S, Doneddu V, et al. BCR-ABL1 kinase inhibits uracil DNA glycosylase UNG2 to enhance oxidative DNA damage and stimulate genomic instability. Leukemia. 2013;27(3):629–34. doi:10.1038/leu.2012.294.
56. Yu C, Rahmani M, Almenara J, Subler M, Krystal G, Conrad D, et al. Histone deacetylase inhibitors promote STI571-mediated apoptosis in STI571- sensitive and -resistant Bcr/Abl+human myeloid leukemia cells. Cancer Res. 2003;63:2118–26.
57. Nimmanapalli R, Fuino L, Bali P, Gasparetto M, Glozak M, Tao J, et al. Histone deacetylase inhibitor LAQ824 both lowers expression and promotes proteasomal degradation of Bcr-Abl and induces apoptosis of imatinib mesylate-sensitive or -refractory chronic myelogenous leukemia- blast crisis cells. Cancer Res. 2003;63:5126–35.
58. Kircher B, Schumacher P, Petzer A, Hoflehner E, Haun M, Wolf AM, et al. Anti-leukemic activity of valproic acid and imatinib mesylate on human Ph+ ALL and CML cells in vitro. Eur J Haematol. 2009;83(1):48–56. doi:10.1111/j.1600-0609.2009.01242.x.
59. Zhang B, Strauss AC, Chu S, Li M, Ho Y, Shiang KD, et al. Effective targeting of quiescent chronic myelogenous leukemia stem cells by histone deacetylase inhibitors in combination with imatinib mesylate. Cancer Cell. 2010;17(5):427–42. doi:10.1016/j.ccr.2010.03.011.
60. Wang Z, Yuan H, Roth M, Stark JM, Bhatia R, Chen WY. SIRT1 deacetylase promotes acquisition of genetic mutations for drug resistance in CML cells. Oncogene. 2013;32(5):589–98. doi:10.1038/onc.2012.83.
61. Li L, Wang L, Li L, Wang Z, Ho Y, McDonald T, et al. Activation of p53 by SIRT1 inhibition enhances elimination of CML leukemia stem cells in combination with imatinib. Cancer Cell. 2012;21(2):266–81. doi:10.1016/j.ccr.2011.12.020.
62. Ng KP, Manjeri A, Lee KL, Huang W, Tan SY, Chuah CT, et al. Physiologic hypoxia promotes maintenance of CML stem cells despite effective BCR-ABL1 inhibition. Blood. 2014;123(21):3316–26. doi:10.1182/blood-2013-07-511907.
63. Ashihara E, Takada T, Maekawa T. Targeting the canonical Wnt/beta-catenin pathway in hematological malignancies. Cancer Sci. 2015;106(6):665–71. doi:10.1111/cas.12655.
64. Jamieson CHM, Ailles LE, Dylla SJ, Muijtjens M, Jones C, Zehnder JL, et al. Granulocyte–macrophage progenitors as candidate leukemic stem cells in blast-crisis CML. N Engl J Med. 2004;351:657–67.
65. Zhang B, Li M, McDonald T, Holyoake TL, Moon RT, Campana D, et al. Microenvironmental protection of CML stem and progenitor cells from tyrosine kinase inhibitors through N-cadherin and Wnt-beta-catenin signaling. Blood. 2013;121(10):1824–38. doi:10.1182/blood-2012-.

66. Briscoe J, Therond PP. The mechanisms of Hedgehog signalling and its roles in development and disease. Nat Rev Mol Cell Biol. 2013;14(7):416–29. doi:10.1038/nrm3598.
67. Dierks C, Beigi R, Guo GR, Zirlik K, Stegert MR, Manley P, et al. Expansion of Bcr-Abl-positive leukemic stem cells is dependent on Hedgehog pathway activation. Cancer Cell. 2008;14(3):238–49. doi:10.1016/j.ccr.2008.08.003.
68. Zhao C, Chen A, Jamieson CH, Fereshteh M, Abrahamsson A, Blum J, et al. Hedgehog signalling is essential for maintenance of cancer stem cells in myeloid leukaemia. Nature. 2009;458(7239):776–9. doi:10.1038/nature07737.
69. Irvine DA, Copland M. Targeting hedgehog in hematologic malignancy. Blood. 2012;119(10):2196–204. doi:10.1182/blood-2011-10-383752.
70. Heidel FH, Bullinger L, Feng Z, Wang Z, Neff TA, Stein L, et al. Genetic and pharmacologic inhibition of beta-catenin targets imatinib-resistant leukemia stem cells in CML. Cell Stem Cell. 2012;10(4):412–24. doi:10.1016/j.stem.2012.02.017.
71. Jin L, Tabe Y, Konoplev S, Xu Y, Leysath CE, Lu H, et al. CXCR4 up-regulation by imatinib induces chronic myelogenous leukemia (CML) cell migration to bone marrow stroma and promotes survival of quiescent CML cells. Mol Cancer Ther. 2008;7(1):48–58. doi:10.1158/1535-7163.MCT-07-0042.
72. Beider K, Darash-Yahana M, Blaier O, Koren-Michowitz M, Abraham M, Wald H, et al. Combination of imatinib with CXCR4 antagonist BKT140 overcomes the protective effect of stroma and targets CML in vitro and in vivo. Mol Cancer Ther. 2014;13(5):1155–69. doi:10.1158/1535-7163.MCT-13-0410.
73. Altman BJ, Jacobs SR, Mason EF, Michalek RD, MacIntyre AN, Coloff JL, et al. Autophagy is essential to suppress cell stress and to allow BCR-Abl-mediated leukemogenesis. Oncogene. 2011;30(16):1855–67. doi:10.1038/onc.2010.561.
74. Helgason GV, Karvela M, Holyoake TL. Kill one bird with two stones: potential efficacy of BCR-ABL and autophagy inhibition in CML. Blood. 2011;118(8):2035–43. doi:10.1182/blood-2011-01-330621.
75. Bellodi C, Lidonnici MR, Hamilton A, Helgason GV, Soliera AR, Ronchetti M, et al. Targeting autophagy potentiates tyrosine kinase inhibitor-induced cell death in Philadelphia chromosome-positive cells, including primary CML stem cells. J Clin Invest. 2009;119(5):1109–23. doi:10.1172/JCI35660.
76. Sillaber C, Mayerhofer M, Bohm A, Vales A, Gruze A, Aichberger KJ, et al. Evaluation of antileukaemic effects of rapamycin in patients with imatinib-resistant chronic myeloid leukaemia. Eur J Clin Investig. 2008;38(1):43–52. doi:10.1111/j.1365-2362.2007.01892.x.
77. Li J, Xue L, Hao H, Han Y, Yang J, Luo J. Rapamycin provides a therapeutic option through inhibition of mTOR signaling in chronic myelogenous leukemia. Oncol Rep. 2012;27(2):461–6. doi:10.3892/or.2011.1502.
78. Ito K, Bernardi R, Morotti A, Matsuoka S, Saglio G, Ikeda Y, et al. PML targeting eradicates quiescent leukaemia-initiating cells. Nature. 2008;453(7198):1072–8. doi:10.1038/nature07016.
79. Chen Y, Hu Y, Zhang H, Peng C, Li S. Loss of the Alox5 gene impairs leukemia stem cells and prevents chronic myeloid leukemia. Nat Genet. 2009;41(7):783–92. doi:10.1038/ng.389.
80. Prost S, Relouzat F, Spentchian M, Ouzegdouh Y, Saliba J, Massonnet G, et al. Erosion of the chronic myeloid leukaemia stem cell pool by PPARgamma agonists. Nature. 2015;525(7569):380–3. doi:10.1038/nature15248.
81. Eechoute K, Sparreboom A, Burger H, Franke RM, Schiavon G, Verweij J, et al. Drug transporters and imatinib treatment: implications for clinical practice. Clin Cancer Res: Off J Am Assoc Cancer Res. 2011;17(3):406–15. doi:10.1158/1078-0432.CCR-10-2250.
82. Hamada A, Miyano H, Watanabe H, Saito H. Interaction of imatinib mesilate with human P-glycoprotein. J Pharmacol Exp Ther. 2003;307(2):824–8. doi:10.1124/jpet.103.055574.
83. Thomas J, Wang L, Clark RE, Pirmohamed M. Active transport of imatinib into and out of cells: implications for drug resistance. Blood. 2004;104(12):3739–45. doi:10.1182/blood-2003-12-4276.

84. Hirayama C, Watanabe H, Nakashima R, Nanbu T, Hamada A, Kuniyasu A, et al. Constitutive overexpression of P-glycoprotein, rather than breast cancer resistance protein or organic cation transporter 1, contributes to acquisition of imatinib-resistance in K562 cells. Pharm Res. 2008;25(4):827–35.
85. Glodkowska-Mrowka E, Mrowka P, Basak GW, Niesiobedzka-Krezel J, Seferynska I, Wlodarski PK, et al. Statins inhibit ABCB1 and ABCG2 drug transporter activity in chronic myeloid leukemia cells and potentiate antileukemic effects of imatinib. Exp Hematol. 2014;42(6):439–47. doi:10.1016/j.exphem.2014.02.006.
86. Iqbal N, Iqbal N. Imatinib: a breakthrough of targeted therapy in cancer. Chemother Res Pract. 2014;2014:357027. doi:10.1155/2014/357027.
87. Breccia M, Molica M, Alimena G. How tyrosine kinase inhibitors impair metabolism and endocrine system function: a systematic updated review. Leuk Res. 2014;38(12):1392–8. doi:10.1016/j.leukres.2014.09.016.
88. Vandyke K, Fitter S, Dewar AL, Hughes TP, Zannettino ACW. Dysregulation of bone remodeling by imatinib mesylate. Blood. 2010;115(4):766–74. doi:10.1182/blood-2009-.
89. Chislock EM, Pendergast AM. Abl family kinases regulate endothelial barrier function in vitro and in mice. PLoS ONE. 2013;8(12):e85231. doi:10.1371/journal.pone.0085231.
90. Hu W, Huang Y. Targeting the platelet-derived growth factor signalling in cardiovascular disease. Clin Exp Pharmacol Physiol. 2015;42(12):1221–4. doi:10.1111/1440-1681.12478.
91. Reddiconto G, Toto C, Palama I, De Leo S, de Luca E, De Matteis S, et al. Targeting of GSK3beta promotes imatinib-mediated apoptosis in quiescent CD34beta chronic myeloid leukemia progenitors, preserving normal stem cells. Blood. 2012;119(10):2335–45. doi:10.1182/blood-2011-06-.
92. Schuster K, Zheng J, Arbini AA, Zhang CC, Scaglioni PP. Selective targeting of the mTORC1/2 protein kinase complexes leads to antileukemic effects in vitro and in vivo. Blood Cancer J. 2011;1(9):e34. doi:10.1038/bcj.2011.30.
93. Janes MR, Limon JJ, So L, Chen J, Lim RJ, Chavez MA, et al. Effective and selective targeting of leukemia cells using a TORC1/2 kinase inhibitor. Nat Med. 2010;16(2):205–13. doi:10.1038/nm.2091.
94. Carayol N, Vakana E, Sassano A, Kaur S, Goussetis DJ, Glaser H, et al. Critical roles for mTORC2- and rapamycin-insensitive mTORC1-complexes in growth and survival of BCR-ABL-expressing leukemic cells. Proc Natl Acad Sci. 2010;107(28):12469–74. doi:10.1073/pnas.1005114107.
95. Naka K, Hoshii T, Muraguchi T, Tadokoro Y, Ooshio T, Kondo Y, et al. TGF-beta-FOXO signalling maintains leukaemia-initiating cells in chronic myeloid leukaemia. Nature. 2010;463(7281):676–80. doi:10.1038/nature08734.
96. Moller GM, Frost V, Melo JV, Chantry A. Upregulation of the TGF beta signalling pathway by Bcr-Abl: implications for haemopoietic cell growth and chronic myeloid leukaemia. FEBS Lett. 2007;581(7):1329–34. doi:10.1016/j.febslet.2007.02.048.
97. Samanta AK, Lin H, Sun T, Kantarjian H, Arlinghaus RB. Janus kinase 2: a critical target in chronic myelogenous leukemia. Cancer Res. 2006;66(13):6468–72. doi:10.1158/0008-5472.CAN-06-0025.
98. Traer E, MacKenzie R, Snead J, Agarwal A, Eiring AM, O'Hare T, et al. Blockade of JAK2-mediated extrinsic survival signals restores sensitivity of CML cells to ABL inhibitors. Leukemia. 2012;26(5):1140–3. doi:10.1038/leu.2011.325.
99. Chen M, Gallipoli P, DeGeer D, Sloma I, Forrest DL, Chan M, et al. Targeting primitive chronic myeloid leukemia cells by effective inhibition of a new AHI-1-BCR-ABL-JAK2 complex. J Natl Cancer Inst. 2013;105(6):405–23. doi:10.1093/jnci/djt006.
100. Gallipoli P, Cook A, Rhodes S, Hopcroft L, Wheadon H, Whetton AD, et al. JAK2/STAT5 inhibition by nilotinib with ruxolitinib contributes to the elimination of CML CD34+ cells in vitro and in vivo. Blood. 2014;124(9):1492–501. doi:10.1182/blood-2013-12-.
101. Neviani P, Harb JG, Oaks JJ, Santhanam R, Walker CJ, Ellis JJ, et al. PP2A-activating drugs selectively eradicate TKI-resistant chronic myeloid leukemic stem cells. J Clin Invest. 2013;123(10):4144–57. doi:10.1172/JCI68951.

102. Neviani P, Perrotti D. SETting OP449 into the PP2A-activating drug family. Clin Cancer Res: Off J Am Assoc Cancer Res. 2014;20(8):2026–8. doi:10.1158/1078-0432.CCR-14-0166.
103. Agarwal A, MacKenzie RJ, Pippa R, Eide CA, Oddo J, Tyner JW, et al. Antagonism of SET using OP449 enhances the efficacy of tyrosine kinase inhibitors and overcomes drug resistance in myeloid leukemia. Clin Cancer Res: Off J Am Assoc Cancer Res. 2014;20(8):2092–103. doi:10.1158/1078-0432.CCR-13-2575.
104. Hegde S, Kaushal N, Ravindra KC, Chiaro C, Hafer KT, Gandhi UH, et al. Delta12-prostaglandin J3, an omega-3 fatty acid–derived metabolite, selectively ablates leukemia stem cells in mice. Blood. 2011;118(26):6909–19. doi:10.1182/blood-2010-.
105. Walker CJ, Oaks JJ, Santhanam R, Neviani P, Harb JG, Ferenchak G, et al. Preclinical and clinical efficacy of XPO1/CRM1 inhibition by the karyopherin inhibitor KPT-330 in Ph1 leukemias. Blood. 2013;122:3034–44. doi:10.1182/blood-2013-04-.
106. Preudhomme C, Guilhot J, Nicolini FE, Guerci-Bresler A, Rigal-Huguet F, Maloisel F, et al. Imatinib plus peginterferon alfa-2a in chronic myeloid leukemia. N Engl J Med. 2010;2511–21.
107. Cortes J, Quintas-Cardama A, Jones D, Ravandi F, Garcia-Manero G, Verstovsek S, et al. Immune modulation of minimal residual disease in early chronic phase chronic myelogenous leukemia: a randomized trial of frontline high-dose imatinib mesylate with or without pegylated interferon alpha-2b and granulocyte-macrophage colony-stimulating factor. Cancer. 2011;117(3):572–80. doi:10.1002/cncr.25438.
108. Talpaz M, Hehlmann R, Quintas-Cardama A, Mercer J, Cortes J. Re-emergence of interferon-alpha in the treatment of chronic myeloid leukemia. Leukemia. 2013;27(4):803–12. doi:10.1038/leu.2012.313.
109. Simonsson B, Gedde-Dahl T, Markevarn B, Remes K, Stentoft J, Almqvist A, et al. Combination of pegylated IFN-alpha2b with imatinib increases molecular response rates in patients with low- or intermediate-risk chronic myeloid leukemia. Blood. 2011;118(12):3228–35. doi:10.1182/blood-2011-02-336685.
110. Goff DJ, Court Recart A, Sadarangani A, Chun HJ, Barrett CL, Krajewska M, et al. A Pan-BCL2 inhibitor renders bone-marrow-resident human leukemia stem cells sensitive to tyrosine kinase inhibition. Cell Stem Cell. 2013;12(3):316–28. doi:10.1016/j.stem.2012.12.011.

Imatinib: Clinical Pharmacology and Therapeutic Results

3

Kazunori Ohnishi

Abstract

Imatinib has a remarkable long-term efficacy in patients with chronic myelogenous leukemia (CML) in the chronic phase. Reported rates of 5-year progression-free survival and overall survival associated with imatinib therapy (400 mg daily) have ranged between 83–94% and 83–97%, respectively. Imatinib is generally well tolerated, and adverse events are typically manageable. Current evidence does not support the extensive use of high-dose imatinib (800 mg daily) as a frontline treatment in patients with CML, and also the excessive dose reductions to less than 300 mg imatinib should be avoided, even in patients who are intolerant to 400 mg imatinib. Addition of pegylated interferon α to imatinib offers additional benefits for CML treatment; however, its addition does not appear to improve PFS or OS. The early molecular response (*BCR-ABL1* transcript level of ≤10% at 3 months) is reportedly associated with improved prognosis in several studies. Furthermore, approximately 40% of patients who exhibited sustained deep molecular response could maintain treatment-free remission after discontinuation of imatinib. Treatment-free remission is now considered to be a new goal of tyrosine kinase inhibitor therapy in patients with CML in the chronic phase.

Keywords

Imatinib • Chronic myelogenous leukemia • Early molecular response • Treatment-free remission

K. Ohnishi (✉)
Japanese Red Cross Aichi Blood Center, 539-3 Minamiyamaguchi-cho, Seto, Aichi 489-8555, Japan
e-mail: k.ohnishi888@gmail.com

T. Ueda (ed.), *Chemotherapy for Leukemia*, DOI 10.1007/978-981-10-3332-2_3

3.1 Introduction

Chronic myelogenous leukemia (CML) is a myeloproliferative neoplasm characterized by the reciprocal chromosomal translocation t(9:22)(q34;q11), which forms the Philadelphia (Ph) chromosome. This translocation generates a novel fusion gene, *BCR-ABL1*, the chimeric protein of which constitutively activates ABL1 tyrosine kinase [1]. Imatinib mesylate (formerly termed CGP 57148B and STI571; Glivec, Novartis, Basel, Switzerland) is the first tyrosine kinase inhibitor (TKI) associated with ABL1, c-kit, and PDGFR and was developed for CML treatment [2]. Imatinib was approved for Ph-positive leukemia treatment in the United States and Japan in May 2001 and November 2001, respectively [3].

Imatinib has shown a remarkable long-term efficacy in CML treatment and is now the standard therapy for this disease. Five-year follow-up data from the International Randomized Study of Interferon and STI571 (IRIS) on newly diagnosed CML in the chronic phase (CP) revealed an 87% complete cytogenetic response (CCyR) rate as the best cumulative response [4]. The estimated 5-year overall survival (OS) was 89%, whereas freedom from progression to accelerated phase (AP) or blast phase (BP) was 93%.

Currently, five highly effective TKIs (first, second, and third generations) are available, and physicians can select the appropriate agent for each patient [5]. Approximately 40% of patients who achieve deep and sustained molecular remission could maintain the same degree of response after discontinuation [6].

3.2 Definition of Responses to TKIs

The definition of hematologic response (HR), cytogenetic response (CyR), and molecular response (MR), as recommended by the European LeukemiaNet (ELN), is shown in Table 3.1 [7]. According to the international scale (IS), molecular response is defined as the ratio of *BCR-ABL1* transcripts to control transcripts [8, 9]. IS was anchored to the average *BCR-ABL1* expression in samples from 30 untreated patients with CML-CP enrolled in the IRIS study, which corresponds to a molecular level of 100%. Several genes are now widely accepted as suitable controls, including *ABL1*, *beta-glucuronidase* (*GUS*), and *BCR*. It is recommended that a sample has at least 10,000 *ABL1* or 24,000 *GUS* copies for minimum quality standards, although the optimal values for *BCR* have not yet been established. Molecular response is expressed as IS or the log reduction of *BCR-ABL1* transcript level as shown in Fig. 3.1. A *BCR-ABL1* expression of ≤0.1% ($MR^{3.0}$) corresponds to major molecular response (MMR).

Table 3.1 Definitions of hematologic, cytogenetic and molecular responses to TKIs

Response	Definitions
Hematologic response (HR)	
Complete hematologic response (CHR)	WBC <10 × 10^9/L
	Platelet count <450 × 10^9/L
	Basophil <5%
	No immature cells
	Spleen nonpalpable
Cytogenetic response (CyR)	
Complete cytogenetic response (CCyR)	No Ph + metaphases
Partial cytogenetic response (PCyR)	1–35% Ph + metaphase
Major cytogenetic response (MCyR)	0–35% Ph + metaphase (CCyR + PCyR)
Molecular response	
Major molecular response (MMR)	*BCR-ABL1* transcript to control transcripts = <0.1% by RQ-PCR (IS) or $MR^{3.0}$ or better
$MR^{3.0}$, $MR^{4.0}$, $MR^{4.5}$, $MR^{5.0}$	3, 4, 4.5, 5 log reduction in *BCR-ABL1* transcript from the standard baseline

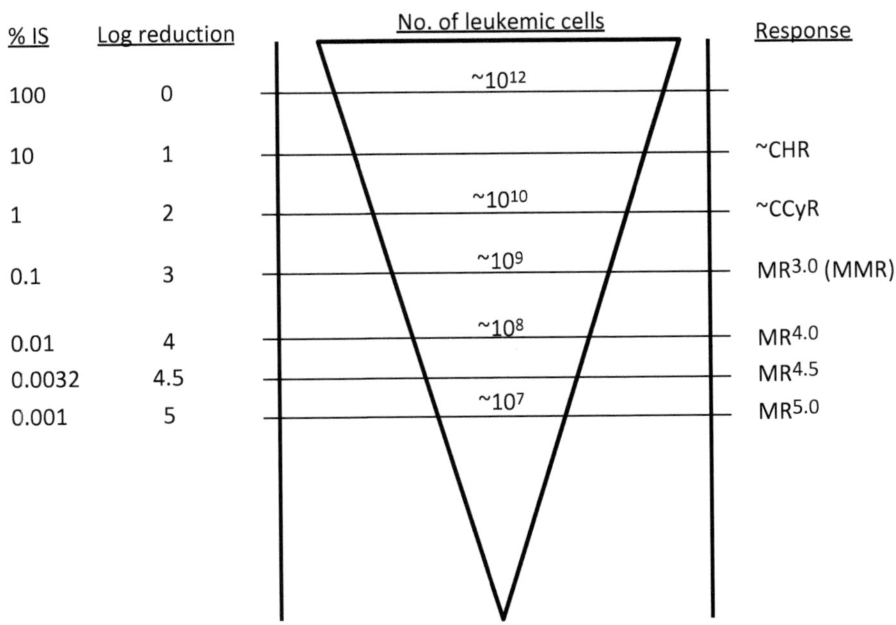

Fig. 3.1 Definitions of response and molecular levels of *BCR-ABL1* transcripts. *IS* international scale, *CHR* complete hematologic response, *CCyR* complete cytogenetic response, *MR* molecular response, *MMR* major molecular response

3.3 Clinical Trials of Imatinib for CML

3.3.1 Phase 1 Study for CML in CP

A phase 1 dose-escalating study of imatinib was conducted from June 1998 [3]. Imatinib was administered orally once daily to 83 patients with CML-CP who were resistant or showed intolerance to treatment with interferon alfa (IFNα). Imatinib was generally well tolerated, although a maximal tolerated dose was not identified despite dose escalation from 25 to 1000 mg. The most common adverse effects included nausea, myalgia, edema, and diarrhea. At a minimum dose of 300 mg/day, imatinib showed cytogenetic response in 29 of the 54 patients, which included 7 patients with CCyR. Further, 400 mg daily dose inhibited the enzymatic activity of BCR-ABL1 in vivo, as demonstrated by decreased phosphorylation of CRKL, a substrate of BCR-ABL1. Therefore, a daily dose of at least 400 mg was recommended for future studies.

3.3.2 Phase 2 Studies for CML in CP, CML in AP, and CML in BP

In a phase 2 study of patients with CML-CP, a total of 532 patients with late-CP CML who failed to respond to IFNα were treated with 400 mg of imatinib daily [10]. Imatinib induced major cytogenetic response (MCyR) in 60% of the 454 patients and complete hematologic response (CHR) in up to 95% of the patients. Over a median follow-up duration of 18 months, the estimated progression-free survival (PFS) and overall survival (OS) was 89% and 95%, respectively. Further, the estimated PFS and OS at 6 years was 61% and 76%, respectively. Incidence of serious adverse events was <6%; hematologic toxic effects were manageable.

In a phase 2 study of imatinib, patients with newly diagnosed CML-AP or CML-BP were treated with 400 or 600 mg imatinib daily and were evaluated for sustained hematologic response (HR) lasting at least 4 weeks. Among the 181 patients with CML-AP, the rate of HR was 82%, and the rate of sustained HR lasting at least 4 weeks was 69% (CHR 34%) [11]. Rates of MCyR and CCyR were 24% and 17%, respectively. The estimated PFS and OS at 12 months was 59% and 74%, respectively.

In 229 patients with CML in myeloid BP, the rate of HR was 52%, and the rate of sustained HR lasting at least 4 weeks was 31% (CHR 9%) [12]. Rates of MCyR and CCyR were 16% and 7%, respectively. The estimated median response duration was 10 months, and the median survival was 6.9 months. Imatinib at an initial dose of 600 mg was associated with a significant improvement in therapeutic efficacy and survival, over that observed with 400 mg dose in patients with CML-AP and CML-BP.

A Japanese phase 2 study of imatinib (600 mg daily) plus chemotherapy (JALSG ALL202 trial) was conducted for newly diagnosed patients ($n = 77$) with Ph-positive acute lymphoblastic leukemia (ALL) [13]. The primary end point was complete remission rate. Complete remission was achieved in 96.2%, while CCyR was achieved in 71.3% patients. The median duration of complete remission was 5.2 months. The estimated 1-year EFS and OS rates were 60% and 76.1%, respectively. The outcomes were significantly better than those of historical controls.

3.3.3 Outcomes of Imatinib Treatment in Newly Diagnosed CML-CP

A prospective, multicenter, phase 3, randomized study [International Randomized Study of Interferon and STI571 (IRIS)] involving newly diagnosed patients with CML-CP ($n = 1016$) was initiated in June 2000 [14]. Patients were randomized to two treatment arms; the imatinib (STI571) group received imatinib 400 mg once daily, and patients in the IFNα + cytarabine group received IFNα (target dose: 5 million units/m^2 per day), and subcutaneous low-dose (20 mg/m^2 per day) cytarabine was added for 10 days every month. Patients were allowed to cross over to the other arm in the event of a lack of response, a loss of response, or development of intolerance to treatment. The primary end point was event-free survival (EFS). Events were defined by the first occurrence of any of the following: death from any cause during treatment, progression to AP or BP, or loss of CHR or MCyR.

Over a median follow-up duration of 18 months, the estimated MCyR was 87.1% and 34.7% in the imatinib and IFNα + cytarabine groups, respectively ($P < 0.001$) [14]. The estimated CCyR was 76.2% and 14.5%, respectively ($P < 0.001$); estimated PFS at 18 months was 96.6% and 79.9%, respectively (*P* < 0.001). Due to the substantial superiority of imatinib detected on interim analysis, the study results were disclosed early and most patients were crossed over to the imatinib arm. Accordingly, this study is now effectively a long-term follow-up study of patients who received imatinib as the initial therapy. After a median follow-up of 60 months, 382 (69%) of the 553 patients randomized to the imatinib arm remained on imatinib, and only 16 (3%) of the 553 patients randomized to IFNα + cytarabine arm remained on the same regimen [4].

In the imatinib group, the cumulative response rate of CCyR at 12 and 60 months was 69% and 87%, respectively. CyR rate and disease progression showed a significant association with Sokal risk. However, once a CCyR was achieved, it appeared to prevent disease progression even in patients with a higher Sokal risk. The estimated rates of EFS and survival without progression to AP/BP at 60 months were 83% and 93%, respectively. The estimated rates of survival without AP/BP at 60 months were 100% in patients who achieved CCyR with MMR at 12 months and 95% in those who achieved CCyR without MMR ($P = 0.007$). Annual rates for all events as well as those of progression to AP/BP declined over time with imatinib therapy. The estimated OS at 60 months was 89%; when the analysis was censored for deaths unrelated to CML, OS rate was estimated to be 95% (Fig. 3.2).

In the most recent update of the IRIS trial, the estimated OS at 8 years was 85% [15]. MMR increased from 24% at 6 months to 39% at 12 months and to a best rate of 86% at 8 years, in a total of 98 patients who were sequentially monitored for *BCR-ABL1* transcript.

In a phase 2 study involving 204 patients with newly diagnosed CML-CP at the Hammersmith Hospital in the United Kingdom, the cumulative incidence of CCyR and MMR at 5 years was 82.7% and 50.1%, respectively [16]. The estimated 5-year OS and PFS was 83.2% and 82.7%, respectively. Twenty-five percent of patients had discontinued imatinib treatment because of unsatisfactory response and/or toxicity by 5 years of treatment. Patients who achieved CCyR at 1 year had a better PFS

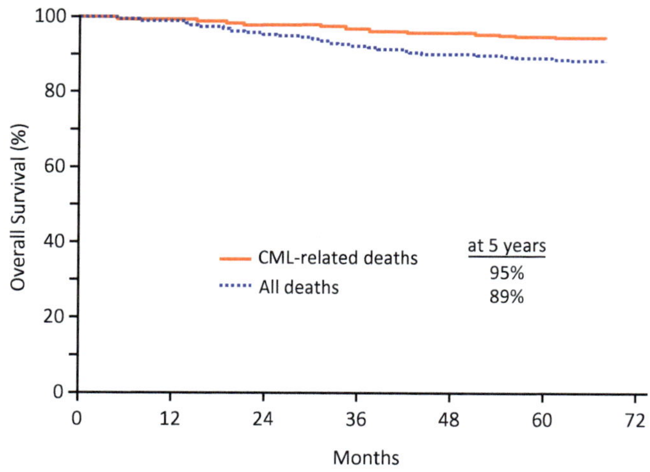

Fig. 3.2 Overall survival in imatinib group in the IRIS trial at a median follow-up of 5 years, on an intention to treat analysis. The estimated 5-year OS (*blue line*) was 89%, and the estimated 5-year OS with deaths associated with only CML (*red line*) was 95% in imatinib group (Adapted from Druker et al. [4]. Copyright © 2006 Massachusetts Medical Society. All rights reserved)

and OS than those who failed to reach CCyR; however, achievement of MMR appeared to confer no further advantage.

A prospective multicenter phase 2 study (CML202 trial) of imatinib therapy in newly diagnosed patients with CML-CP was performed in Japan Adult Leukemia Study Group (JALSG) [17]. Over a median follow-up of 65 months, the estimated 7-year OS and EFS in 481 evaluable patients were 93% and 87%, respectively. Cumulative incidence of MMR at 18 months and 7 years from the start of imatinib was 39% and 79%, respectively. Figure 3.3 represents the survivals of newly diagnosed patients with CML before and after imatinib era in JALSG studies [17–19].

In newly diagnosed patients with CML-CP treated with 400 mg imatinib, the reported rates of CCyR and MMR at 1 year ranged from 49% to 77% and from 18% to 58%, respectively [7]. Over a minimum duration of 5 years, PFS ranged between 83% and 94%, and OS ranged between 83% and 97% (Table 3.2). The proportion of patients who continued to receive imatinib treatment at 3–5 years from initiation ranged between 63% and 79%, while 50% were continuing treatment after 8 years. However, differences in the definition of PFS and EFS used in these studies should be taken into account while comparing the long-term outcomes in these studies. In some studies, data on patients who were taken off therapy for reasons other than progression were censored. Kantarjian et al. proposed that any instance of toxicity or death from any cause, on or off therapy, should be counted as an event to calculate EFS and PFS [20].

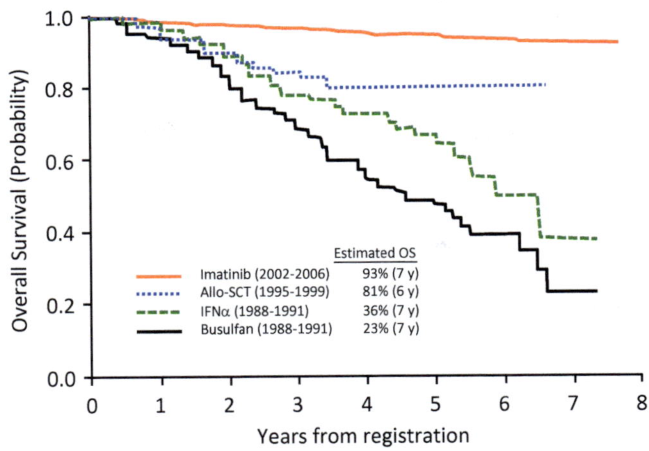

Fig. 3.3 Therapeutic advances in newly diagnosed patients with CML-CP based on JALSG studies. This chart illustrates the survivals of adult patients with newly diagnosed CML-CP who were prospectively enrolled in JALSG studies from 1988 to 2006. From 1988 to 1991, 170 patients were enrolled in a phase 3 study that was conducted to compare the effect of IFNα with that of busulfan. The estimated 7-year rates of OS were 36% in IFNα group ($n = 85$, *green line*) and 23% in busulfan group ($n = 85$, *black line*), respectively (Adapted from Ohnishi et al. [18]). From 1995 to 1999, 257 patients were enrolled in a prospective study to investigate the optimal indication of SCT. The estimated 6-year OS (*blue line*) of patients younger than 50 years who received allo-SCT was 81% ($n = 82$) (Adapted from Ohnishi et al. [19]). From 2002 to 2006, 489 patients were enrolled in CML202 trial to examine the efficacy of imatinib therapy. The estimated 7-year OS (*red line*) was 93% (Adapted from Ohnishi et al. [17])

Table 3.2 Long-term outcomes of first-line treatment of imatinib for newly diagnosed patients with CML-CP in clinical studies

Study/source	Imatinib dose, mg	No. of patients	CCyR % Best rate	MMR % Best rate	OS %	PFS %	EFS %	At year
IRIS [4, 15]	400	553	83	86	85	92	81	8
Hammersmith hospital [16]	400	204	83	50	83	83	81[a]	5
JALSG CML202 [17]	400[b]	481	90	79	93	93	87	7

[a]Event as defined in the IRIS trial: 81%; event as defined as the probability of stable cytogenetic response: 63%

[b]The mean daily dose during the first 24 months of treatment: = >360 mg ($n = 294$), 270–359 mg ($n = 90$) and less than 270 mg ($n = 67$)

3.4 Adverse Events

The most common adverse events of imatinib 400 mg reported from the IRIS trial [4] and the Japanese CML202 trial [17] were edema (peripheral and periorbital edema) (60% and 49%), muscle cramps (49% and 17%), diarrhea (45% and 16%), nausea (50% and 22%), musculoskeletal pain (47% and 21%), rash (40% and 40%), fatigue (39% and 24%), and headache (37% and 8%), respectively. Incidence of grade 3 or 4 adverse events in both trials was neutropenia (17%, 18%), thrombocytopenia (9%, 12%), anemia (4%, 6%), and elevated liver enzymes (5%, 4%), respectively. Several types of vascular adverse events have been reported in patients receiving second- or third-generation BCR-ABL1 TKIs [21]. However, imatinib exhibits a favorable long-term safety profile. The vascular safety of imatinib therapy is well documented and occurrence of congestive heart failure has been rare (1.7%) [22]. Newly occurring or worsening grade 3 or 4 hematologic or biochemical adverse events were infrequent both after 2 and 4 years of treatment. Imatinib is generally well tolerated; most adverse events were grade 1 or 2 in severity and tended to be most frequent in the first year of treatment. Discontinuation of imatinib for drug-related adverse events was required in <4% of patients over a median follow-up duration of 60 months.

3.5 Dosing Issue

The recommended starting dose of imatinib for patients with CML-CP is 400 mg/day, while that for patients with CML-AP or BP is 600 mg/day. Efficacy evaluation of imatinib 800 mg/day was performed in a phase 3, randomized study (TOPS trial). Newly diagnosed patients with CML-CP were treated with either 800 mg/day or 400 mg/day of imatinib [23, 24]. The primary end point was MMR at 12 months. MMR rates were similar in both treatment arms at 12 months (51.6% vs. 50.2%; $P = 0.77$) and 42 months (75.8% vs. 79.0%; $P = 0.48$). Further, no significant between-group difference was observed with respect to EFS, PFS, or OS. However, patients who tolerated more than 600 mg/day of imatinib showed a higher response rate.

In the ELN study, 216 patients with newly diagnosed CML at high Sokal risk were randomly assigned to receive imatinib 800 or 400 mg/day for at least 1 year [25]. The primary end point of CCyR at 12 months was comparable between the two treatment arms, as were the OS, PFS, and EFS. In the high-dose arm, the median average daily dose was 720 mg (range: 350–800 mg).

In a phase 2 study (TIDEL trial) of higher-dose imatinib, patients with newly diagnosed CML-CP initiated on imatinib 600 mg/day were shifted to 800 mg/day, if the prespecified response criteria were not met [26]. The primary end points were MMR, MCyR, and CCyR at 2 years. Both TIDEL trial and IRIS trial showed comparable MMR rates at 12 months (47% and 40%, respectively). However, the MMR at 24 months was higher in TIDEL trial (73% vs. 55% in the IRIS trial). Superior response in patients who were able to tolerate imatinib at 600 mg suggests that early dose intensity may be critical to achieve optimal response in CML-CP.

Overall, the current body of evidence alone does not justify extensive use of higher-dose imatinib (800 mg daily) as a frontline therapy in patients with CML-CP. Indeed, treatment adherence appears to be more important than initiation of treatment at a higher dose.

Subgroup analyses of a Japanese phase 2 study (CML202 trial) were performed according to the mean daily dose during the first 24 months of treatment: ≥360 mg (400 mg group; $n = 294$), 270–359 mg (300 mg group; $n = 90$) and <270 mg (200 mg group; $n = 67$). This was because imatinib dosage was reduced in many patients due mainly to adverse events [17]. No significant between-group differences were observed in OS and EFS between the 300- and 400-mg groups. These results indicate that long-term outcomes in small, elderly, and/or female patients who received 300 mg imatinib daily were similar to those who received 400 mg/day. However, cumulative rates of cytogenetic (92% vs. 98%; $P = 0.018$) or molecular response (78% vs. 87%, $P = 0.017$) at 7 years in the 300-mg group were inferior to those in the 400-mg group. Further, survival and efficacy was markedly inferior in the 200-mg group. Therefore, excessive dose reduction (<300 mg/day) should be avoided even in patients who are intolerant to imatinib 400 mg/day or in those who have a small body size.

3.6 Imatinib and Interferon α Combination

IFNα can induce sustained cytogenetic response in some patients with CML-CP [27]. Furthermore, Essers et al. reported that acute stimulation with IFNα activates dormant hematopoietic stem cells, while chronic stimulation leads to their exhaustion [28]. In a German CML Study IV, a randomized 5-arm trial designed to optimize imatinib therapy, 465 patients were randomized to imatinib alone or imatinib plus IFNα 2a or 2b [29]. Imatinib + IFNα failed to show superiority over imatinib monotherapy with respect to MMR and 3-year OS.

In a French phase 3 study (SPIRIT trial), 636 newly diagnosed patients with CML-CP were randomly assigned to receive imatinib (400 mg daily) alone, imatinib (400 mg) plus cytarabine or pegylated interferon (peginterferon) α-2a (90 μg weekly), or imatinib 600 mg daily alone [30]. The primary end points were EFS, PFS, and OS. At 12 months, the rate of molecular response was significantly higher in the imatinib + peginterferon α-2a group than that in imatinib 400 mg alone group (30% vs. 14%; $P = 0.001$). However, the combination was associated with substantial toxic effect, because of which peginterferon α was discontinued in 46% of the patients.

The Nordic randomized phase 2 study compared imatinib (400 mg daily) monotherapy with imatinib plus peginterferon α-2b (50 μg weekly) after imatinib induction in patients with CML-CP with low and intermediate Sokal risk [31]. The primary end point of MMR rate at 12 months was significantly higher in the former group, when compared with imatinib-alone group (82% vs. 54%, $P = 0.002$). Peginterferon α-2b was discontinued in 61% of patients in the combination arm. Therefore, the combination of peginterferon α with imatinib, despite the increase in associated toxicity, seems to enhance deep molecular response rates and should offer more possibilities for TKI therapy. These results suggested that addition of peginterferon-α added value to imatinib treatment but were not associated with superior PFS or OS.

3.7 Pharmacokinetics of Imatinib Therapy

Oral bioavailability of imatinib is 98%, and its half-life is approximately 20 h. Therefore, imatinib is administered orally in a once daily regime in patients with CML. Imatinib is metabolized mainly by CYP3A4 isoenzyme. The pharmacokinetics of imatinib tends to show considerable interpatient variability [32]. The mean plasma trough level of imatinib at day 28 was slightly higher in females than that in males (1078 ± 515 ng/mL vs. 921 ± 531 ng/mL). A weak correlation of imatinib trough levels with body weight, body surface area, and the age of patients was observable. However, Larson et al. suggested that effects of these factors on imatinib trough levels are not likely to be clinically significant due to the large interpatient variability in plasma trough concentrations.

The imatinib trough levels were significantly higher in patients who achieved CCyR than those who did not (mean, 1009 ng/mL vs. 812 ng/mL, $P = 0.01$). Thus, an imatinib trough level of ˃1000 ng/mL appears to be important for achievement of CcyR. Picard et al., too, reported a threshold of 1002 ng/mL to achieve MMR [33].

3.8 Prognostic Factors

Predictive variables for risk of progression and probability of drug discontinuation are required for patients with CML. Three prognostic classifications are currently available, and two of these (the Sokal score and the Euro [Hasford] score) have been used in studies of TKIs [34, 35]. However, the Sokal score was developed for patients treated with conventional chemotherapy, while the Euro score was based on IFNα therapy. In the European Treatment and Outcome Study for CML (EUTOS), a new prognostic risk score based on a study of 2060 imatinib-treated patients was developed to predict the probability of achieving CCyR within 18 months (Table 3.3) [36]. The EUTOS score relies on the percentage of

Table 3.3 Risk scores for CML-CP

Risk score	Calculation	Risk definition by calculation
Sokal score [34]	Exp 0.0116 × (age − 43.4) + 0.0345 × (spleen − 7.51) + 0.188 × [(platelet count/700)^2 − 0.563] + 0.0887 × (blast cells − 2.10)	Low risk: < 0.8 Intermediate risk: 0.8–1.2 High risk: >1.2
Euro (Hasford) score [35]	0.666 when age = >50 year + (0.042 × spleen) + 1.0956 when platelet count > 1500 × 10^9/L + (0.0584 × blast cells) + 0.20399 when basophils >3 % + (0.0413 × eosinophils) × 100	Low risk: = <780 Intermediate risk: 781–1480 High risk: >1480
EUTOS score [36]	(7 x basophils) + (4 x spleen)	Low risk: = <87 High risk: >87

Age is in years. Spleen is in centimeters below the costal margin (maximum distance). Blast cells, eosinophils, and basophils are in percents of peripheral blood differential basophils and spleen size to differentiate high-risk from low-risk patients. Other variables (age, platelet count, blast cells, and eosinophils) used in the previous classifications were later shown not to affect the response to imatinib. The EUTOS score predicted that 34% of high-risk patients would fail to achieve a CCyR in 18 months and also predicted a significant difference in PFS (82% for high-risk vs. 90% for low-risk patients, $P = 0.006$).

In the German CML Study IV, the relationship between comorbidities at diagnosis and overall prognosis were assessed using the Charlson Comorbidity Index (CCI) [37]. Age was associated with a higher CCI score in 863 patients, while comorbidities had an impact on OS. However, comorbidities had no negative effect on response rates and progression to advanced phases. Therefore, OS may not be appropriate for assessment of outcome measures for TKI therapy in CML-CP.

As biological variables, translocation type (standard and variant), additional chromosomal alteration (del der 9, trisomy 8, isochromosome 17, additional loss of material from 22q, and double Ph), transcript type, and baseline *BCR-ABL1* kinase domain mutations have been reported. Regarding the leukemic stem cell burden, Mustjoki et al. reported a correlation between the proportion of Ph-positive cells in $CD34^+$ $CD38^-$ fraction at diagnosis and the cytogenetic and molecular response [38].

Novel biological prognostic biomarkers for clonal evolution of CML have been identified by use of gene expression profiles, whole exome sequencing, and protein-level profiling.

Radich et al. identified 3000 genes that showed a significant association with the disease phase on DNA microarray analysis [39]. Their findings suggest the progression of CP CML to advanced phase CML as a two-step process. Patients with gene expression patterns of advanced disease may benefit from more aggressive therapies. Recently, targeted deep sequencing has been performed in Ph-positive clones, and mutations of *ASXL1*, *DNMT3A*, *RUNX1*, and *TET2* have been identified [40]. These *BCR-ABL1*-independent gene mutations in patients with CML may be important cofactors in the clonal evolution of CML.

3.9 Monitoring the Response to Treatment of TKIs

Monitoring the response to imatinib requires absolute and differential blood counts, cytogenetic tests, and molecular testing for *BCR-ABL1* transcript level and for *ABL1* tyrosine kinase domain mutations [7]. According to ELN recommendations for imatinib therapy, blood counts and differentials are required frequently during the first 3 months until CHR has been confirmed. Cytogenetic testing is required at 3 and 6 months, every 6 months thereafter until confirmation of CCyR, and every 12 months thereafter. Real-time quantitative polymerase chain reaction (RQ-PCR) for assessment of *BCR-ABL1* transcript levels is recommended every 3 months until MMR has been achieved and confirmed and, at least, every 6 months thereafter (Table 3.4).

Table 3.4 Evaluation of response to first-line TKIs at each time point (months) in ELN recommendations 2013 and the NCCN guidelines for CML version 2.2017

	Optimal		Warning		Failure	
Months	ELN	NCCN	ELN	NCCN	ELN	NCCN
Baseline	NA *a	NA	High risk or CCA/ Ph+ *b, Major route *c	NA	NA	NA
3	*BCR-ABL1* =<10% *d and/or Ph+ =< 35%	*BCR-ABL1*= <10%	*BCR-ABL1* >10% and/or Ph+ 36–95%	*BCR-ABL1* >10%*e	No CHR and/or Ph+ >95%	*BCR-ABL1* >10% *e
6	*BCR-ABL1* <1% and/or Ph+ 0%	*BCR-ABL1* =<10%	*BCR-ABL1* 1–10% and/or Ph+ 1–35%	NA	*BCR-ABL1* >10% and/or Ph+ >35%	*BCR-ABL1* >10%
12	*BCR-ABL1* =<0.1%	*BCR-ABL1* <1%	*BCR-ABL1* >0.1–1%	*BCR-ABL1* 1–10%	*BCR-ABL1* >1% and/or Ph+ >0	*BCR-ABL1* >10%
Then, at any time	*BCR-ABL1* =<0.1%	*BCR-ABL1* <0.1%	CCA/Ph– (–7 or 7q–) *f	*BCR-ABL1* 0.1 – <1%	Loss of CHR, Loss of CCyR Confirmed loss of MMR Mutations CCA/Ph+	*BCR-ABL1* > = 1%

*a NA: not applicable
*b CCA/Ph+: clonal chromosomal abnormalities in Ph + cells
*c Major route: trisomy 8, trisomy Ph (+der(22)t(9;22)(q34;q11)), isochromosome 17 (i(17)(q10), trisomy 19, and ider(22)(q10)t(9;22)(q34;q11))
*d RQ-PCR values expressed using the IS
*e Patients with *BCR-ABL1* only slightly >10% at 3 months and/or with a steep decline from baseline have generally favorable outcomes. It is important to interpret the value at 3 months before making drastic change
*f CCA/Ph-: clonal chromosomal abnormalities in Ph- cells

Before investigation of the causes of imatinib failure, potential issues with treatment compliance and drug interactions should be ruled out. *BCR-ABL1* kinase domain point mutations are detectable in about 50% of patients who experience treatment failure and in those showing progression on direct sequencing (a sensitivity of 10–20%). Currently, the mutations can be identified with more sensitive techniques.

3.10 Prognosis Based on Response

Prognosis according to the response to imatinib is assessed by correlations between molecular response to imatinib and progression-free survival (PFS) or overall survival (OS), based on the landmark analyses of imatinib therapy (Table 3.4). The most widely used time points are 3, 6, and 12 months [7, 9, 41].

The early molecular response (EMR) is typically used to indicate *BCR-ABL1* transcript level after 3 months of therapy. Marin et al. reported first that *BCR-ABL1* expression ≤9.84% IS at 3 months was associated with a higher probability of 8-year PFS and OS in patients with CML-CP treated with imatinib (Fig. 3.4) [42]. Branford et al. reported significantly superior outcomes among patients with *BCR-ABL1* ≤10% IS at 3 months. Furthermore, patients with *BCR-ABL1* halving time of >76 days among those with *BCR-ABL1* >10% IS at 3 months achieved significantly inferior outcomes as compared to that in patients with *BCR-ABL1* halving time ≤76 days [43]. Similarly, in a subgroup analysis of the German CML IV study dataset, a half-log reduction in *BCR-ABL1* transcripts at 3 months was identified as

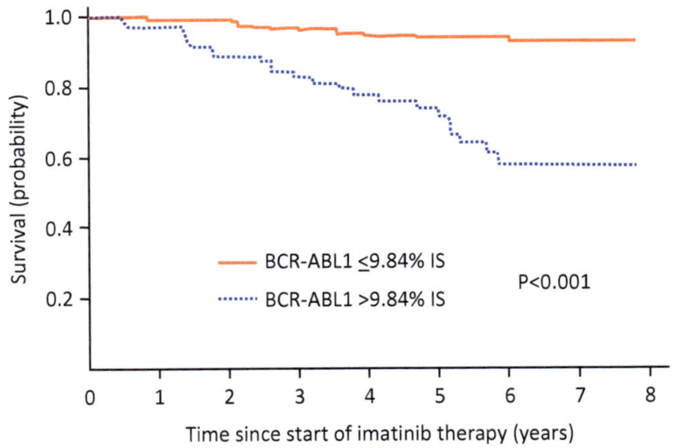

Fig. 3.4 Landmark analysis of overall survival with imatinib 400 mg therapy on the basis of *BCR-ABL1* level at 3 months at the Hammersmith hospital. The estimated 8-year OS was 93.3% in patients with *BCR-ABL1* transcript level ≤9.84% at 3 months (*red line*) and 56.9% in patients with *BCR-ABL1* level transcript level >9.84% at 3 months (*blue line*), ($P < 0.001$). (Adapted from Marin et al. [42]. Reprinted with permission.)

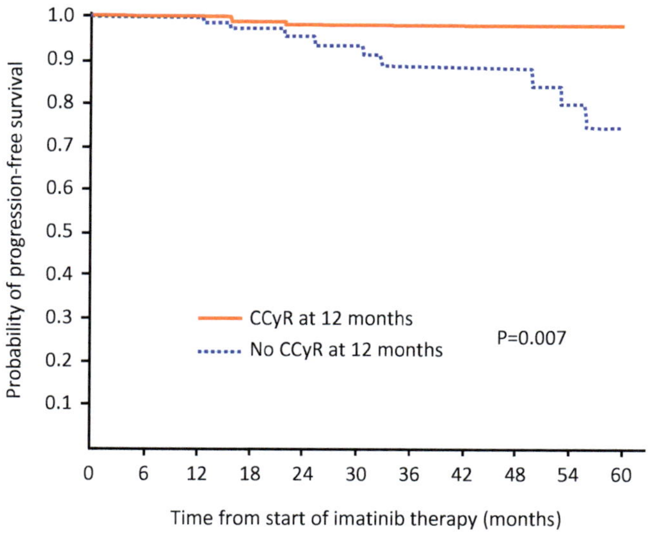

Fig. 3.5 Landmark analysis of progression-free survival on the basis of cytogenetic response to imatinib at 1 year at the Hammersmith hospital. The patients who had achieved CCyR (*red line*) had a better 5-year PFS than those who had not (*blue line*) (96% vs 74%; $P = 0.007$) and also better OS. Achieving MMR conferred no further advantage (Adapted from de Lavallade et al. [16]. Reprinted with permission. © (2006) American Society of Clinical Oncology. All rights reserved)

the most accurate predictor of 5-year OS [44]. EMR was reported also to be prognostically critical in several sub-analyses in the imatinib arm in the comparative studies of second-generation TKI. Therefore, the ELN recommendations and the National Comprehensive Cancer Network (NCCN) guidelines for CML have defined *BCR-ABL1* =<10% IS at 3 months as indicative of optimal. However, these results were not based on the prospective intervention studies but on subgroup analyses of each trial. Furthermore, Kim et al. showed that achieving MMR at 6 months overcame the EMR failure at 3 months [45]. Therefore, a single measurement of *BCR-ABL1* transcripts level at 3 months is not sufficient to define failure that may merit a change of treatment, whereas two tests (at 3 and 6 months) are more supportive of the need to change the treatment [7, 41]. MMR (*BCR-ABL1* ≤0.1% IS) at 12 months has been associated with PFS and OS in several prospective studies of TKIs; ELN, too, recommends MMR at 12 months as an optimal indicator [7]. However, the NCCN guidelines employ use of CCyR (0.1% to <1% *BCR-ABL1* IS) as an optimal measure of response at 12 months, based on several studies that suggest MMR not to be of prognostic significance in patients who achieve CCyR at 12 months (Fig. 3.5) [16]. On the other hand, since the achievement of MMR at 18 months was significantly associated with EFS compared to patients with >0.1 to <1% *BCR-ABL1* IS [46], the NCCN guidelines recommend <0.1% *BCR-ABL1* IS at 18 months.

3.11 Resistance to Imatinib

Development of resistance to imatinib is multifactorial [47, 48]. Imatinib is administered orally. Therefore, metabolism of imatinib is influenced by absorption in the gastrointestinal tract, by enzymatic inactivation, plasma-protein binding, and cellular drug influx and efflux. In the leukemic cells, gene amplification of *BCR-ABL1*, mutations of *ABL1* tyrosine kinase domain, and clonal evolution are involved in the evolution of resistance. Quiescent leukemic stem cells may remain even if deep molecular response was achieved, and more than half of patients relapsed after discontinuation of imatinib.

CYP3A4 is mainly responsible for imatinib metabolism. Therefore, drug interaction should be considered in clinical practice. Imatinib binds to serum protein by 89–96%, mainly to albumin, and also to alpha-1 acid glycoprotein (AGP). However, AGP is now considered unlikely as the cause of imatinib resistance because the amount of imatinib bound to AGP is much lower than that bound to albumin. Regarding drug transporters, overexpression of ATP-binding cassette subfamily B member 1 (ABCB1) linked to imatinib efflux and lower expression of human organic cation transporter-1 (hOCT-1) linked to imatinib influx are also thought to be potentially linked to mechanism of development of resistance to imatinib [49, 50]. However, the role of drug transporters in clinical resistance requires confirmation.

Primary cytogenetic resistance to imatinib is reported in 15–25% of newly diagnosed patients with CML-CP. Overexpression of BCR-ABL1 was shown to cause resistance. However, *BCR-ABL-1* gene amplification or increased BCR-ABL1 expression are less frequently involved. Mutations in *BCR-ABL1* tyrosine kinase domain are reported as the most common mechanism of secondary resistance to imatinib [47]. Mutations in ATP-binding loop (P-loop) are reported to be associated with poor response to imatinib therapy. The presence of T315I mutation (the gate keeper position) was reported as the highest resistance to imatinib. Among *BCR-ABL1* mutations resistant to imatinib, 43% were less sensitive mutations to the second-generation TKIs, including 14% with T315I [51].

Several recent studies have shown that adherence to imatinib was a significant determinant of therapeutic response. Noens et al. found that one third of 169 patients were considered to be nonadherent to imatinib and that treatment adherence was associated with high rates of optimal response and CCyR [52]. In another study, adherence ($\leq 90\%$ or $>90\%$) was strongly associated with the 6-year probability of MMR (28.4% vs. 94.5%, respectively; $P < 0.0001$) and that of complete molecular response (CMR) (0% vs. 43.8%, respectively; $P = 0.002$) [53]. In this study, the multivariate analysis identified adherence and hOCT1 expression level were the only independent predictors of achievement of MMR. Further, poor adherence to imatinib therapy was an important factor that contributed to cytogenetic relapse and treatment failure.

3.12 Treatment-Free Remission

Studies have shown that some patients that exhibit a deep and sustained molecular response to imatinib may discontinue TKI therapy without molecular relapse. In the prospective, multicenter, non-randomized Stop Imatinib (STIM) study, imatinib treatment was discontinued in CML patients who showed a sustained CMR ($MR^{5.0}$ or better and undetectable transcripts on quantitative RT-PCR) for at least 2 years [6]. Molecular relapse was defined as detection of *BCR-ABL1* transcripts on quantitative RT-PCR with loss of $MR^{5.0}$. At 12 months after discontinuation, the probability of persistent CMR among these 69 patients was 41%. All patients who relapsed responded to reintroduction of imatinib. In the updated analysis of STIM study, the overall probability of sustained CMR at 6 and 60 months was 43% and 38%, and low-intermediate Sokal risk and longer duration of imatinib therapy were predictive of improved prognosis after discontinuation [54].

A multicenter observational study (A-STIM [According to Stop Imatinib]) was conducted to evaluate persistence of MMR in 80 patients with CML-CP who had stopped imatinib after prolonged CMR (same definition as in the STIM study) [55]. Molecular relapse was defined as loss of MMR (>0.1% *BCR-ABL1* IS). The estimated cumulative incidence of MMR loss was 35% and 36% at 12 and 24 months, respectively. Cumulative incidence of molecular relapse (based on STIM definition) was 51% and 54% at 12 and 24 months, respectively (Fig. 3.6). Median time to second CMR was estimated at 7.3 months in re-treated patients. Fluctuation of *BCR-ABL1* transcript levels below the MMR threshold was observed in 31% of

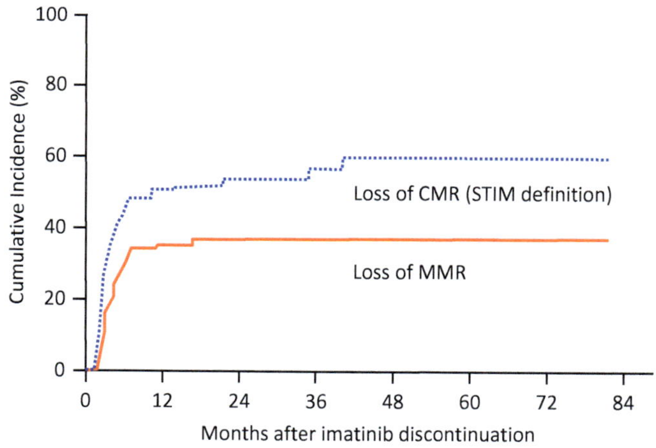

Fig. 3.6 Cumulative incidence of molecular relapse after imatinib discontinuation in patients with CML-CP in A-STIM trial. Cumulative incidence of molecular relapse using STIM definition (*blue line*) was 51% at 12 months and 54% at 24 months. Cumulative incidence of molecular relapse of MMR loss (*red line*) was 35% at 12 months and 36% at 24 months (Adapted from Rousselot et al. [55]. Reprinted with permission. © (2014) American Society of Clinical Oncology. All rights reserved)

patients after imatinib discontinuation. Patients previously treated with IFNα showed a trend toward a lower rate of MMR loss by 24 months as compared to that in patients treated with first-line imatinib (28.8% vs. 44.7%; $P = 0.061$).

In an Australian prospective TWISTER study, 40 patients with CML-CP who had sustained CMR ($MR^{4.5}$) on imatinib for at least 2 years were discontinued for imatinib [56]. Molecular relapse was defined as loss of MMR. At 24 months, the actual estimate of sustained MMR rate was 47.1%. In the 21 patients who were treated with IFNα before imatinib, a shorter duration of IFNα treatment before imatinib was significantly associated with risk of relapse.

In a Japanese retrospective study, 50 patients who had discontinued imatinib for at least 6 months were evaluated [57]. Sustained CMR rate after discontinuation of imatinib was estimated to be 47%. Imatinib dose intensity and prior IFNα administration were independent predictors of molecular recurrence within 12 months on multivariate analysis.

Thus, treatment-free remission (TFR) is now considered as an appropriate end point in studies of CML therapy because significant difference in OS has not been observed in recent clinical trials. All discontinuation studies showed that most recurrences occur within the first 6 months of discontinuation. It is conceivable that the time to recurrence would correlate with the amount of residual CML and that long-term TKI therapy may exhaust the CML clone.

3.13 Mathematical Models of Dynamics of CML

Molecular monitoring of leukemic cell burden during imatinib therapy for CML showed a biphasic decline of *BCR-ABL1* transcript levels and a rapid relapse upon treatment discontinuation. Two mathematical models have been proposed. Michor et al. used a four-compartment model to explain the kinetics of the molecular response to imatinib, with the assumption that imatinib has no substantial effect on leukemic stem cells [58]. The dynamics of their mathematical model are as follows: Leukemic stem cells expand exponentially at a slow rate. Imatinib reduces the rate at which leukemic stem cells produce progenitors. Hence, the abundance of leukemic progenitors declines once treatment is initiated. Similarly, imatinib reduces the rate at which leukemic progenitors produce differentiated cells. The abundance of differentiated leukemic cells shows a biphasic decline. On discontinuation of imatinib, the leukemic cells proliferate rapidly because the leukemic stem cells are not depleted. Resistant leukemic stem cells might expand faster than original leukemic stem cells.

Roeder et al. applied a self-organizing stem cell concept to *BCR-ABL1*-positive CML [59]. This model assumes that imatinib treatment modulates the competitive properties of *BCR-ABL1*-positive cells, i.e., imatinib selectively inhibits proliferation of *BCR-ABL1*-positive cells and causes degradation of proliferating stem cells. The model predicts that the malignant cell population can indeed be eradicated by continuous long-term imatinib administration, if no resistance occurs.

3.14 Guidelines for CML

ELN recommendations and the NCCN guidelines are widely used for treatment of CML [7, 41]. According to ELN recommendations, the responses are categorized as "optimal" or "failure" as follows [7]: Optimal response is associated with the best long-term outcome, wherein there is no indication for a change in that treatment. Failure implies that the patient should receive a different treatment to limit the risk of progression. Failures are distinguished as either primary (failure to achieve a given response at a given time) or secondary (loss of response). Between optimal and failure, there is an intermediate zone, previously referred to as "suboptimal" and now designated as "warning." Warning implies that the characteristics of the disease and the response to treatment require more frequent monitoring to permit timely changes in therapy to prevent treatment failure.

The criteria for categorization of the response to imatinib and other TKIs as the first-line treatment are summarized in Table 3.4. First of all, phase 3 studies comparing imatinib with second-generation TKIs (nilotinib and dasatinib) have shown a superiority of second-generation TKIs with significant differences in response but not with respect to outcomes. Therefore, both imatinib and second-generation TKIs are recommended as first-line treatments. Secondly, in evaluation of response, the value of molecular response after 12 months of treatment are controversial, therefore, there are the differences between the ELN and the NCCN recommendations. Furthermore, if TFR is accepted as the goal of TKI therapy, these evaluations will be changed appropriately. Thirdly, the guidelines currently recommend that a patient with CML who is responding optimally to TKI continues indefinitely treatment at the standard recommended dose. Discontinuation of TKI therapy outside of a clinical trial should be considered in the selected patients under the strict molecular monitoring.

For patients with newly diagnosed CML-AP, imatinib (600 mg daily) or second-generation TKIs are recommended. Allogeneic hematopoietic stem cell transplantation should be considered based on the response to TKIs. For patients with newly diagnosed CML-BP or those with Ph-positive ALL, high dose of imatinib (800 mg daily) or second-generation TKIs combined with appropriate chemotherapy, followed by allogeneic hematopoietic stem cell transplantation is recommended.

3.15 Conclusion

In conclusion, imatinib therapy has markedly improved outcomes for patients with CML-CP. Survival of patients who continue on imatinib is comparable to that of the general population. Currently, five highly effective TKIs are available; a third-generation TKI, ponatinib has been shown to be effective against resistant mutations including T315I, although vascular adverse events are a key limitation. Evidence from two randomized trials of imatinib versus second-generation TKIs justify placing nilotinib and dasatinib in the frontline setting but do not justify the exclusion of imatinib. Furthermore, the long-term safety of imatinib therapy has been established; therefore, imatinib is still used as a first-line TKI.

Recent studies have shown that in a subset of patients showing sustained molecular response to imatinib, TKI therapy may be discontinued without the risk of molecular relapse. Thus, TFR is considered as an appropriate end point. Socioeconomic factors may vary widely with patients in clinical practice. Especially, drug prices of TKIs are too high, and patients are more likely to be nonadherent to TKIs. It is critical to reduce treatment costs for TKI therapies.

References

1. Druker BJ. Translation of the Philadelphia chromosome into therapy for CML. Blood. 2008;112(13):4808–17. doi:10.1182/blood-2008-07-077958.
2. Deininger M, Buchdunger E, Druker BJ. The development of imatinib as a therapeutic agent for chronic myeloid leukemia. Blood. 2005;105(7):2640–53. doi:10.1182/blood-2004-08-3097.
3. Druker BJ, Talpaz M, Resta DJ, Peng B, Buchdunger E, Ford JM, et al. Efficacy and safety of a specific inhibitor of the BCR-ABL tyrosine kinase in chronic myeloid leukemia. N Engl J Med. 2001;344(14):1031–7. doi:10.1056/nejm200104053441401.
4. Druker BJ, Guilhot F, O'Brien SG, Gathmann I, Kantarjian H, Gattermann N, et al. Five-year follow-up of patients receiving imatinib for chronic myeloid leukemia. N Engl J Med. 2006;355(23):2408–17. doi:10.1056/NEJMoa062867.
5. Larson RA. Is there a best TKI for chronic phase CML? Hematol Am Soc Hematol Educ Program. 2015;2015(1):250–6. doi:10.1182/asheducation-2015.1.250.
6. Mahon FX, Rea D, Guilhot J, Guilhot F, Huguet F, Nicolini F, et al. Discontinuation of imatinib in patients with chronic myeloid leukaemia who have maintained complete molecular remission for at least 2 years: the prospective, multicentre Stop Imatinib (STIM) trial. Lancet Oncol. 2010;11(11):1029–35. doi:10.1016/s1470-2045(10)70233-3.
7. Baccarani M, Deininger MW, Rosti G, Hochhaus A, Soverini S, Apperley JF, et al. European LeukemiaNet recommendations for the management of chronic myeloid leukemia: 2013. Blood. 2013;122(6):872–84. doi:10.1182/blood-2013-05-501569.
8. Cross NC, White HE, Colomer D, Ehrencrona H, Foroni L, Gottardi E, et al. Laboratory recommendations for scoring deep molecular responses following treatment for chronic myeloid leukemia. Leukemia. 2015;29(5):999–1003. doi:10.1038/leu.2015.29.
9. Deininger MW. Molecular monitoring in CML and the prospects for treatment-free remissions. Hematol Am Soc Hematol Educ Program. 2015;2015(1):257–63. doi:10.1182/asheducation-2015.1.257.
10. Kantarjian H, Sawyers C, Hochhaus A, Guilhot F, Schiffer C, Gambacorti-Passerini C, et al. Hematologic and cytogenetic responses to imatinib mesylate in chronic myelogenous leukemia. N Engl J Med. 2002;346(9):645–52. doi:10.1056/NEJMoa011573.
11. Talpaz M, Silver RT, Druker BJ, Goldman JM, Gambacorti-Passerini C, Guilhot F, et al. Imatinib induces durable hematologic and cytogenetic responses in patients with accelerated phase chronic myeloid leukemia: results of a phase 2 study. Blood. 2002;99(6):1928–37.
12. Sawyers CL, Hochhaus A, Feldman E, Goldman JM, Miller CB, Ottmann OG, et al. Imatinib induces hematologic and cytogenetic responses in patients with chronic myelogenous leukemia in myeloid blast crisis: results of a phase II study. Blood. 2002;99(10):3530–9.
13. Yanada M, Takeuchi J, Sugiura I, Akiyama H, Usui N, Yagasaki F, et al. High complete remission rate and promising outcome by combination of imatinib and chemotherapy for newly diagnosed BCR-ABL-positive acute lymphoblastic leukemia: a phase II study by the Japan Adult Leukemia Study Group. J Clin Oncol. 2006;24(3):460–6. doi:10.1200/jco.2005.03.2177.

14. O'Brien SG, Guilhot F, Larson RA, Gathmann I, Baccarani M, Cervantes F, et al. Imatinib compared with interferon and low-dose cytarabine for newly diagnosed chronic-phase chronic myeloid leukemia. N Engl J Med. 2003;348(11):994–1004. doi:10.1056/NEJMoa022457.
15. Deininger M, O'Brien SG, Guilhot F, Goldman JM, Hochhaus A, Hughes TP, et al. International randomized study of interferon vs STI571 (IRIS) 8-year follow up: sustained survival and low risk for progression or events in patients with newly diagnosed chronic myeloid leukemia in chronic phase (CML-CP) treated with imatinib. Blood. 2009;114(22):1126. (abstract)
16. de Lavallade H, Apperley JF, Khorashad JS, Milojkovic D, Reid AG, Bua M, et al. Imatinib for newly diagnosed patients with chronic myeloid leukemia: incidence of sustained responses in an intention-to-treat analysis. J Clin Oncol. 2008;26(20):3358–63. doi:10.1200/jco.2007.15.8154.
17. Ohnishi K, Nakaseko C, Takeuchi J, Fujisawa S, Nagai T, Yamazaki H, et al. Long-term outcome following imatinib therapy for chronic myelogenous leukemia, with assessment of dosage and blood levels: the JALSG CML202 study. Cancer Sci. 2012;103(6):1071–8. doi:10.1111/j.1349-7006.2012.02253.x.
18. Ohnishi K, Tomonaga M, Kamada N, Onozawa K, Kuramoto A, Dohy H, et al. A long term follow-up of a randomized trial comparing interferon-alpha with busulfan for chronic myelogenous leukemia. The Kouseisho Leukemia Study Group. Leuk Res. 1998;22(9):779–86.
19. Ohnishi K, Ino A, Kishimoto Y, Usui N, Shimazaki C, Ohtake S, et al. Multicenter prospective study of interferon alpha versus allogeneic stem cell transplantation for patients with new diagnoses of chronic myelogenous leukemia. Int J Hematol. 2004;79(4):345–53.
20. Kantarjian H, O'Brien S, Jabbour E, Shan J, Ravandi F, Kadia T, et al. Impact of treatment end point definitions on perceived differences in long-term outcome with tyrosine kinase inhibitor therapy in chronic myeloid leukemia. J Clin Oncol. 2011;29(23):3173–8. doi:10.1200/jco.2010.33.4169.
21. Moslehi JJ, Deininger M. Tyrosine kinase inhibitor-associated cardiovascular toxicity in chronic myeloid leukemia. J Clin Oncol. 2015;33(35):4210-8. doi:10.1200/JCO.2015.62.4718.
22. Atallah E, Durand JB, Kantarjian H, Cortes J. Congestive heart failure is a rare event in patients receiving imatinib therapy. Blood. 2007;110(4):1233–7. doi:10.1182/blood-2007-01-070144.
23. Cortes JE, Baccarani M, Guilhot F, Druker BJ, Branford S, Kim DW, et al. Phase III, randomized, open-label study of daily imatinib mesylate 400 mg versus 800 mg in patients with newly diagnosed, previously untreated chronic myeloid leukemia in chronic phase using molecular end points: tyrosine kinase inhibitor optimization and selectivity study. J Clin Oncol. 2010;28(3):424–30. doi:10.1200/jco.2009.25.3724.
24. Baccarani M, Druker BJ, Branford S, Kim DW, Pane F, Mongay L, et al. Long-term response to imatinib is not affected by the initial dose in patients with Philadelphia chromosome-positive chronic myeloid leukemia in chronic phase: final update from the Tyrosine Kinase Inhibitor Optimization and Selectivity (TOPS) study. Int J Hematol. 2014;99(5):616–24. doi:10.1007/s12185-014-1566-2.
25. Baccarani M, Rosti G, Castagnetti F, Haznedaroglu I, Porkka K, Abruzzese E, et al. Comparison of imatinib 400 mg and 800 mg daily in the front-line treatment of high-risk, Philadelphia-positive chronic myeloid leukemia: a European LeukemiaNet Study. Blood. 2009;113(19):4497–504. doi:10.1182/blood-2008-12-191254.
26. Hughes TP, Branford S, White DL, Reynolds J, Koelmeyer R, Seymour JF, et al. Impact of early dose intensity on cytogenetic and molecular responses in chronic- phase CML patients receiving 600 mg/day of imatinib as initial therapy. Blood. 2008;112(10):3965–73. doi:10.1182/blood-2008-06-161737.
27. Ohnishi K, Ohno R, Tomonaga M, Kamada N, Onozawa K, Kuramoto A, et al. A randomized trial comparing interferon-alpha with busulfan for newly diagnosed chronic myelogenous leukemia in chronic phase. Blood. 1995;86(3):906–16.
28. Essers MA, Offner S, Blanco-Bose WE, Waibler Z, Kalinke U, Duchosal MA, et al. IFNalpha activates dormant haematopoietic stem cells in vivo. Nature. 2009;458(7240):904–8. doi:10.1038/nature07815.

29. Hehlmann R, Muller MC, Lauseker M, Hanfstein B, Fabarius A, Schreiber A, et al. Deep molecular response is reached by the majority of patients treated with imatinib, predicts survival, and is achieved more quickly by optimized high-dose imatinib: results from the randomized CML-study IV. J Clin Oncol. 2014;32(5):415–23. doi:10.1200/jco.2013.49.9020.
30. Preudhomme C, Guilhot J, Nicolini FE, Guerci-Bresler A, Rigal-Huguet F, Maloisel F, et al. Imatinib plus peginterferon alfa-2a in chronic myeloid leukemia. N Engl J Med. 2010;363(26):2511–21. doi:10.1056/NEJMoa1004095.
31. Simonsson B, Gedde-Dahl T, Markevarn B, Remes K, Stentoft J, Almqvist A, et al. Combination of pegylated IFN-alpha2b with imatinib increases molecular response rates in patients with low- or intermediate-risk chronic myeloid leukemia. Blood. 2011;118(12): 3228–35. doi:10.1182/blood-2011-02-336685.
32. Larson RA, Druker BJ, Guilhot F, O'Brien SG, Riviere GJ, Krahnke T, et al. Imatinib pharmacokinetics and its correlation with response and safety in chronic-phase chronic myeloid leukemia: a subanalysis of the IRIS study. Blood. 2008;111(8):4022–8. doi:10.1182/blood-2007-10-116475.
33. Picard S, Titier K, Etienne G, Teilhet E, Ducint D, Bernard MA, et al. Trough imatinib plasma levels are associated with both cytogenetic and molecular responses to standard-dose imatinib in chronic myeloid leukemia. Blood. 2007;109(8):3496–9. doi:10.1182/blood-2006-07-036012.
34. Sokal JE, Cox EB, Baccarani M, Tura S, Gomez GA, Robertson JE, et al. Prognostic discrimination in "good-risk" chronic granulocytic leukemia. Blood. 1984;63(4):789–99.
35. Hasford J, Pfirrmann M, Hehlmann R, Allan NC, Baccarani M, Kluin-Nelemans JC, et al. A new prognostic score for survival of patients with chronic myeloid leukemia treated with interferon alfa. Writing Committee for the Collaborative CML Prognostic Factors Project Group. J Natl Cancer Inst. 1998;90(11):850–8.
36. Hasford J, Baccarani M, Hoffmann V, Guilhot J, Saussele S, Rosti G, et al. Predicting complete cytogenetic response and subsequent progression-free survival in 2060 patients with CML on imatinib treatment: the EUTOS score. Blood. 2011;118(3):686–92. doi:10.1182/blood-2010-12-319038.
37. Saussele S, Krauss MP, Hehlmann R, Lauseker M, Proetel U, Kalmanti L, et al. Impact of comorbidities on overall survival in patients with chronic myeloid leukemia: results of the randomized CML study IV. Blood. 2015;126(1):42–9. doi:10.1182/blood-2015-01-617993.
38. Mustjoki S, Richter J, Barbany G, Ehrencrona H, Fioretos T, Gedde-Dahl T, et al. Impact of malignant stem cell burden on therapy outcome in newly diagnosed chronic myeloid leukemia patients. Leukemia. 2013;27(7):1520–6. doi:10.1038/leu.2013.19.
39. Radich JP, Dai H, Mao M, Oehler V, Schelter J, Druker B, et al. Gene expression changes associated with progression and response in chronic myeloid leukemia. Proc Natl Acad Sci U S A. 2006;103(8):2794–9. doi:10.1073/pnas.0510423103.
40. Schmidt M, Rinke J, Schafer V, Schnittger S, Kohlmann A, Obstfelder E, et al. Molecular-defined clonal evolution in patients with chronic myeloid leukemia independent of the BCR-ABL status. Leukemia. 2014;28(12):2292–9. doi:10.1038/leu.2014.272.
41. NCCN Guidelines chronic myeloid leukemia version 2.2017 [database on the Internet] 2017. Available from: http://www.nccn.org/professionals/physician_gls/f_guidelines.asp. Accessed 21 Feb 2017.
42. Marin D, Ibrahim AR, Lucas C, Gerrard G, Wang L, Szydlo RM, et al. Assessment of BCR-ABL1 transcript levels at 3 months is the only requirement for predicting outcome for patients with chronic myeloid leukemia treated with tyrosine kinase inhibitors. J Clin Oncol. 2012;30(3):232–8. doi:10.1200/jco.2011.38.6565.
43. Branford S, Yeung DT, Parker WT, Roberts ND, Purins L, Braley JA, et al. Prognosis for patients with CML and >10% BCR-ABL1 after 3 months of imatinib depends on the rate of BCR-ABL1 decline. Blood. 2014;124(4):511–8. doi:10.1182/blood-2014-03-566323.
44. Hanfstein B, Shlyakhto V, Lauseker M, Hehlmann R, Saussele S, Dietz C, et al. Velocity of early BCR-ABL transcript elimination as an optimized predictor of outcome in chronic myeloid leukemia (CML) patients in chronic phase on treatment with imatinib. Leukemia. 2014;28(10):1988–92. doi:10.1038/leu.2014.153.

45. Kim DD, Hamad N, Lee HG, Kamel-Reid S, Lipton JH. BCR/ABL level at 6 months identifies good risk CML subgroup after failing early molecular response at 3 months following imatinib therapy for CML in chronic phase. Am J Hematol. 2014;89(6):626–32. doi:10.1002/ajh.23707.
46. Hughes TP1, Hochhaus A, Branford S, Müller MC, Kaeda JS, Foroni L et al. Long-term prognostic significance of early molecular response to imatinib in newly diagnosed chronic myeloid leukemia: an analysis from the International Randomized Study of Interferon and STI571 (IRIS). Blood. 2010;116(19):3758–65. doi:10.1182/blood-2010-03-273979.
47. Mauro MJ. Defining and managing imatinib resistance. Hematol Am Soc Hematol Educ Program. 2006:219–25. doi:10.1182/asheducation-2006.1.219.
48. Apperley JF. Part I: Mechanisms of resistance to imatinib in chronic myeloid leukaemia. Lancet Oncol. 2007;8(11):1018–29. doi:10.1016/s1470-2045(07)70342-x.
49. Mahon FX, Deininger MW, Schultheis B, Chabrol J, Reiffers J, Goldman JM, et al. Selection and characterization of BCR-ABL positive cell lines with differential sensitivity to the tyrosine kinase inhibitor STI571: diverse mechanisms of resistance. Blood. 2000;96(3):1070–9.
50. White DL, Saunders VA, Dang P, Engler J, Zannettino AC, Cambareri AC, et al. OCT-1-mediated influx is a key determinant of the intracellular uptake of imatinib but not nilotinib (AMN107): reduced OCT-1 activity is the cause of low in vitro sensitivity to imatinib. Blood. 2006;108(2):697–704. doi:10.1182/blood-2005-11-4687.
51. Branford S, Melo JV, Hughes TP. Selecting optimal second-line tyrosine kinase inhibitor therapy for chronic myeloid leukemia patients after imatinib failure: does the BCR-ABL mutation status really matter? Blood. 2009;114(27):5426–35. doi:10.1182/blood-2009-08-215939.
52. Noens L, van Lierde MA, De Bock R, Verhoef G, Zachee P, Berneman Z, et al. Prevalence, determinants, and outcomes of nonadherence to imatinib therapy in patients with chronic myeloid leukemia: the ADAGIO study. Blood. 2009;113(22):5401–11. doi:10.1182/blood-2008-12-196543.
53. Marin D, Bazeos A, Mahon FX, Eliasson L, Milojkovic D, Bua M, et al. Adherence is the critical factor for achieving molecular responses in patients with chronic myeloid leukemia who achieve complete cytogenetic responses on imatinib. J Clin Oncol. 2010;28(14):2381–8. doi:10.1200/jco.2009.26.3087.
54. Etienne G, Guilhot J, Rea D, Rigal-Huguet F, Nicolini F, Charbonnier A et al. Long-term follow-up of the French Stop Imatinib (STIM1) Study in patients with chronic myeloid leukemia. J Clin Oncol. 2017;35(3):298–305. doi:10.1200/JCO.2016.68.2914.
55. Rousselot P, Charbonnier A, Cony-Makhoul P, Agape P, Nicolini FE, Varet B, et al. Loss of major molecular response as a trigger for restarting tyrosine kinase inhibitor therapy in patients with chronic-phase chronic myelogenous leukemia who have stopped imatinib after durable undetectable disease. J Clin Oncol. 2014;32(5):424–30. doi:10.1200/jco.2012.48.5797.
56. Ross DM, Branford S, Seymour JF, Schwarer AP, Arthur C, Yeung DT, et al. Safety and efficacy of imatinib cessation for CML patients with stable undetectable minimal residual disease: results from the TWISTER study. Blood. 2013;122(4):515–22. doi:10.1182/blood-2013-02-483750.
57. Takahashi N, Kyo T, Maeda Y, Sugihara T, Usuki K, Kawaguchi T, et al. Discontinuation of imatinib in Japanese patients with chronic myeloid leukemia. Haematologica. 2012;97(6):903–6. doi:10.3324/haematol.2011.056853.
58. Michor F, Hughes TP, Iwasa Y, Branford S, Shah NP, Sawyers CL, et al. Dynamics of chronic myeloid leukaemia. Nature. 2005;435(7046):1267–70. doi:10.1038/nature03669.
59. Roeder I, Horn M, Glauche I, Hochhaus A, Mueller MC, Loeffler M. Dynamic modeling of imatinib-treated chronic myeloid leukemia: functional insights and clinical implications. Nat Med. 2006;12(10):1181–4. doi:10.1038/nm1487.

Dasatinib, Nilotinib, Bosutinib, Ponatinib, and Other TKIs

4

Shinya Kimura

Abstract

ABL tyrosine kinase inhibitor (TKI) imatinib mesylate has led to a marked change in the treatment of chronic myeloid leukemia (CML). However, resistance and intolerance to imatinib are frequently reported, particularly in patients with advanced-stage disease; this leads to around 30% of CML patients discontinuing imatinib treatment. Point mutations within the *ABL* kinase domain, which interfere with imatinib binding, are the most critical cause of imatinib resistance. To overcome this, the second-generation ATP-competing ABL TKIs such as dasatinib, nilotinib, bosutinib, and bafetinib have been developed. Despite promising clinical results of these, a common mutation, T315I, is not effectively targeted by any of the second-generation ABL TKIs. Therefore, a third-generation ABL TKI, ponatinib, was developed and shows good clinical efficacy against CML cells harboring the T315I mutation. Thus, treatments for CML are progressing rapidly, and further evolution is expected.

Keywords

Chronic myeloid leukemia • BCR-ABL • Tyrosine kinase inhibitor

S. Kimura (✉)
Division of Hematology, Respiratory Medicine and Oncology, Department of Internal Medicine, Faculty of Medicine, Saga University, 5-1-1 Nabeshima, Saga 849-8501, Japan
e-mail: shkimu@cc.saga-u.ac.jp

T. Ueda (ed.), *Chemotherapy for Leukemia*, DOI 10.1007/978-981-10-3332-2_4

4.1 Introduction

Binding of adenosine triphosphate (ATP) to the ATP-binding pocket within the ABL kinase domain is essential for activation of the chimeric BCR-ABL protein; this process underlies the pathogenesis of CML. Imatinib mesylate (Fig. 4.1a) is a tyrosine kinase inhibitor (TKI) that binds to the ATP-binding pocket within the ABL kinase domain, thereby competitively inhibiting the binding of ATP. As such,

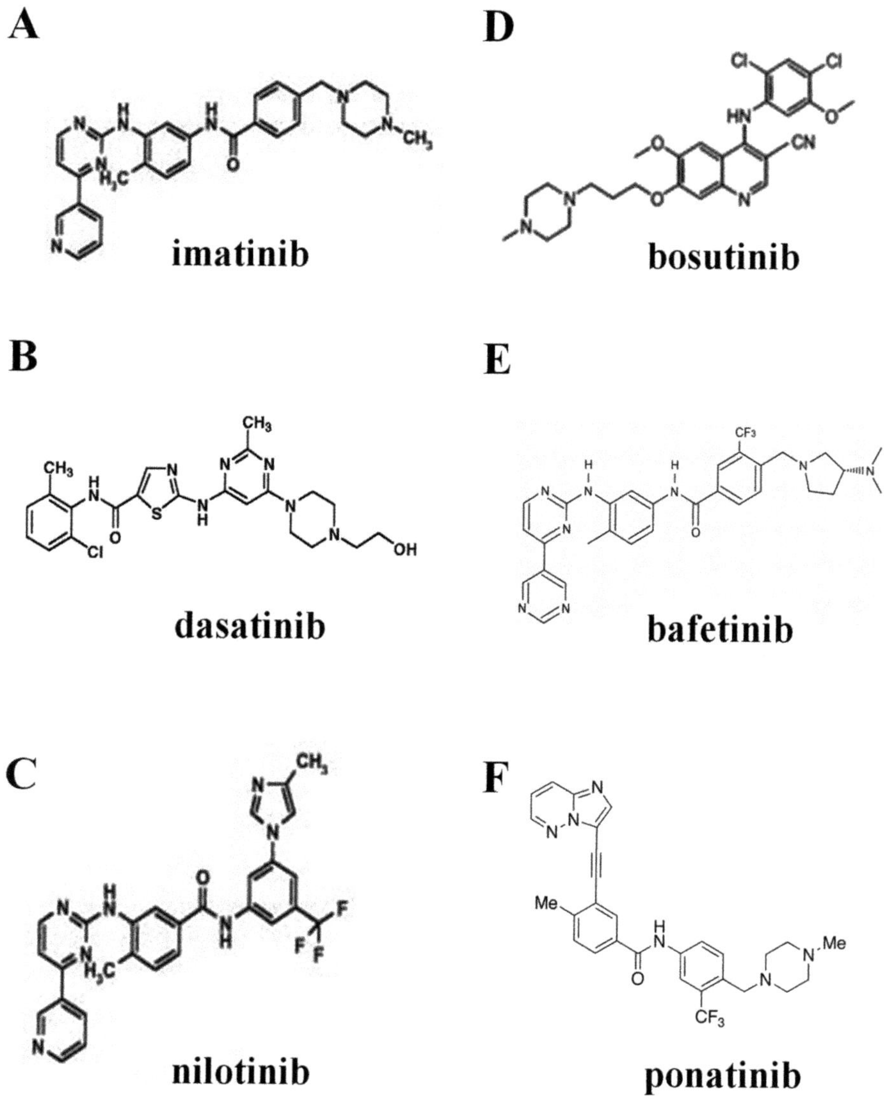

Fig. 4.1 Chemical structures of ABL tyrosine kinases. **a** Imatinib mesylate, **b** dasatinib, **c** nilotinib, **d** bosutinib, **e** bafetinib, **f** ponatinib

imatinib mesylate has led to a marked change in the treatment of chronic myeloid leukemia (CML) [1]. However, resistance and intolerance to imatinib are frequently reported, particularly in patients with advanced-stage disease [2, 3]; this leads to around 30% of CML patients discontinuing imatinib treatment [4].

Point mutations within the *ABL* kinase domain, which interfere with imatinib binding, are the most critical cause of imatinib resistance [5, 6]. To overcome this, four second-generation ATP-competing ABL TKIs, dasatinib [7], nilotinib [8], bosutinib [9], and bafetinib [10], have been developed. Studies show that dasatinib and nilotinib are more effective than imatinib when used to treat naive CML patients in the chronic phase (CP) of the disease [11, 12]. Despite promising clinical results, a common mutation, T315I, is not effectively targeted by any of the second-generation ABL TKIs [13]. Therefore, a third-generation ABL TKI, ponatinib, was developed and shows good clinical efficacy against CML cells harboring the T315I mutation [14]. Thus, treatments for CML are progressing rapidly, and further evolution is expected.

TKIs are classified as Type I (imatinib, nilotinib, bafetinib, and ponatinib), which completely occupy the ATP-binding pocket, and Type II (dasatinib and bosutinib), which partially occupy the ATP-binding pocket (Fig. 4.2) [15]. Type I ABL TKIs bind to the kinase domain of ABL only when the domain adopts an inactive or "closed" conformation. Conversely, Type II ABL TKIs bind to the kinase domain of ABL when the domain adopts the active or "open" conformation [16]. For this reason, Type II ABL TKIs are generally more potent, but less specific, than Type I ABL TKIs.

4.2 Second-Generation ABL TKIs

4.2.1 Dasatinib (Sprycel®)

4.2.1.1 Structure and Preclinical Studies

The chemical formula of dasatinib (Fig. 4.1b) is $C_{22}H_{26}ClN7O_2S$, and its molecular weight is 488 g/mol. The International Union of Pure and Applied Chemistry (IUPAC) name for dasatinib is *N*-(2-chloro-6-methylphenyl)-2-[[6-[4-(2-hydroxyethyl)piperazin-1-yl]-2-methylpyrimidin-4-yl]amino]-1,3-thiazole-5-carboxamide. Dasatinib was developed as a SRC family kinase (SFK) inhibitor. Its affinity for the ABL kinase domain is 325-fold higher than that of imatinib; this was achieved by modifying the piperazinyl ethanol based on thiazole [7]. Imatinib forms six hydrogen bonds with the ATP-binding pocket, while dasatinib forms only two. Also, dasatinib inhibits more than 50 tyrosine kinases, including BCR-ABL, all nine SFKs (SRC, LCK, LYN, FGR, YES, FYN, HCK, BLK, and FRK), c-KIT, EPHA2, and PDGFR-β, suggesting that its specificity is relatively low. Although dasatinib is effective against most mutated BCR-ABLs, its effect on BCR-ABL harboring T315I/A, F317 L/V, V299 L, Q252H, and E255K/V mutations is limited (Fig. 4.3) [7, 17, 18].

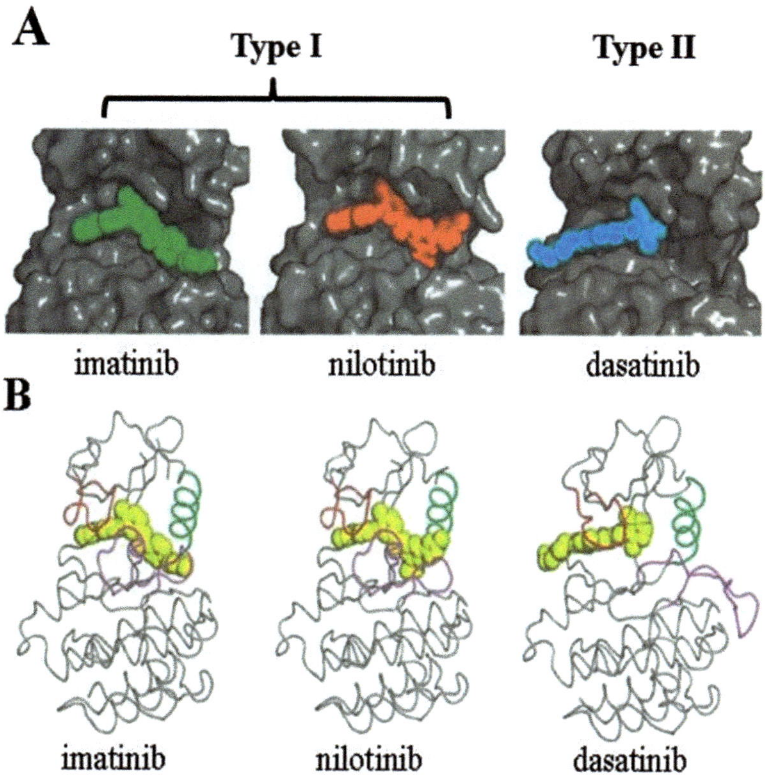

Fig. 4.2 Structure of ABL complexed with imatinib, nilotinib, and dasatinib. **a** Crystal structures of ABL kinase complexed with imatinib (*green*), nilotinib (*red*), and dasatinib (*blue*). Residues from the nucleotide-binding loop (P-loop) and activation loop (A-loop) are omitted from the surface calculation to improve clarity. **b** Comparison of the different binding modes of imatinib (*left*), nilotinib (*middle*), and dasatinib (*right*). The positions of the P-loop (*red*) and A-loop (*magenta*) vary according to whether the kinase is in an active conformation [in which the P-loop adopts an extended conformation and the N-terminal end of the activation loop adopts a "DFG-in" conformation (*right*)] or an inactive conformation [in which the P-loop is bent over the inhibitor and the N-terminal end of the activation loop adopts a "DFG-out" conformation (*left* and *middle*)]. Imatinib and nilotinib block the kinase in an inactive conformation. The *green* helix is helix C, which often moves between the active and inactive states (Adapted and modified from 15)

4.2.1.2 Pharmacokinetics

The T_{max} (the time at which the maximum serum concentration, C_{max}, is observed) of dasatinib is estimated to be approximately 0.5 h. Both dasatinib and the total radioactivity plasma concentration decrease rapidly, with an elimination half-life ($T_{1/2}$) of less than 4 h [19]. Because the $T_{1/2}$ of dasatinib is very short, the initial recommendation is that it be administered in twice-daily (bis in die; BID) doses. However, a once-daily (quaque die; QD) dose of 100 mg is as effective as 70 mg BID and has fewer adverse effects [20]. Thus, dasatinib is usually administered to adults with chronic phase CML (CML-CP) at a dose of 100 mg QD. This suggests that

		IC_{50} fold increase (WT = 1)			
		Bosutinib	Imatinib	Dasatinib	Nilotinib
	Parental	38.31	10.78	> 50	38.43
	WT	1	1	1	1
P-LOOP	L248V	2.97	3.54	5.11	2.80
	G250E	4.31	6.86	4.45	4.56
	Q252H	0.81	1.39	3.05	2.64
	Y253F	0.96	3.58	1.58	3.23
	E255K	9.47	6.02	5.61	6.69
	E255V	5.53	16.99	3.44	10.31
C-Helix	D276G	0.60	2.18	1.44	2.00
	E279K	0.95	3.55	1.64	2.05
ATP binding region (drug contact sites)	V299L	26.10	1.54	8.65	1.34
	T315I	45.42	17.50	75.03	39.41
	F317L	2.42	2.60	4.46	2.22
SH2-contact	M351T	0.70	1.76	0.88	0.44
Substrate binding region (drug contact sites)	F359V	0.93	2.86	1.49	5.16
A-LOOP	L384M	0.47	1.28	2.21	2.33
	H396P	0.43	2.43	1.07	2.41
	H396R	0.81	3.91	1.63	3.10
	G398R	1.16	0.35	0.69	0.49
C terminal lobe	F486S	2.31	8.10	3.04	1.85

Sensitive	≤2
Moderately resistant	2.01-4
Resistant	4.01-10
Highly resistant	> 10

Fig. 4.3 IC_{50} values for bosutinib, imatinib, dasatinib, and nilotinib against 18 mutated forms of BCR/ABL expressed in Ba/F3-transfected cells. IC_{50}, relative concentration that inhibits 50%; *WT* wild type, *P-loop* phosphate-binding loop, *ATP* adenosine triphosphate, *SH2* Src homology 2, *A-loop* activation loop (Adapted from 18)

inhibiting ABL kinase for only several hours per day is enough to prevent CML progression and that constitutive suppression of multiple kinases might induce a greater number of adverse effects [20]. We also showed that a 2 h exposure of CML cells to another second-generation ABL TKI, bafetinib, was enough to inhibit proliferation [21].

With respect to its interaction with other agents, a previous study showed that dose-adjusted area under the concentration-time curve (AUC) for dasatinib over the first 4 h of a 12 h dosage interval ($AUC_{[0-4]}$) in patients taking an H_2 receptor antagonist or proton pump inhibitor (PPI) was significantly lower than that in patients not taking an acid suppressant [22]. Also, CYP3A4 inhibitors may increase the levels of dasatinib in the system. Thus, clinicians should consider reducing the dose of dasatinib if a patient is also taking CYP3A4 inhibitors. By contrast, CYP3A4 inducers may reduce the systemic levels of dasatinib. Thus, it may be necessary to increase the dose when CYP3A4 inducers are used simultaneously [23].

4.2.1.3 Clinical Effects

A phase 2 clinical trial in which 387 imatinib-resistant/intolerant patients with CML-CP received 70 mg of dasatinib BID (140 mg/day) was performed, and a complete cytogenetic response [CCyR: a state in which the Philadelphia (Ph) chromosome was not detected] was achieved in 49% of cases [24].

Another clinical trial [the dasatinib versus imatinib study in treatment-naive CML patients (DASISION) trial] examined the use of first-line dasatinib immediately after a diagnosis of CML. Dasatinib (100 mg QD) or imatinib (400 mg QD) was administered to previously untreated patients with CML-CP: a CCyR was observed in 77% and 66% of cases, respectively, after 12 months. Also, a major molecular response [MMR: a ≥3 log reduction in *BCR-ABL* mRNA levels as measured by real-time quantitative PCR (RQ-PCR)] was observed in 46% and 28% of cases, respectively. The time to MMR was significantly shorter in the dasatinib group (Table 4.1a) [11].

Dasatinib is indicated not only for CML but also for Ph chromosome-positive acute lymphoblastic leukemia (Ph^+ALL). Patients with newly diagnosed Ph^+ALL received dasatinib induction therapy for 84 days, which is combined with steroids

Table 4.1 Clinical effects of first-line dasatinib and nilotinib

a. Dassision (dasatinib)				b. ENESTnd (nilotinib)				
		Imatinib	Dasatinib			Imatinib	Nilotinib	Nilotinib
		400 mg QD	100 mg QD			400 mg QD	300 mg BID	400 mg BID
CCyR				CCyR				
	3 M	31%	54%					
	6 M	59%	73%		6 M	45%	67%	63%
	9 M	67%	78%					
	12 M	72%	83%		12 M	65%	80%	78%
MMR				MMR				
	3 M	0.40%	8%		3 M	1.00%	9%	5%
	6 M	8%	27%		6 M	12%	33%	30%
	9 M	18%	39%		9 M	18%	43%	38%
	12 M	28%	46%		12 M	22%	44%	43%
Progression to AP/BP		3.50%	1.90%	Progression to AP/BP		4%	<1%	<1%

CCyR complete cytogenetic response, *MMR* major molecular response, *AP* accelerated phase, *BP* blastic phase, *QD* once a day, *BID* twice a day for the first 32 days and intrathecal chemotherapy. At 20 months, overall survival was 69.2%, and disease-free survival was 51.1%. In adults with Ph⁺ALL, induction treatment with dasatinib plus steroids leads to a complete hematologic response (CHR) in virtually all patients irrespective of age, with good compliance, no deaths, and a rapid debulking of the neoplastic clone [25]. When 34 patients with relapsed Ph^+ALL or CML-lymphoid blast crisis (CML-LB) were treated with a combination of dasatinib and hyper-CVAD, 84% achieved CCyR after one cycle of therapy. Overall, 42% of patients achieved a complete molecular response (CMR: defined as *bcr-abl* mRNA negativity as measured by RQ-PCR), and 35% had a MMR [26].

Imatinib does not prevent central nervous system (CNS) relapse due to poor penetration through the blood-brain barrier [27]. Although dasatinib is a substrate of P glycoprotein (as is imatinib) [28], the high potency of dasatinib means that residual concentrations in the CNS are sufficient to prevent the proliferation of CML cells. Thus, dasatinib has therapeutic potential for the management of intracranial leukemic disease and shows substantial clinical activity in patients who experience CNS relapse while receiving imatinib therapy [29].

4.2.1.4 Adverse Effects

Pleural effusion and thrombocytopenia are observed slightly more frequently, and edema, gastrointestinal symptoms, muscle-related symptoms, and rash are observed less frequently, with dasatinib than with imatinib [11]. Dasatinib-induced platelet dysfunction can cause clinically significant bleeding [30]. Adverse effects such as colitis and pleuritis are common and are preceded by large granular lymphocyte (LGL) lymphocytosis [31]. Recent reports of pulmonary arterial hypertension in those taking dasatinib have raised concerns about the long-term sequelae of drugs that may need to be administered for decades [32].

4.2.1.5 Indications and Usage

Dasatinib is indicated for the treatment of adult patients with newly diagnosed CML-CP, for adults with all phases of CML[-CP/accelerated (AP)/blastic phase (BP)] showing resistance or intolerance to prior therapy (including imatinib), and for adults with Ph^+ALL showing resistance or intolerance to prior therapy. A dose of 100 mg QD is recommended for CML-CP patients, whereas 140 mg QD is recommended for patients with CML-AP/BP or Ph^+ALL. Dasatinib is administered orally, either with or without food.

4.2.1.6 Immunoeffects

A subset of patients treated with dasatinib show an increased number of LGL, and the outcome is reported to be more favorable in such patients [33]. Generally, the greater the dose of dasatinib, the higher the incidence of LGL lymphocytosis. This is thought to be due to direct stimulation of LGL proliferation or to inhibition of LGL-suppressing regulatory T cells (Tregs) by dasatinib [34]; however, the mechanistic details are unclear.

Dasatinib induces a rapid, dose-dependent, and substantial mobilization of non-leukemic lymphocytes and monocytes in the blood, peaking 1–2 h after oral intake;

the blood counts closely mirror the plasma concentration of the drug. A previous study showed preferential mobilization of natural killer (NK), NKT, B, and $\gamma\delta^+$ T cells, coupled with more effective transmigration of leukocytes through an endothelial cell layer, along with improved NK cell cytotoxicity [35].

4.2.1.7 Stop Studies

Only one dasatinib stop study [the dasatinib discontinue (DADI) trial] has been published [36]. Dasatinib treatment subsequent to imatinib was discontinued after confirmation of a stable deep molecular response (DMR; defined as *bcr-abl* mRNA negativity as measured by RQ-PCR) for more than 1 year. At a median follow-up of 20 months after discontinuation, the estimated treatment-free remission (TFR) rates were 49% at 6 months and 48% at 12 months (Fig. 4.4a). The TFR rate at 12 months was significantly poorer in imatinib-resistant patients (8%) than in other patients (58%) ($p = 0.0001$) (Fig. 4.4b). The high NK cell and low $\gamma\delta^+$ T cell and $CD4^+$ Tregs ($CD25^+CD127^{low}$) counts observed before discontinuation were significantly correlated with successful discontinuation of therapy. All molecularly relapsed patients returned to DMR within 6 months after the reintroduction of dasatinib. These findings suggested that discontinuation of dasatinib after sustained DMR for more than 1 year is feasible, particularly in patients without a prior history of imatinib resistance.

4.2.2 Nilotinib (Tasigna®)

4.2.2.1 Structure and Preclinical Studies

The chemical formula of nilotinib (Fig. 4.1c) is $C_{28}H_{22}F_3N_7O$, and its molecular weight is 530 g/mol. The IUPAC name is 4-methyl-*N*-[3-(4-methyl-1*H*-imidazol -1-yl)-5-(trifluoromethyl)phenyl]-3-[(4-pyridin-3-ylpyrimidin-2-yl)amino]benzamide. Structural modification of imatinib (to generate nilotinib) led to a 30-fold increase in anti-CML activity. Nilotinib forms four hydrogen bonds with the ATP-binding pocket, and it suppresses ABL, PDGFR, and c-KIT activity, but not SFK activity. The affinity of imatinib for PDGFR and c-KIT is stronger than that for ABL, whereas the affinity of nilotinib for ABL is stronger than that for other kinases. Thus, nilotinib has higher specificity for ABL than imatinib and other TKIs, including dasatinib and bosutinib [8]. Although nilotinib is effective against most forms of mutated ABL (except T315I), its effects against ABL harboring E255K/V, Y253F/H, Q252H, and F359 V are limited (Fig. 4.3) [8, 17, 18].

4.2.2.2 Pharmacokinetics

The T_{max} of nilotinib is 3 h, and the $T_{1/2}$ following multiple daily dosing is approximately 17 h, which is much longer than that of dasatinib. One important issue with nilotinib is that the type and quantity of food affect its absorption. When administered after a high-fat meal, the AUC of nilotinib in CML patients increases by 50% [37].

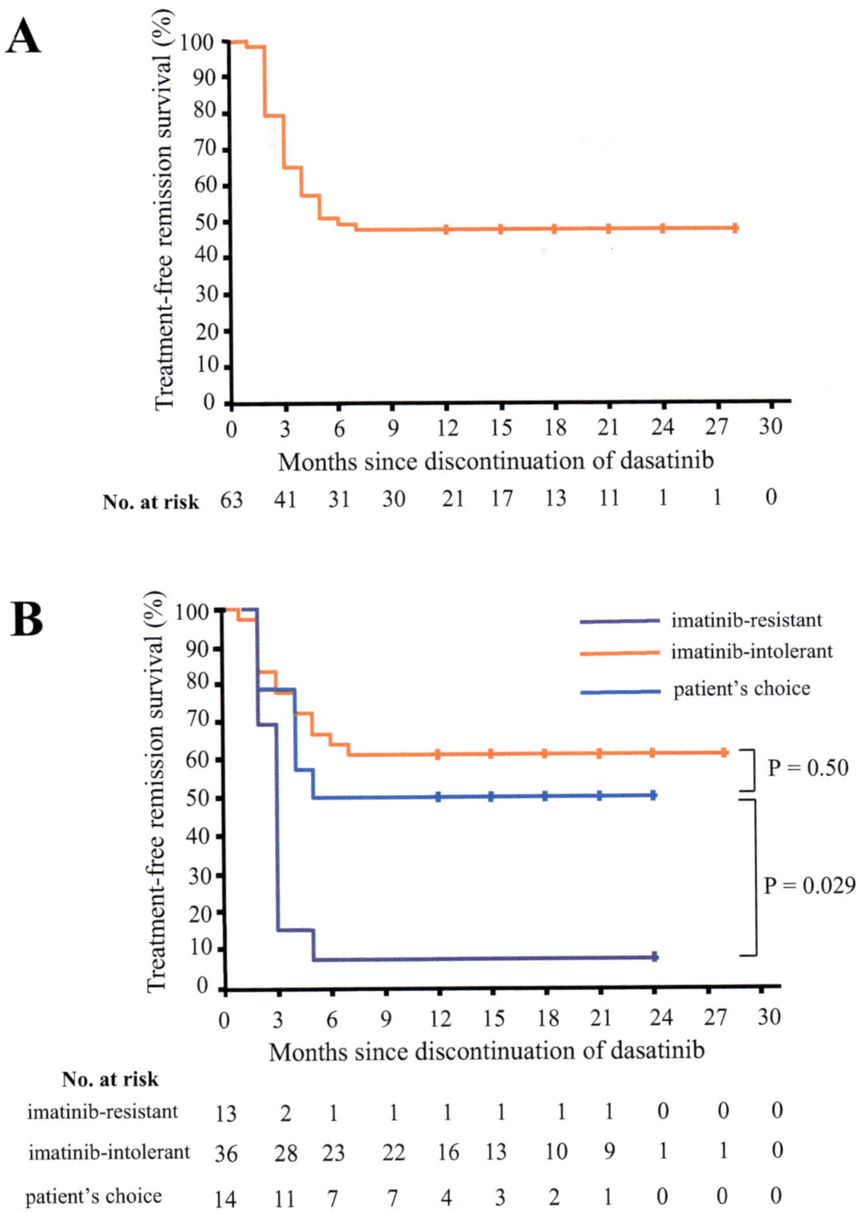

Fig. 4.4 Kaplan-Meier estimates of treatment-free survival in patients with chronic myeloid leukemia after discontinuation of dasatinib. **a** For all 63 patients, the estimated treatment-free remission rate was 49% (95% CI, 36–61%) at 6 months and 48% (95% CI, 35–59%) at 12 months. **b** Treatment-free remission rates based on the reasons for switching patients from imatinib to dasatinib (Adapted from 36)

Nilotinib is a competitive inhibitor of cytochromes CYP3A4, CYP2C8, CYP2C9, and CYP2D6 [38]. Single-dose or repeated-dose administration of nilotinib results in weak and moderate inhibition of CYP3A, respectively [39]. Thus, care must be taken when it is administered in combination with other agents that affect CYPs. In addition, PPIs cause a modest reduction in the rate and extent of nilotinib absorption [40]. With respect to transporters, OCT-1-mediated influx may be a key determinant of the molecular response to imatinib; however, it is unlikely to impact cellular uptake and patient responses [41].

4.2.2.3 Clinical Effects

In a phase 2 open-label study, 400 mg of nilotinib was administered BID to patients with CML-CP after imatinib failure or intolerance. At 6 months, the rate of major cytogenetic response (McyR, Ph ≤35%) was 48% and that of CCyR was 31%. Nilotinib was effective in patients harboring BCR-ABL mutations associated with imatinib resistance (except T315I) and also in patients with a resistance mechanism that was independent of BCR-ABL mutations [42].

Another study reviewed the outcome of 420 patients with CML post-imatinib failure (resistance-recurrence in 374; toxicity in 46). The estimated 3 year survival rates were 72% in 88 patients who progressed to the chronic phase, 30% in 130 patients who progressed to the AP, 7% in 156 patients who progressed to the BP, and 75% in 37 CP patients who were imatinib intolerant [43].

The Efficacy and Safety in Clinical Trials – Newly Diagnosed Patients (ENESTnd) study examined patients with previously untreated CML-CP. Patients received nilotinib at 300 or 400 mg BID or imatinib at 400 mg QD. After 12 months, the MMR rate was 44% in the nilotinib 300 mg BID group, 43% in the nilotinib 400 mg BID group, and 22% in the imatinib group (Table 4.1b) [12].

Another study reported that, after a priming procedure with peginterferon α-2a (90 μg per week for 1 month), CML patients received peginterferon α-2a (45 μg per week) combined with nilotinib (600 mg daily) up until 24 months after interferon initiation. At 12 months, 17% of patients had achieved more than 4.5 log reduction of *BCR-ABL* mRNA determined RQ-PCR (MR4.5). Despite substantial toxicity, most patients remained on the study drugs for more than 1 year [44].

Imatinib and dasatinib have been registered for the treatment of Ph^+ALL. Nilotinib has also been tested as a second-line drug and can offer an alternative to patients who fail to respond to a first-line drug [45]. The combination of nilotinib and high-dose cytotoxic drugs is feasible, achieving a high cumulative CMR and hematologic relapse-free survival rates [46].

4.2.2.4 Adverse Effects

In a phase 2 trial involving imatinib-resistant/imatinib-intolerant CML-CP patients, grade 3 or higher side effects, including thrombocytopenia, neutropenia, and increased levels of bilirubin and lipase, were observed. Cross-intolerance with imatinib was rare [42]. The ENESTnd study revealed no significant difference between imatinib and nilotinib in terms of safety. Rash, headache, and mild increases in liver and pancreatic enzyme levels were observed slightly more frequently in patients receiving nilotinib, but edema, muscle convulsions, and neutropenia were observed less frequently [12].

Recent reports show that nilotinib may be associated with an increased risk of vascular adverse events, including peripheral artery occlusive disease (PAOD) [47, 48]. Despite this, the risk of developing PAOD while on TKI therapy is unclear, and causality has not been established. A retrospective cohort analysis examined the rates of PAOD in CML-CP patients treated with imatinib or nilotinib or with non-tyrosine kinase-based therapy. Nilotinib was associated with higher rates of PAOD than imatinib [49]. Although the underlying mechanisms remain unknown, patients should be screened for PAOD and other vascular risk factors such as diabetes mellitus prior to starting nilotinib and again during therapy.

4.2.2.5 Indication and Usage

Nilotinib is indicated for the treatment of adult patients with newly diagnosed CML-CP and for the treatment of CML-CP/AP in adults resistant or intolerant to prior therapies, including imatinib. Nilotinib should be taken BID at approximately 12 h intervals and on an empty stomach. No food should be consumed for at least 2 h before and for at least 1 h after the drug is taken. Newly diagnosed CML-CP patients should receive 300 mg BID nilotinib, and those with resistant or intolerant CML-CP/AP should receive 400 mg BID.

4.2.2.6 Immunoeffects

Nilotinib inhibits the proliferation and suppressive capacity of Tregs in a dose-dependent manner. However, the production of cytokines by Tregs and $CD4^{+}CD25^{-}$ T cells is only inhibited at high concentrations of nilotinib (i.e., doses exceeding the mean therapeutic serum concentration of the drug). Nilotinib does not hamper Tregs function at clinically relevant doses [50].

4.2.2.7 Stop Studies

Several nilotinib stop studies, such as ENEStop [51], ENESTFreedom [52], and NILSt [53], are ongoing.

4.2.3 Bosutinib (Bosulif®)

4.2.3.1 Structure and Preclinical Studies

The chemical formula of bosutinib (Fig. 4.1d) is $C_{26}H_{29}Cl_2N_5O_3$, and its molecular weight is 530 g/mol. The IUPAC name is 4-[(2,4-dichloro-5-methoxyphenyl) amino]-6-methoxy-7-[3-(4-methylpiperazin-1-yl)propoxy] quinolone-3-carbonitrile. The affinity of bosutinib for ABL is about 50-fold higher than that of imatinib, and it shows characteristically weak inhibitory activity against c-KIT and PDGFR, which can sometimes cause adverse effects in patients treated with imatinib. The affinity of bosutinib for ABL is weaker than that of dasatinib, while that of bosutinib for SFKs (including SRC, LYN, HCK, and FYN) is almost ten times higher than that of dasatinib. However, bosutinib has only a very weak inhibitory effect on other

SFKs, including YES, LCK, FGR, and BLK [9]. A conserved water-mediated hydrogen bond network defines the kinase selectivity of bosutinib [54].

Although bosutinib is effective against most mutant BCR-ABLs (except T315I), its effects against BCR-ABL harboring E255K/V or V299 L are limited (Fig. 4.3) [9, 18, 55].

4.2.3.2 Pharmacokinetics

A study showed that treatment with single and multiple doses of bosutinib resulted in slow absorption, with a median time to T_{max} of 4–6 h and a $T_{1/2}$ from 13 to 22 h [56]. Preliminary assessments showed that the C_{max} increased by ~2.52-fold and the AUC by ~2.28-fold when bosutinib (200 mg) was administered with food rather than under fasting conditions; administration of 400 mg of bosutinib with food increased the AUC by ~1.5-fold. Under fed conditions, bosutinib exposure was linear, and the dose was proportional, and the C_{max} increased by ~1.5-fold. The $T_{1/2}$ supports a once-daily dosing regimen [57].

Bosutinib interacts with potent CYP3A4 inhibitors [58]; thus, care is needed when it is used in combination with other agents that affect CYPs. Bosutinib absorption may be reduced when coadministered with lansoprazole or other PPIs. Caution should be used in such cases as subtherapeutic exposure to bosutinib may limit its clinical antitumor activity; short-acting antacids are recommended instead of PPIs [58].

Nilotinib and dasatinib are high-affinity substrates for ABCG2, which mediates cancer cell resistance to these compounds. Both nilotinib and dasatinib interact with ABCB1; however, this leads to resistance against dasatinib alone. Neither ABCB1 nor ABCG2 induced resistance to bosutinib. At relatively higher concentrations, both TKIs inhibit both transporters [28].

4.2.3.3 Clinical Effects

The safety and efficacy of bosutinib have been assessed in a phase 1/2 study that enrolled 288 CML patients that were resistant or intolerant to imatinib [59]; later, another 119 CML-CP patients that were resistant or intolerant to nilotinib or dasatinib were enrolled after these agents had been approved [60]. The dose escalation phase of this trial determined that the recommended phase 2 dose of bosutinib was 500 mg QD. During the phase 2 portion of this trial (median follow-up, 24 months), 86% of CP patients achieved CHR and 53% achieved McyR. A phase 1/2, nonrandomized clinical trial revealed similar responses across all BCR-ABL kinase domain mutations when compared with wild-type BCR-ABL, with the exception of the highly resistant T315I mutation. Patients with the bosutinib-resistant V299 L mutation were not included in the study [59].

Another study examined the long-term efficacy and safety of bosutinib (500 mg/day) in adults with imatinib-resistant/intolerant CML-CP. The cumulative McyR rate was 59%, and the Kaplan-Meier probability of maintaining McyR at 4 years was 75%. The cumulative incidence of nontreatment progression/death at 4 years was 19%. Significant baseline predictors of both McyR and CCyR at 3 and 6 months included a prior cytogenetic response to imatinib, baseline McyR, prior interferon therapy, <6 months' duration from diagnosis to initiation of imatinib treatment, and no interferon treatment prior to imatinib [61].

The efficacy of bosutinib for patients treated with bosutinib as a fourth-line drug has also been reported. The probability of either maintaining or improving the CCyR response was 56.6%, and 36.7% of patients achieved or maintained their baseline MMR. Even in patients without baseline CCyR, the probability of obtaining CCyR, MMR, and MR4.5 was 13%, 11%, and 14%, respectively. Bosutinib appears to be an appropriate treatment option for patients who are resistant or intolerant to first-, second-, and third-line TKIs [62]. When bosutinib was used as a third-line drug to treat Japanese CML patients, the cumulative McyR rate by week 24 was 18%, and the cumulative MMR rate was 18%; no transformations occurred [63].

The Bosutinib Efficacy and Safety in Newly Diagnosed CML (BELA) trial involved patients with previously untreated CML-CP. The cumulative MMR rates in the BELA trial were 59% for bosutinib and 49% for imatinib [64].

4.2.3.4 Adverse Effects

The most common treatment-emergent adverse event is mild/moderate, typically self-limiting, diarrhea. Grade 3/4 non-hematologic adverse events (>2% of patients) included elevated ALT levels (10% of patients), diarrhea (9%), rash (9%), and vomiting (3%) [59]. The BELA study revealed that certain gastrointestinal adverse events were more common with bosutinib than with imatinib (e.g., diarrhea and vomiting), as were elevated alanine aminotransferase and aspartate aminotransferase levels and pyrexia. Edema, musculoskeletal problems, increased creatine phosphokinase levels, and leukopenia were significantly less common in patients receiving bosutinib. Diarrhea was typically transient, mostly grade 1/2, and occurred early during treatment; however, it was manageable with antidiarrheal medication. The higher rates of elevated aminotransferase in patients receiving bosutinib were managed by altering the dose and/or the prescription of concomitant medication [65].

A meta-analysis based on ten randomized clinical trials revealed that dasatinib, nilotinib, and ponatinib increased the risk of vascular occlusive events in patients with CML when compared with imatinib. There was no significant difference between bosutinib and imatinib [66].

4.2.3.5 Indication and Usage

Bosutinib is indicated for the treatment of adult patients with all-phase CML(-CP/AP/BC) that is resistant or intolerant to prior therapy. The recommended dose of bosutinib is 500 mg QD to be taken with food. Dose escalation to 600 mg QD should be considered for patients who do not reach CHR by week 8 or CCyR by week 12 and do not have grade 3 or greater adverse reactions. Dose reduction to 200 mg QD is recommended for patients with hepatic impairment (at baseline).

4.2.3.6 Immunoeffects

Unlike dasatinib, bosutinib does not induce LGL expansion [35].

4.2.3.7 Stop Studies

Several stop studies using combinations of second-generation ABL TKIs are ongoing. However, to my knowledge, no stop study has focused only on bosutinib.

4.2.4 Bafetinib (Formerly INNO-406)

Bafetinib (Fig. 4.1e) was developed preclinically in Japan, and phase 1 has been completed successfully in CML patients that are resistant/intolerant to other TKIs. Since bafetinib has not yet been approved, it will be discussed only briefly here. Bafetinib simultaneously inhibits ABL and LYN, and its activity against ABL is about 55-fold greater than that of imatinib. While it is also effective against most mutants, it has no effect on the T315I mutant [10, 17]. A phase 1 trial revealed few serious adverse effects, and the drug was effective for some dasatinib-resistant patients [67]. Interestingly, bafetinib may also be effective in patients with Parkinson's disease [68].

4.3 Third-Generation ABL TKIs

4.3.1 Ponatinib (Iclusig®)

4.3.1.1 Structure and Preclinical Studies

The chemical formula of ponatinib (Fig. 4.1f) is $C_{29}H_{27}F_3N_6O$, and its molecular weight is 533 g/mol. The IUPAC name is 3-(2-imidazo[1,2-b]pyridazin-3-ylethynyl) -4-methyl-*N*-[4-[(4-methylpiperazin-1-yl)methyl]-3-(trifluoromethyl)phenyl]benzamide. Ponatinib was designed using a computational and structure-based drug design platform, and it inhibits the enzymatic activity of BCR-ABL with very high potency and broad specificity. Ponatinib was intended to target not only native BCR-ABL but also isoforms that carry mutations that confer resistance to treatment with existing TKIs, including the T315I mutation for which no effective therapy exists [69]. Ponatinib is a multi-targeted kinase inhibitor that suppresses more than 60 kinases, including ABL, PDGFR, c-KIT, SFK, VEGFR, and FGFR activities [14, 70]. Ponatinib is effective against most mutant BCR-ABLs, including T315I; therefore, it is often referred to as a pan-BCR-ABL TKI. It avoids the conformational effects of T315I due to its long and flexible carbon-carbon triple bond (Fig. 4.5) [14]. At present, ponatinib is the only ABL TKI that is effective against the T315I mutation. However, caution is needed, as it may be ineffective against compound mutations [71].

4.3.1.2 Pharmacokinetics

The T_{max} of ponatinib is approximately 4 h, and the $T_{1/2}$ is 22 h. A daily dose of 30 mg achieves steady-state trough plasma concentrations that exceed 40 nM, a concentration sufficient to inhibit the viability of cells expressing all BCR-ABL

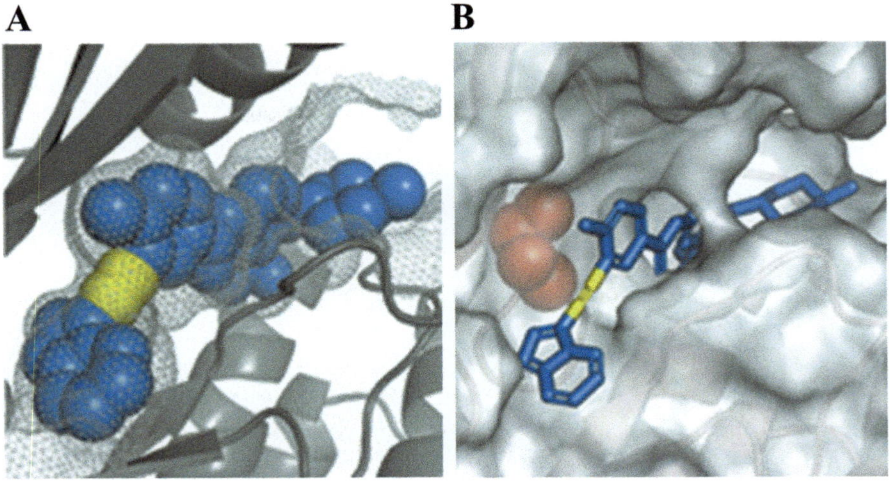

Fig. 4.5 Structure of ponatinib. **a** Ponatinib (represented by *blue* and *yellow* space-filling spheres) shows optimal fit with the binding cavity of AVL-T315I (indicated by a mesh pattern). **b** The triple bond (*yellow*) is a unique structural feature of ponatinib (*blue*). This bond allows the drug to avoid the mutant gatekeeper residue I315 (Represented by *red* space-filling spheres) (Adapted from 72)

mutants, including the T315I gatekeeper mutant [72]. Food does not affect the single-dose pharmacokinetics of ponatinib [73].

The drug is metabolized (partially) by CYP3A4. Caution should be exercised when prescribing ponatinib concurrently with strong CYP3A4 inhibitors; indeed, a dose reduction to 30 mg QD (from the 45 mg QD starting dose) could be considered [74]. Although coadministration of lansoprazole led to a modest, albeit statistically significant, reduction in the C_{max} of ponatinib, the systemic dose of ponatinib did not change. The findings suggest that no dose adjustment is necessary when ponatinib is administered along with drugs that increase gastric pH [75].

4.3.1.3 Clinical Effects

The Ponatinib Ph⁺ALL and CML Evaluation (PACE) study, which examined 267 patients with chronic phase CML, found that 56% showed a major cytogenetic response (51% of patients that were resistant to or experienced unacceptable side effects with dasatinib or nilotinib and 70% of patients harboring the T315I mutation), 46% showed a complete cytogenetic response (40% and 66%, respectively, of those in the above two subgroups), and 34% showed a MMR (27% and 56%, respectively, of those in the above two subgroups). Responses were observed regardless of baseline BCR-ABL kinase domain mutation status, and all were durable; the estimated rate of a sustained major cytogenetic response of at least 12 months was 91%. No single BCR-ABL mutation conferring resistance to ponatinib was detected. Among 83 patients with CML-AP, 55% showed a major hematologic response, and 39% showed an McyR. Among the 62 patients with CML-BP, 31% showed a major hematologic response, and 23% showed an McyR. Among 32 patients with Ph⁺ALL,

41% showed a major hematologic response, and 47% showed an McyR [76]. Subanalysis of the PACE trial revealed that McyR was achieved regardless of baseline mutation status. Responses were also observed in patients with mutations other than T315I (e.g., E255V, F359 V, or Y253H).

Fifty-one CML patients were treated with first-line ponatinib; of these, 43 were started on 45 mg of ponatinib daily, and eight were started on 30 mg daily. Overall, 43 (94%) of 46 evaluable patients achieved a CCyR at 6 months [77]. However, the study was terminated on June 18, 2014, at the recommendation of the FDA, due to concerns about the increased risk of thromboembolism.

The impact of the T315I mutation on prognosis after treatment with ponatinib is still unclear. Zabriskie reported that T315I-inclusive compound mutants confer high-level resistance to TKIs, including ponatinib [78]. Parker et al. reported that low-level mutations were detectable by sensitive mass spectrometry prior to ponatinib initiation (baseline) in 15% of TKI-resistant patients (including 4% of patients harboring low-level T315I). Most, however, did not undergo clonal expansion during ponatinib treatment; moreover, no specific individual mutations were associated with an inferior outcome. Ponatinib may prove to be particularly advantageous for patients harboring multiple TKI-resistant mutations that are detectable by mass spectrometry [79].

4.3.1.4 Adverse Effects

Common adverse events noted in the PACE study included thrombocytopenia (37% of patients), rash (34%), dry skin (32%), and abdominal pain (22%). Serious arterial thrombotic events were observed in 9% of patients; these events were considered to be treatment related in 3%. In total, 12% of patients discontinued treatment due to an adverse event [76].

A clinical trial of ponatinib as a first-line treatment showed that the most common toxicity-related effects were skin related (69%). Increased lipase levels were also noted in 63% of patients. Cardiovascular events (mainly hypertension) occurred in 49% of patients. Grade 3/4 myelosuppression occurred in 29% of patients, and 10% of patients developed cerebrovascular or vaso-occlusive disease. Finally, 85% of patients underwent treatment interruption at some point, and 88% required a dose reduction [77].

4.3.1.5 Indication and Usage

Ponatinib is indicated for the treatment of adult patients with all-phase CML(-CP/AP/BP) that is resistant or intolerant to prior ABL tyrosine TKI therapy or Ph^+ALL that is resistant or intolerant to prior TKI therapy. The dose is 45 mg QD with or without food. The dose should be modified or interrupted in cases of hematologic and non-hematologic toxicity.

4.3.1.6 Immunoeffects

At present, no data regarding ponatinib-induced immune responses have been published.

4.3.1.7 Stop Studies

The SPIRIT 3 study, which includes a ponatinib stop, is ongoing [80].

4.4 Fourth-Generation ABL TKIs

4.4.1 PF-114

PF-114 is a novel, orally available selective pan-BCR-ABL inhibitor that targets T315I and suppresses models of advanced Ph^+ ALL. PF-114 is more selective than dasatinib or ponatinib. It efficiently inhibits all tested BCR-ABL mutants in both cellular and biochemical assays when used at doses of 10–100 nM. Like ponatinib, it suppresses the development of new resistance mutations in a mutation assay based on Ba/F3 cells [81]. A clinical trial of PF-114 is being planned.

4.5 Conclusion

The advent of imatinib, followed by the second-generation (dasatinib, nilotinib, and bosutinib) and third-generation (ponatinib) variants, has led to a marked improvement in the treatment and prognosis of CML. Further evolution of treatment is surely expected. However, if we are to provide treatments tailor-made to fit individual CML patients, more agents with different activity profiles are required.

References

1. Druker BJ. Perspectives on the development of imatinib and the future of cancer research. Nat Med. 2009;15:1149–52.
2. Druker BJ, Sawyers CL, Kantarjian H, et al. Activity of a specific inhibitor of the BCR-ABL tyrosine kinase in the blast crisis of chronic myeloid leukemia and acute lymphoblastic leukemia with the Philadelphia chromosome. N Engl J Med. 2001;344:1038–42.
3. Ottmann OG, Druker BJ, Sawyers CL, et al. A phase 2 study of imatinib in patients with relapsed or refractory Philadelphia chromosome-positive acute lymphoid leukemias. Blood. 2002;100:1965–71.
4. Quintás-Cardama A, Kantarjian H, Cortes J. Imatinib and beyond – exploring the full potential of targeted therapy for CML. Nat Rev Clin Oncol. 2009;6:535–43.
5. Gorre ME, Mohammed M, Ellwood K, et al. Clinical resistance to STI-571 cancer therapy caused by BCR-ABL gene mutation or amplification. Science. 2001;293:876–80.
6. Deininger M, Buchdunger E, Druker BJ. The development of imatinib as a therapeutic agent for chronic myeloid leukemia. Blood. 2005;105:2640–53.
7. Shah NP, Tran C, Lee FY, et al. Overriding imatinib resistance with a novel ABL kinase inhibitor. Science. 2004;305:399–401.
8. Weisberg D, Manley PW, Breitenstein W, et al. Characterization of AMN107, a selective inhibitor of native and mutant Bcr-Abl. Cancer Cell. 2005;7:129–41.
9. Golas JM, Arndt K, Etienne D, et al. SKI-606, a 4-anilino-3-quinolinecarbonitrile dual inhibitor of Src and Abl kinases, is a potent antiproliferative agent against chronic myelogenous

leukemia cells in culture and causes regression of K562 xenografts in nude mice. Cancer Res. 2003;3:375–81.
10. Kimura S, Naito H, Segawa H, et al. NS-187, a potent and selective dual Bcr-Abl/Lyn tyrosine kinase inhibitor, is a novel agent for imatinib-resistant leukemia. Blood. 2005;106:3948–54.
11. Kantarjian H, Shah NP, Hochhaus A, et al. Dasatinib versus imatinib in newly diagnosed chronic-phase chronic myeloid leukemia. N Engl J Med. 2010;362:2260–70.
12. Saglio G, Kim DW, Issaragrisil S, et al. Nilotinib versus imatinib for newly diagnosed chronic myeloid leukemia. N Engl J Med. 2010;362:2251–9.
13. Kimura S, Ando T, Kojima K. BCR-ABL point mutations and TKI treatment in CML patients. J Hematol Transf. 2014;2:1022–33.
14. O'Hare T, Shakespeare WC, Zhu X, et al. AP24534, a pan-BCR-ABL inhibitor for chronic myeloid leukemia, potently inhibits the T315I mutant and overcomes mutation-based resistance. Cancer Cell. 2009;16:401–12.
15. Weisberg E, Manley PW, Sandra W, et al. Structure of ABL in complex with imatinib, nilotinib and dasatinib. Nat Rev Cancer. 2007;7:345–56.
16. Asaki T, Sugiyama Y, Hamamoto T, et al. Design and synthesis of 3-substituted benzamide derivatives as Bcr-Abl kinase inhibitors. Bioorg Med Chem Lett. 2006;16:1421–5.
17. Deguchi Y, Kimura S, Ashihara E, et al. Comparison of imatinib, dasatinib, nilotinib and INNO-406 in imatinib-resistant cell lines. Leuk Res. 2008;32:980–3.
18. Redaelli S, Piazza R, Rostagno R, et al. Activity of bosutinib, dasatinib, and nilotinib against 18 imatinib-resistant BCR/ABL mutants. J Clin Oncol. 2009;27:469–71.
19. Christopher LJ, Cui D, Wu C, et al. Metabolism and disposition of dasatinib after oral administration to humans. Drug Metab Dispos. 2008;36:1357–64.
20. Shah NP, Kantarjian HM, Kim DW, et al. Intermittent target inhibition with dasatinib 100 mg once daily preserves efficacy and improves tolerability in imatinib-resistant and -intolerant chronic-phase chronic myeloid leukemia. J Clin Oncol. 2008;26:3204–12.
21. Yokota A, Kimura S, Masuda S, et al. INNO-406, a novel BCR-ABL/Lyn dual tyrosine kinase inhibitor, suppresses the growth of Ph^+ leukemia cells in the central nervous system and cyclosporine A augments its in vivo activity. Blood. 2007;109:306–14.
22. Takahashi N, Miura M, Niioka T, et al. Influence of H_2-receptor antagonists and proton pump inhibitors on dasatinib pharmacokinetics in Japanese leukemia patients. Cancer Chemother Pharmacol. 2012;69:999–1004.
23. Wang L, Christopher LJ, Cui D, et al. Identification of the human enzymes involved in the oxidative metabolism of dasatinib: an effective approach for determining metabolite formation kinetics. Drug Metab Dispos. 2009;36:1828–39.
24. Hochhaus A, Baccarani M, Deininger M, et al. Dasatinib induces durable cytogenetic responses in patients with chronic myelogenous leukemia in chronic phase with resistance or intolerance to imatinib. Leukemia. 2008;22:1200–6.
25. Foa R, Vitale A, Vignetti M, et al. Dasatinib as first-line treatment for adult patients with Philadelphia chromosome-positive acute lymphoblastic leukemia. Dasatinib as first-line treatment for adult patients with Philadelphia chromosome-positive acute lymphoblastic leukemia. Blood. 2011;118:6521–8.
26. Benjamini O, Dumlao TL, Kantarjian H, et al. Phase II trial of hyper CVAD and dasatinib in patients with relapsed Philadelphia chromosome positive acute lymphoblastic leukemia or blast phase chronic myeloid leukemia. Am J Hematol. 2014;89:282–7.
27. Pfeifer H, Wassmann B, Hofmann WK, et al. Risk and prognosis of central nervous system leukemia in patients with Philadelphia chromosome-positive acute leukemias treated with imatinib mesylate. Clin Cancer Res. 2003;9:4674–81.
28. Hegedus C, Ozvegy-Laczka C, Apati A, et al. Interaction of nilotinib, dasatinib and bosutinib with ABCB1 and ABCG2: implications for altered anti-cancer effects and pharmacological properties. Br J Pharmacol. 2009;158:1153–64.
29. Porkka K, Koskenvesa P, Lundán T, et al. Dasatinib crosses the blood-brain barrier and is an efficient therapy for central nervous system Philadelphia chromosome-positive leukemia. Blood. 2008;112:1005–12.

30. Quintás-Cardama A, Han X, Kantarjian H, et al. Tyrosine kinase inhibitor-induced platelet dysfunction in patients with chronic myeloid leukemia. Blood. 2009;114:261–3.
31. Mustjoki S, Ekblom M, Arstila TP, et al. Clonal expansion of T/NK-cells during tyrosine kinase inhibitor dasatinib therapy. Leukemia. 2009;23:1398–405.
32. Mosleji JJ, Deininger M. Tyrosine Kinase inhibitor-associated cardiovascular toxicity in chronic myeloid leukemia. J Clin Oncol. 2015;33:4210–8.
33. Kim DH, Kamel-Reid S, Chang H, et al. Natural killer or natural killer/T cell lineage large granular lymphocytosis associated with dasatinib therapy for Philadelphia chromosome positive leukemia. Haematologica. 2009;94:135–9.
34. Fei F, Yu Y, Schmitt A, Rojewski MT, et al. Dasatinib inhibits the proliferation and function of CD4+CD25+ regulatory T cells. Br J Haematol. 2009;144:195–205.
35. Mustjoki S, Auvinen K, Kreutzman A, et al. Rapid mobilization of cytotoxic lymphocytes induced by dasatinib therapy. Leukemia. 2013;27:914–24.
36. Imagawa J, Tanaka H, Okada M, et al. Discontinuation of dasatinib in chronic myeloid leukaemia patients who have maintained deep molecular response for more than 1 year: the prospective, multicentre Dasatinib Discontinuation (DADI) Trial. Lancet Haematol. 2015;2:e528–3.
37. Tanaka C, Yin OQ, Sethuraman V, et al. Clinical pharmacokinetics of the BCR-ABL tyrosine kinase inhibitor nilotinib. Clin Pharmacol Ther. 2010;87:197–203.
38. Deremer DL, Ustun C, Natarajan K. Nilotinib: a second-generation tyrosine kinase inhibitor for the treatment of chronic myelogenous leukemia. Clin Ther. 2008;30:1956–75.
39. Zhang H, Sheng J, Ko JH, et al. Inhibitory effect of single and repeated doses of nilotinib on the pharmacokinetics of CYP3A substrate midazolam. J Clin Pharmacol. 2015;55:401–8.
40. Yin OQ, Gallagher N, Fischer D, et al. Effect of the proton pump inhibitor esomeprazole on the oral absorption and pharmacokinetics of nilotinib. J Clin Pharmacol. 2010;50:960–7.
41. White DL, Saunders VA, Dang P, et al. OCT-1-mediated influx is a key determinant of the intracellular uptake of imatinib but not nilotinib (AMN107): reduced OCT-1 activity is the cause of low in vitro sensitivity to imatinib. Blood. 2006;108:697–704.
42. Kantarjian HM, Giles F, Gattermann N, et al. Nilotinib (formerly AMN107), a highly selective BCR-ABL tyrosine kinase inhibitor, is effective in patients with Philadelphia chromosome-positive chronic myelogenous leukemia in chronic phase following imatinib resistance and intolerance. Blood. 2007;110:3540–6.
43. Kantarjian H, O'Brien S, Talpaz M, et al. Outcome of patients with Philadelphia chromosome-positive chronic myelogenous leukemia post-imatinib mesylate failure. Cancer. 2007;109:1556–60.
44. Nicolini FE, Etienne G, Dubruille V, et al. Nilotinib and peginterferon alfa-2a for newly diagnosed chronic-phase chronic myeloid leukaemia (NiloPeg): a multicentre, non-randomised, open-label phase 2 study. Lancet Haematol. 2015;2:e37–46.
45. Ottmann OG, Larson RA, Kantarjian HM, et al. Phase II study of nilotinib in patients with relapsed or refractory Philadelphia chromosome – positive acute lymphoblastic leukemia. Leukemia. 2013;27:1411–3.
46. Kim DY, Joo YD, Lim SN, et al. Nilotinib combined with multiagent chemotherapy for newly diagnosed Philadelphia-positive acute lymphoblastic leukemia. Blood. 2015;126:746–56.
47. Aichberger KJ, Herndlhofer S, Schernthaner GH, et al. Progressive peripheral arterial occlusive disease and other vascular events during nilotinib therapy in CML. Am J Hematol. 2011;86:533–9.
48. Kim TD, Rea D, Schwarz M, et al. Peripheral artery occlusive disease in chronic phase chronic myeloid leukemia patients treated with nilotinib or imatinib. Leukemia. 2013;27:1316–21.
49. Giles FJ, Mauro MJ, Hong F, et al. Rates of peripheral arterial occlusive disease in patients with chronic myeloid leukemia in the chronic phase treated with imatinib, nilotinib, or non-tyrosine kinase therapy: a retrospective cohort analysis. Leukemia. 2013;27:1310–5.
50. Fei F, Yu Y, Schmitt A, et al. Effects of nilotinib on regulatory T cells: the dose matters. Mol Cancer. 2010;9:22–31.
51. https://clinicaltrials.gov/ct2/show/NCT01698905
52. https://clinicaltrials.gov/ct2/show/NCT01784068

53. https://upload.umin.ac.jp/cgi-open-bin/ctr/ctr.cgi?function=brows&action=brows&type=summary&recptno=R000008409&language=J
54. Levinson NM, Boxer SG. A conserved water-mediated hydrogen bond network defines bosutinib's kinase selectivity. Nat Chem Biol. 2014;10:127–32.
55. Daud AI, Krishnamurthi SS, Saleh MN, et al. Phase I study of bosutinib, a src/abl tyrosine kinase inhibitor, administered to patients with advanced solid tumors. Clin Cancer Res. 2012;18:1092–100.
56. Abbas R, Hug BA, Leister C, et al. A phase I ascending single-dose study of the safety, tolerability, and pharmacokinetics of bosutinib (SKI-606) in healthy adult subjects. Cancer Chemother Pharmacol. 2012;69:221–7.
57. Abbas R, Hug BA, Leister C, et al. Effect of ketoconazole on the pharmacokinetics of oral bosutinib in healthy subjects. J Clin Pharmacol. 2011;51:1721–7.
58. Abbas R, Leister C, Sonnichensen D. A clinical study to examine the potential effect of lansoprazole on the pharmacokinetics of bosutinib when administered concomitantly to healthy subjects. Clin Drug Invest. 2013;33:589–95.
59. Cortes JE, Kantarjian HM, Brummendorf TH, et al. Safety and efficacy of bosutinib (SKI-606) in chronic phase Philadelphia chromosome-positive chronic myeloid leukemia patients with resistance or intolerance to imatinib. Blood. 2011;118:4567–76.
60. Khoury HJ, Cortes JE, Kantarjian HM, et al. Bosutinib is active in chronic phase chronic myeloid leukemia after imatinib and dasatinib and/or nilotinib therapy failure. Blood. 2012;119:3403–12.
61. Brümmendorf TH, Cortes JE, Khoury HJ, et al. Factors influencing long-term efficacy and tolerability of bosutinib in chronic phase chronic myeloid leukaemia resistant or intolerant to imatinib. Br J Haematol. 2016;172:97–110.
62. García-Gutiérrez V, Martinez-Trillos A, Lopez Lorenzo JL, et al. Bosutinib shows low cross intolerance, in chronic myeloid leukemia patients treated in fourth line. Results of the Spanish compassionate use program. Am J Hematol. 2015;90:429–33.
63. Nakaseko C, Takahashi N, Ishizawa K, et al. A phase 1/2 study of bosutinib in Japanese adults with Philadelphia chromosome-positive chronic myeloid leukemia. Int J Hematol. 2015;101:154–64.
64. Brümmendorf TH, Cortes JE, de Souza CA, et al. Bosutinib versus imatinib in newly diagnosed chronic-phase chronic myeloid leukaemia: results from the 24-month follow-up of the BELA trial. Br J Haematol. 2015;168:69–81.
65. Gambacorti-Passerini C, Cortes JE, Lipton JH, et al. Safety of bosutinib versus imatinib in the phase 3 BELA trial in newly diagnosed chronic phase chronic myeloid leukemia. Am J Hematol. 2014;89:947–53.
66. Douxfils J, Haguet H, Mullier F, et al. Association between BCR-ABL tyrosine kinase inhibitors for chronic myeloid leukemia and cardiovascular events, major molecular response, and overall survival: a systematic review and meta-analysis. JAMA Oncol. 2016. doi:10.1001/jamaoncol.2015.5932.
67. Kantarjian H, le Coutre P, Cortes J, et al. Phase I study of INNO-406, a dual Abl/Lyn kinase inhibitor, in Philadelphia chromosome-positive leukemias post-imatinib resistance or intolerance. Cancer. 2010;16:2665–72.
68. Imam SZ, Trickler W, Kimura S, et al. Neuroprotective efficacy of a new brain-penetrating C-Abl inhibitor in a murine Parkinson's disease model. PLoS One. 2013;8:e65129.
69. Zhou T, Commodore L, Huang WS, et al. Structural mechanism of the Pan-BCR-ABL inhibitor ponatinib (AP24534): lessons for overcoming kinase inhibitor resistance. Chem Biol Drug Des. 2011;77:1–11.
70. Gozgit JM, Wong MJ, Moran L, et al. Ponatinib (AP24534), a multitargeted pan-FGFR inhibitor with activity in multiple FGFR-amplified or mutated cancer models. Mol Cancer Ther. 2012;11:690–9.
71. Khorashad JS, Kelley TW, Szankasi P, et al. BCR-ABL1 compound mutations in tyrosine kinase inhibitor-resistant CML: frequency and clonal relationships. Blood. 2013;121:489–98.

72. Cortes JE, Kantarjian H, Shah NP, et al. Ponatinib in refractory Philadelphia chromosome-positive leukemias. N Engl J Med. 2012;367:2075–88.
73. Narasimhan NI, Dorer DJ, Niland K, et al. Effects of food on the pharmacokinetics of ponatinib in healthy subjects. J Clin Pharm Ther. 2013;38:440–4.
74. Narasimhan NI, Dorer DJ, Niland K, et al. Effects of ketoconazole on the pharmacokinetics of ponatinib in healthy subjects. J Clin Pharmacol. 2013;53:974–81.
75. Narasimhan NI, Dorer DJ, Davis J, et al. Evaluation of the effect of multiple doses of lansoprazole on the pharmacokinetics and safety of ponatinib in healthy subjects. Clin Drug Investig. 2014;34:723–9.
76. Cortes JE, Kim DW, Pinilla-Ibarz J, et al. A phase 2 trial of ponatinib in Philadelphia chromosome-positive leukemias. N Engl J Med. 2013;369:1783–96.
77. Jain P, Kantarjian H, Jabbour E, et al. Ponatinib as first-line treatment for patients with chronic myeloid leukaemia in chronic phase: a phase 2 study. Lancet Haematol. 2015;2:e376–83.
78. Zabriskie MS, Eide CA, Tantravahi SK, et al. BCR-ABL1 compound mutations combining key kinase domain positions confer clinical resistance to ponatinib in Ph chromosome-positive leukemia. Cancer Cell. 2014;26:428–42.
79. Parker WT, Yeung DT, Yeoman AL, et al. The impact of multiple low-level BCR-ABL1 mutations on response to ponatinib. Bolld. 2016;127:1870–80.
80. EudraCT number 2012-005696-14.
81. Mian AA, Rafiei A, Haberbosch I, et al. PF-114, a potent and selective inhibitor of native and mutated BCR/ABL is active against Philadelphia chromosome-positive (Ph+) leukemias harboring the T315I mutation. Leukemia. 2015;29:1104–14.

Part II

New Antibodies for Leukemia

Rituximab and Alemtuzumab for Chronic Lymphocytic Leukemia: Basic Results and Pharmacokinetics

5

Katsuki Sugiyama

Abstract

Rituximab is a chimeric anti-CD20 monoclonal antibody (mAb) and the first mAb to be approved for use in the treatment of cancer. The proposed mechanisms of action of rituximab include antibody-dependent cellular cytotoxicity (ADCC), complement-dependent cytotoxicity (CDC), and induction of apoptosis. The influences of CD20 expression level, circulating soluble CD20, Fcγ receptor (FcγR) polymorphisms, complement regulatory proteins, and C1qA-276 polymorphisms on susceptibility and resistance to rituximab have been previously described. In a pharmacokinetic study, from the first to the fourth or eighth weekly dose of rituximab, post-infusion serum concentrations increased and steady-state serum concentrations were not reached. The combined use of rituximab and fludarabine, bendamustine, lenalidomide, or histone deacetylase inhibitors may be one of the optimal solutions for overcoming rituximab resistance in the treatment of chronic lymphocytic leukemia (CLL). The characteristic toxicities of rituximab are infusion reactions, late-onset neutropenia, hepatitis B virus reactivation, and opportunistic infections.

Alemtuzumab is a humanized anti-CD52 mAb and the first mAb to be approved for use in the treatment of CLL. The proposed mechanisms of action of alemtuzumab include ADCC, CDC, and induction of apoptosis. The influences of CD52 expression level, circulating soluble CD52, FcγR polymorphisms, and cytogenetic abnormalities on susceptibility and resistance to alemtuzumab have been previously described. In a pharmacokinetic study, systemic clearance decreased with repeated administration of alemtuzumab due to decreased receptor-mediated clearance. The combined use of alemtuzumab and fludarabine, cyclophosphamide, or rituximab may be one of the optimal solutions for overcoming alemtuzumab resistance in the treatment of CLL. The characteristic

K. Sugiyama (✉)
Division of Clinical Oncology and Hematology, Department of Internal Medicine, The Jikei University School of Medicine, 3-25-8 Nishi-shimbashi, Minato-ku, Tokyo 105-8461, Japan
e-mail: katsuki@jikei.ac.jp

T. Ueda (ed.), *Chemotherapy for Leukemia*, DOI 10.1007/978-981-10-3332-2_5

toxicities of alemtuzumab are infusion reactions, opportunistic infections, and cytopenia.

Keywords
Rituximab • Alemtuzumab • Monoclonal antibody • Chronic lymphocytic leukemia

5.1 Introduction

Monoclonal antibodies (mAbs) are increasingly being used in the treatment of patients with cancer. MAbs are proteins directed against specific antigens that are uniquely expressed on tumor cells or more highly expressed on tumor cells compared with normal cells [1]. Rituximab and alemtuzumab are the most commonly used mAbs in the treatment of chronic lymphocytic leukemia (CLL). This chapter will review the current understanding of these mAbs, including the mechanisms of action and resistance, pharmacokinetics, and toxicities.

5.2 Rituximab

5.2.1 Development of Rituximab

5.2.1.1 Background and Features

Rituximab (IDEC-C2B8) is a recombinant chimeric anti-CD20 monoclonal antibody (mAb) containing human immunoglobulin G (IgG) 1 heavy chain and human kappa light chain constant regions, as well as murine immunoglobulin heavy and light chain variable regions (Fig. 5.1) [2]. Rituximab binds to CD20 expressed on normal and malignant B cells and leads to B-cell depletion. A high-affinity murine anti-CD20 mAb (IDEC-2B8) was initially identified, and subsequently, a mouse/human chimeric antibody, IDEC-C2B8, was constructed. It has been shown that the chimeric mAb has specificity and affinity equivalent to that of the native-murine parent [3]. The fragment crystallizable (Fc) region from human IgG1 was selected for prolongation of serum $t_{1/2}$ because of less human anti-mouse antibody (HAMA) development, its ability to mediate antibody-dependent cellular cytotoxicity (ADCC) with human effector cells, and complement-dependent cytotoxicity (CDC) in the presence of human complement serum [3, 4]. It is the first mAb to be approved for use in the treatment of cancer and represents an important advance in the treatment of CLL and B-cell non-Hodgkin's lymphomas (NHLs).

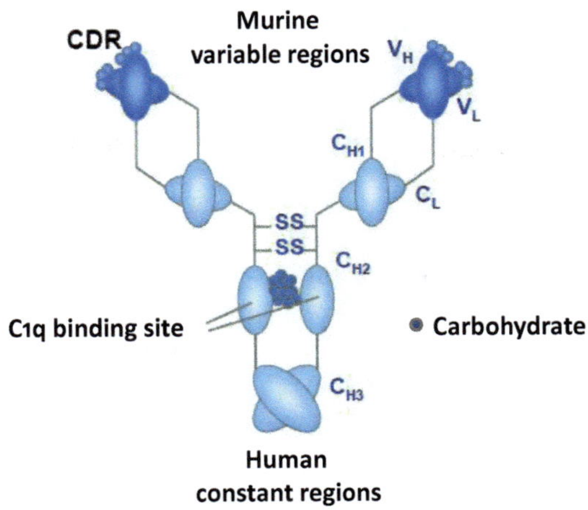

Fig. 5.1 Chimeric structure of rituximab. Rituximab is a chimeric anti-CD20 monoclonal antibody containing human IgG1 heavy chain and human kappa light chain constant regions and murine immunoglobulin heavy and light chain variable regions. The molecular formula is C_{6426} H_{9900} N_{1700} O_{2008} S_{44} and the molecular weight is 144,510 daltons. *CDR* complementarity determining region, V_H variable regions of heavy chains, V_L variable regions of light chains, C_H constant regions of heavy chains, C_L constant regions of light chains, *C1q* complement component 1, q subcomponent

5.2.1.2 CD20 Antigen

The CD20 antigen is a 33- to 37-kDa non-glycosylated phosphoprotein with four transmembrane-spanning regions. Although the physiological functions of CD20 have yet to be clarified, it is thought to play an important role in B-cell activation, differentiation, proliferation, and signal transduction. CD20 is expressed on the surface of normal precursor and mature B cells, but not normal B stem cells or plasma cells [5, 6].

5.2.1.3 Favorable Features of CD20 as a Target Antigen

The CD20 antigen is highly expressed on the cellular surface membrane of most B-lymphocyte tumors making it a rational target in the treatment of CLL and B-cell NHLs. CD20 is stable on the membrane of the B cells and is not internalized following the binding of rituximab. It is also not shed or secreted into the circulation in normal individuals resulting in no detectable soluble CD20 serum levels, which might block targeting of the antibody to B-lymphocyte tumors. Since CD20 is not expressed on the normal B stem cells or plasma cells, they are spared from the direct antibody effects resulting in normal mature B cells that can proliferate even after rituximab-induced depletion of B cells. CD20 is not expressed on non-hematopoietic tissues where it could interfere with the antibody [3, 5, 6].

5.2.2 Mechanism of Action of Rituximab

Although the exact or predominant mechanism of how rituximab binding to CD20 results in cytotoxicity has yet to be completely clarified, the proposed mechanisms of action of rituximab include ADCC, CDC, and induction of apoptosis.

5.2.2.1 ADCC

ADCC is mediated by immune effector cells binding to rituximab-coated B cells. This requires rituximab to bind through the Fc region to Fc receptors for IgG (FcγRs) on immune effector cells, such as natural killer (NK) cells, monocytes, macrophages, and granulocytes [3]. ADCC is better mediated through the IgG1 constant region, and polymorphisms in the genes encoding FcγRs may affect the response to rituximab therapy [5].

5.2.2.2 CDC

Rituximab can recruit components of the complement cascade through the Fc region. The first step is the binding of C1q components to the Fc region. C1q activation triggers the classical complement cascade, which leads to the generation of the membrane attack complex that causes direct lysis of the B cells by disrupting the cell membrane [3]. CDC is better mediated through the IgG1 constant region, and it has been demonstrated that CDC by rituximab correlates not only with the CD20 expression level but also with segregation of CD20 into specialized microdomains on the plasma membrane known as lipid rafts [7].

5.2.2.3 Apoptosis

Upon CD20 cross-linking after rituximab treatment, induction of apoptosis involving activation of caspase-9, caspase-3, and poly-adenosine diphosphate ribose polymerase (PARP) cleavage has been described in primary CLL cells, and downregulation of the antiapoptotic proteins XIAP and Mcl-1 has been described as well [8]. In addition, downregulation of the antiapoptotic protein bcl-2 by rituximab treatment has been observed in some B-cell lines [9]. Furthermore, it has been suggested that the transactivation of src family tyrosine kinases and subsequent increase of the intracellular calcium level upon CD20 translocation into lipid rafts are another proposed mechanism of action of rituximab-induced apoptosis [10, 11]. Additive and synergistic effects between rituximab- and chemotherapy-induced apoptosis have been observed suggesting that rituximab-induced apoptosis uses a final pathway similar to chemotherapeutic agents, leading to the use of combined chemoimmunotherapy regimens.

5.2.3 Susceptibility and Resistance to Rituximab

5.2.3.1 CD20 Expression

It has been observed that the CD20 expression level correlates with rituximab-mediated CDC. There are some in vitro data showing that CDC is more rapidly and efficiently induced by rituximab in cells with a higher CD20 expression level [12]. Therefore, loss or down modulation of CD20 may impact the efficacy of rituximab. As mentioned previously, CD20 is not shed or internalized following the binding of rituximab in normal individuals. However, it has been demonstrated that shaving/trogocytosis of CD20 is mediated by FcγR on acceptor cells, such as NK cells, monocytes, or macrophages in patients with CLL [13]. It has also been demonstrated that type I (rituximab-like) mAb-induced antigenic modulation occurs as a result of internalization of type I (rituximab-like) mAb-CD20 complexes by the B cells themselves in several cell lines [14] and the internalization is augmented by FcγRIIb [15]. In addition, CLL and mantle cell lymphoma (MCL) samples demonstrate more rapid internalization than follicular lymphoma (FL) and diffuse large B-cell lymphoma (DLBCL) [16], suggesting that internalization may explain the differing sensitivity of B-cell malignancies to rituximab.

5.2.3.2 Circulating Soluble CD20 (sCD20)

High levels of sCD20 are present in the plasma of patients with CLL. Plasma sCD20 has been shown to compete with cell surface CD20 for rituximab binding and significantly diminish the binding of rituximab to the surface of CLL cells [16]. It has been reported that response to rituximab is correlated with dose in patients with CLL, suggesting that rituximab dosing may be adjusted according to sCD20 level [17].

5.2.3.3 FcγR Polymorphisms

The influence of FcγR polymorphisms on rituximab-mediated ADCC has been previously described. There are three classes of FcγR: FcγRI (CD64), FcγRII (CD32), and FcγRIII (CD16). The polymorphism in FcγRIIIa consisting of a valine (V) or a phenylalanine (F) in amino acid position 158 results in a different affinity for IgG1-FcγRIIIa binding. The FcγRIIIa-158V homozygous genotype (V/V) has a greater affinity for human IgG1 than V/F or F/F. Patients with follicular lymphoma with the V/V genotype have a better clinical response to rituximab than patients with V/F or F/F. The polymorphism in FcγRIIa consisting of a histidine (H) or an arginine (R) in amino acid position 131 also results in a different affinity for IgG1-FcγRIIa binding, with better clinical results for FcγRIIa-131H homozygous patients. However, not all results demonstrate that these polymorphisms are clinically relevant [18–20]. It has been described that FcγRIIIa and FcγRIIa polymorphisms do not predict the clinical response to rituximab in patients with CLL [21].

5.2.3.4 Complement Regulatory Proteins

The role of complement regulatory proteins such as CD46, CD55, and CD59 in rituximab-mediated CDC has been previously described. Expression of high levels of CD46 or CD55 prevents the activity of C3 convertase, whereas expression of CD59 prevents the assembly of the active membrane attack complex, resulting in interference of completion of the complement cascade. There are some in vitro data showing that complement regulatory proteins may play an important role in rituximab-mediated CDC [22–24]. Currently, however, there is little in vivo data

Table 5.1 Pharmacokinetic parameters of rituximab

Number of weekly doses of 375 mg/m^2	*n*	–	AUC (μg · h/ml)	C_{max} (μg/ml)	$t_{1/2}$ (h)	CL (L/h)	MRT (h)	Vd (L)
Four	8	Mean	118,237	194.3	387.8	0.0437	517	11.16
		SD	49,963	54.5	176.6	0.0601	232	3.00
Eight	15	Mean	502,147	445.2	393.6	0.0122	568	6.13
		SD	174,273	103.0	185.2	0.0038	267	1.55

AUC area under the curve, C_{max} maximum concentration, $t_{1/2}$ elimination half-life, *CL* clearance, *MRT* mean residence time, *Vd* volume of distribution, *h* hours

showing that CD46, CD55, or CD59 expression level correlates with response to rituximab.

5.2.3.5 C1qA-276 Polymorphism

The influence of the C1qA-276 polymorphism on rituximab-mediated CDC has also been previously described [20, 25]. However, there are very few data indicating that the polymorphism predicts response to rituximab.

5.2.4 Pharmacokinetics of Rituximab

Table 5.1 shows pharmacokinetic parameters, and Fig. 5.2 shows a serum concentration over time plot in patients with B-cell non-Hodgkin lymphoma, who received four or eight weekly doses of intravenous rituximab 375 mg/m^2. From the first to the fourth or eighth intravenous infusion of rituximab, post-infusion mean serum concentrations increased and almost doubled. Steady-state serum concentrations of rituximab were not reached following four or eight weekly infusions. In addition, patients still had detectable rituximab concentrations in their serum several months after the end of treatment. Serum levels of free rituximab were measured by enzyme-linked immunosorbent assay (ELISA) [26].

5.2.4.1 Distribution

It has been demonstrated that rituximab is widely distributed in body organs. By gamma camera measurements, radioactivity was detected in the heart, liver, lungs, spleen, and kidneys of patients with relapsed NHL who received iodine-131-labeled rituximab. The ratios of tumor to whole-body radioactivity increased over time, whereas those of organ to whole body decreased, indicating evidence of specific antibody binding [27]. It has been reported that rituximab levels in cerebrospinal fluid were detected after infusions with a C_{max} of 0.55 μg/ml compared with a C_{max} of 400 μg/ml in peripheral blood [28].

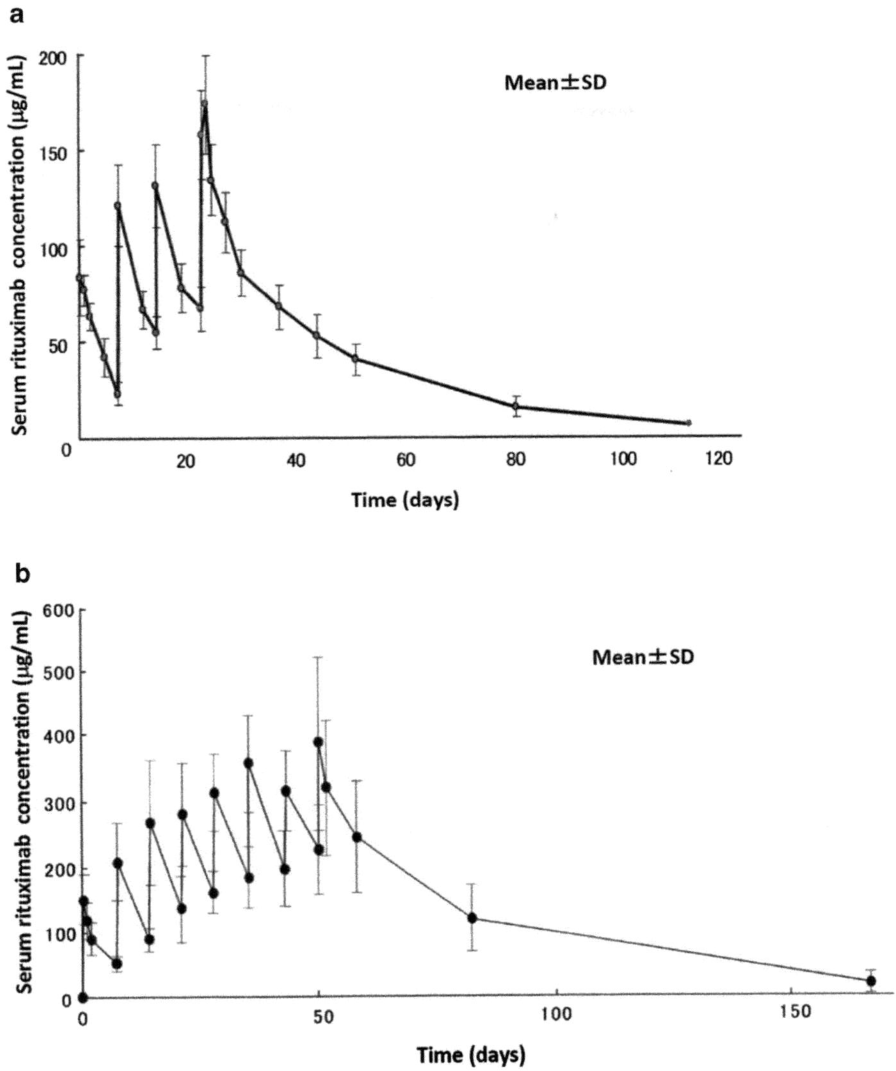

Fig. 5.2 Pharmacokinetics of rituximab. Mean serum rituximab concentrations as a function of time following four weekly infusions of 375 mg/m^2 (**a**, $n = 8$) or eight weekly infusions of 375 mg/m^2 (**b**, $n = 15$). From the first to the fourth or eighth intravenous infusion of rituximab, post-infusion mean serum concentrations increased with time, and steady-state serum concentrations were not reached following four or eight weekly infusions

5.2.4.2 Metabolism

Little is known about the mechanisms of rituximab metabolism. It is speculated that rituximab is degraded by a nonspecific catabolism of proteins in the liver and other organs.

5.2.4.3 Excretion

It has been demonstrated that radioactivity was excreted mainly through the kidneys in patients with relapsed NHL who received iodine-131-labeled rituximab. The percentage of radioactivity excreted in the urine was almost 50% at the time of the whole-body half-life [27].

5.2.5 Overcoming Rituximab Resistance

5.2.5.1 Rituximab in Combination with Other Agents

The combined use of rituximab and other agents with different mechanisms of action may be one of the optimal solutions for overcoming rituximab resistance.

Fludarabine

It has been demonstrated that there is synergistic activity between rituximab and fludarabine, a purine analog agent, against a follicular lymphoma cell line. Fludarabine has been shown to induce downregulation of complement regulatory proteins CD46 and CD55 without significantly altering CD20 expression, resulting in enhancing rituximab-mediated CDC [29]. Although rituximab and fludarabine have demonstrated just an additive cytotoxic effect in primary CLL cells, the combination therapy of rituximab and fludarabine has already given positive results in the treatment of patients with CLL.

Bendamustine

It has been demonstrated that there is synergistic activity between rituximab and bendamustine, an alkylating agent, against primary CLL cells in vitro. Bendamustine has been shown to synergistically induce the proapoptotic effects of rituximab that may depend on caspase-7 and caspase-8 activation, but not p53 or caspase-3 [30]. Practically, it has been reported that the combination therapy of rituximab and bendamustine is active in patients with previously untreated, relapsed, or refractory CLL [31, 32].

Lenalidomide

It has been demonstrated that there is synergistic activity between rituximab and lenalidomide, an immunomodulatory agent, against CLL and B-NHL cells in vitro. It has been shown that lenalidomide enhances NK cell-mediated ADCC of rituximab-treated primary CLL cells that have been treated previously with fludarabine plus cyclophosphamide and that this enhanced NK cell-mediated ADCC is associated with enhanced granzyme B and Fas ligand expression [33]. It has also been demonstrated that lenalidomide repairs defective T-cell immune synapse formation, a characteristic of CLL, and enhances NK cell-mediated ADCC of rituximab-treated CLL cells [34, 35]. However, it has been demonstrated that lenalidomide promotes internalization of CD20 in CLL cells, resulting in decreased expression of cell surface CD20 [36]. These studies suggest that lenalidomide may act synergistically to enhance rituximab-mediated anti-CLL activity if alternative sequences of administration are optimized. Practically, it has been reported that the combination therapy of rituximab and lenalidomide is active in patients with relapsed or refractory CLL [37].

Histone Deacetylase (HDAC) Inhibitors

It has been demonstrated that HDAC inhibitors augment the cytotoxic activity of rituximab by increasing the surface expression of CD20 on lymphoma cells. Valproic acid and romidepsin have been shown to increase CD20 expression at protein and mRNA levels in B-cell lymphoma cell lines with relatively low expression of cell surface CD20, resulting in enhanced rituximab-mediated CDC [38, 39]. Entinostat has also been shown to increase CD20 expression at protein and mRNA levels in rituximab-sensitive or rituximab-resistant B-cell lymphoma cell lines and enhance rituximab activity in vivo [40]. However, these findings have not yet been extended to clinical trials in CLL.

5.2.5.2 Treatment with Other Anti-CD20 Monoclonal Antibodies

The use of other anti-CD20 mAbs, such as ofatumumab, obinutuzumab, tositumomab, ^{90}Y-ibritumomab tiuxetan, and ^{131}I-tositumomab, is another optimal solution for overcoming rituximab resistance.

5.2.6 Characteristic Toxicities and Management

5.2.6.1 Infusion Reactions

Infusion reactions are one of the most commonly occurring adverse reactions with rituximab. Infusion reactions are mediated by cytokine release (cytokine release syndrome), not by immunoglobulin E (IgE) (type 1 hypersensitivities). When cytokines, such as tumor necrosis factor-α (TNF-α), interferon-γ (IFN-γ), or interleukin-6 (IL-6), are released into the circulation from cells targeted by rituximab as well as immune effector cells recruited to the area, systemic symptoms such as rigor, fever, headache, nausea, sweating, itching, skin rash, cough, fatigue, hypertension, hypotension, tachycardia, angioedema, facial edema, hypoxemia, bronchospasm, pulmonary infiltrates, interstitial pneumonia, acute respiratory distress syndrome, myocardial infarction, ventricular fibrillation, and myocardial shock can occur. Infusion reactions usually occur within 30–120 min, most often with the first infusion. The symptoms are generally mild to moderate in severity and manageable in most patients. A slow initial rate of infusion is recommended to reduce the risk of infusion reactions. Prophylactic administrations of histamine antagonists (diphenhydramine) and antipyretic analgesics (acetaminophen) are also recommended. Steroids (hydrocortisone) should be considered in patients receiving rituximab not already in combination with steroids [41, 42].

5.2.6.2 Late-Onset Neutropenia (LON)

LON is a recognized late complication of rituximab-combined chemotherapy, occurring at least 4 weeks after treatment. The incidence of LON has been reported at about 25%, and a high incidence of LON has been reported in patients treated with an intensive primary chemotherapy regimen, such as high-dose therapy followed by stem cell transplantation [43]. LON has been attributed to rituximab, but the mechanism for developing LON remains unclear. It has been suggested that perturbation of stromal-derived factor-1 (SDF-1) during B-cell recovery following rituximab treatment retards neutrophil emergence from the bone marrow. SDF-1 is a chemokine required for early B-cell development and retention of the B-lineage and granulocytic precursors in the bone marrow microenvironment [44]. It has been demonstrated that the FcγRIIIa 158 V/V and V/F polymorphisms are associated with developing LON. This suggests that in patients with a high-affinity genotype, depletion of B cells may be more profound, subsequently stimulating increased bone marrow lymphopoiesis and resulting in less effective granulopoiesis [45]. The clinical course of LON was generally self-limited and not associated with severe infections.

5.2.6.3 Hepatitis B Virus Reactivation

Reactivation of hepatitis B virus (HBV) infection is a well-recognized complication in hepatitis B surface antigen (HBsAg)-positive cancer patients when they undergo cytotoxic chemotherapy. However, HBV reactivation has been reported to occur not only in HBsAg-positive patients but also in patients with a resolved HBV infection who are negative for HBsAg but positive for antibodies against the hepatitis B core antigen (anti-HBc) and/or antibodies against the hepatitis B surface antigen (anti-HBs) undergoing cytotoxic chemotherapy. HBV reactivation has been previously reported to be much less common in patients with resolved HBV, but with the recent increase in the use of rituximab, reports have increased. Since HBV reactivation in patients with resolved HBV is associated with a higher risk of fulminant hepatic failure, patients with resolved HBV receiving rituximab should be closely monitored with HBV DNA for a more prolonged period of time, even after completion of rituximab, so as to promptly start administration of nucleoside/nucleotide analogs to prevent HBV reactivation [46–50].

5.2.6.4 Opportunistic Infections

It has been observed that opportunistic infections, such as pneumocystis jiroveci pneumonia (PCP) or some viral infections, increase in patients receiving rituximab. However, the exact influence of rituximab on incidence of infection is still controversial. It has been suggested that, although rituximab by itself does not increase the incidence or change the spectrum of infections in hematologic patients, a possible influence of concomitant immunosuppressive medication such as chemotherapy and/or significant doses of glucocorticoids on the frequency of infections may be present. Screening and/or prophylaxis should be considered in patients receiving rituximab in combination with other immunosuppressive medications to minimize infectious complications. Sulfamethoxazole-trimethoprim prophylaxis against PCP is generally recommended [51].

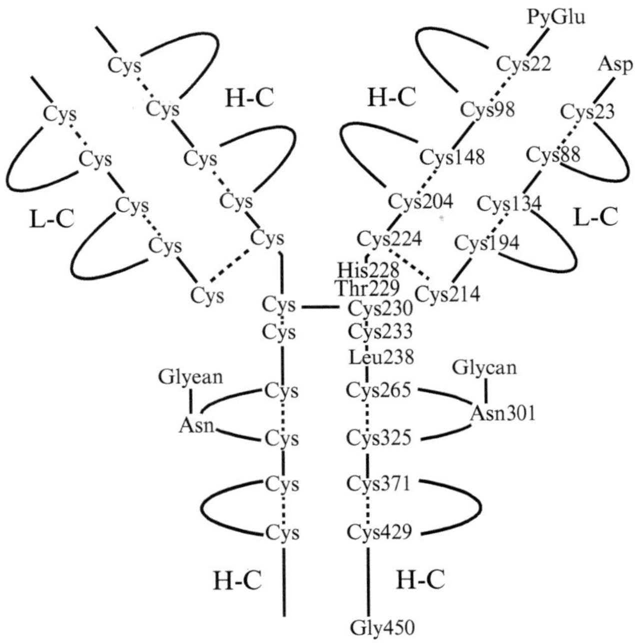

Fig. 5.3 Structure of alemtuzumab. Alemtuzumab is a recombinant anti-CD52 humanized IgG1 kappa monoclonal antibody constructed by genetic engineering using the hypervariable regions from murine antihuman CD52 IgG2a antibodies. The molecular formula is C_{6468} H_{10066} N_{1732} O_{2005} S_{40}, and the molecular weight is approximately 150,000 daltons. *H-C* heavy chains, *L-C* light chains

5.3 Alemtuzumab

5.3.1 Development of Alemtuzumab

5.3.1.1 Background and Features

Alemtuzumab (Campath-1H) is a recombinant anti-CD52 humanized IgG1 kappa mAb (Fig. 5.3) [52]. A murine immunoglobulin M (IgM) antibody (Campath-1M) was initially selected, followed by a murine IgG2b antibody (Campath-1G) that demonstrated clinical activity in refractory CLL, even in patients who had failed Campath-1M [53]. Subsequently, a reshaped human IgG1 antibody, Campath-1H, was constructed by genetic engineering using the hypervariable regions from Campath-1G and found to have equivalent or superior activity to Campath-1G in vivo [54]. Alemtuzumab is the first mAb to be approved for use in the treatment of CLL.

5.3.1.2 CD52 Antigen

The CD52 antigen is a 21- to 28-kDa heavily glycosylated membrane-anchored glycoprotein with a short sequence of only 12 amino acids. Although the physiological functions of CD52 have yet to be clarified, it is thought to mediate a variety of biological effects such as the promotion of cell-cell adhesion, protection of the cell from environmental insult, activation of T-regulatory cells, and signal transduction. CD52 is highly expressed on all B and T lymphocytes at various stages of differentiation, except plasma cells, as well as on granulocytes, monocytes, macrophages, eosinophils, NK cells, and dendritic cells. The only other site of expression is in the male reproductive tract [55–57].

5.3.1.3 Favorable Features of CD52 as a Target Antigen

The CD52 antigen seems to be highly expressed on lymphocyte tumor cells, particularly in T-cell prolymphocytic leukemia (T-PLL), followed by CLL, with lower levels of expression on normal lymphocytes [58]. CD52 is not expressed on hematopoietic stem cells, plasma cells, erythrocytes, or platelets. Therefore, they are spared from the direct antibody effects [55–57].

5.3.2 Mechanism of Action of Alemtuzumab

Although the mechanism of action of alemtuzumab has yet to be clarified, proposed mechanisms of action of alemtuzumab include ADCC, CDC, and induction of apoptosis. ADCC is mediated by immune effector cells binding to alemtuzumab-coated cells, and this requires alemtuzumab to bind through the Fc region to FcγRs on immune effector cells. CDC is mediated by the recruitment of components of the complement cascade through the Fc region. Both ADCC and CDC are better mediated through the IgG1 constant region [55–57]. Alemtuzumab has been shown to induce not only caspase-dependent apoptosis but also caspase-independent and lipid raft-dependent apoptosis in primary CLL cells [59].

5.3.3 Susceptibility and Resistance to Alemtuzumab

5.3.3.1 CD52 Expression

It has been shown that patients who fail to respond to alemtuzumab have a lower CD52 expression, whereas the highest expression values are found in patients with a major response to alemtuzumab, suggesting that the level of CD52 expression correlates with alemtuzumab treatment [58].

5.3.3.2 Circulating Soluble CD52 (sCD52)

It has been demonstrated that high levels of sCD52 are present in the plasma of patients with CLL. Plasma sCD52 has been shown to be able to form immune complexes with alemtuzumab, resulting in reducing the serum concentration of alemtuzumab, and may influence the efficacy of alemtuzumab treatment. These findings suggest that patients with CLL and high sCD52 levels may require a higher dose of alemtuzumab [60].

Table 5.2 Pharmacokinetic parameters of alemtuzumab

Dose (mg)	Timing	–	C_{max} (μg/ml)	t_{max} (h)	$AUC_{0-24\,h}$ (μg · h/ml)	$AUC_{0-56\,h}$ (μg · h/ml)	CL (L/h)	V_z (L/kg)	V_{ss} (L/kg)	$t_{1/2z}$ (h)	MRT (h)
10	First	*n*	8	8	7	–	–	–	–	–	–
		Mean	0.8	4.97	6.58	–	–	–	–	–	–
		SD	0.2	6.85	4.31	–	–	–	–	–	–
30	First	*n*	22	22	17	8	8	8	8	8	8
		Mean	2.7	2.61	24.4	58.5	17.39	0.113	0.111	10.65	14.62
		SD	1.9	0.43	23.5	49.3	18.12	0.037	0.041	10.05	14.11
	Last	*n*	21	21	–	21	21	16	16	16	16
		Mean	10.2	4.71	–	404	2.00	0.252	0.185	147.5	163.8
		SD	5.8	10.40	–	326	1.63	0.168	0.084	82.5	103.2

C_{max} maximum concentration, t_{max} maximum drug concentration time, *AUC* area under the curve, *CL* clearance, V_z volume of distribution at terminal phase, V_{ss} volume of distribution at steady state, $t_{1/2z}$ terminal-phase elimination half-life, *MRT* mean residence time, *h* hours

5.3.3.3 FcγR Polymorphisms

Although the influence of FcγR polymorphisms on mAb-mediated ADCC has been described, FcγRIIIa and FcγRIIa polymorphisms may not predict the clinical response to alemtuzumab in CLL patients [61].

5.3.3.4 Cytogenetic Abnormalities

It has been reported that alemtuzumab is effective in a subgroup of patients with high-risk cytogenetic abnormalities such as del(17p13.1) and del(11q22.3) [62].

5.3.4 Pharmacokinetics of Alemtuzumab

Table 5.2 shows pharmacokinetic parameters, and Fig. 5.4 shows a serum concentration over time plot in patients with previously treated CLL. Patients received the recommended dose and schedule of intravenous (IV) alemtuzumab, which is comprised of a 2-h IV infusion with a starting dose of 3 mg on day 1, 10 mg on day 2, and 30 mg three times weekly for a total of 8–12 weeks. Alemtuzumab pharmacokinetics displayed nonlinear elimination kinetics. After the last 30 mg dose, the mean volume of distribution at the steady state was 0.18 L/kg (range 0.1–0.4 L/kg). Systemic clearance decreased with repeated administration due to decreased receptor-mediated clearance, that is to say, loss of CD52 receptors in the periphery. After 12 weeks of dosing, patients exhibited a sevenfold increase in mean AUC. Mean half-life was 11 h (range 2–32 h) after the first 30 mg dose and was 6 days (range 1–14 days) after the last 30 mg dose. Serum levels of free alemtuzumab were measured by ELISA [63].

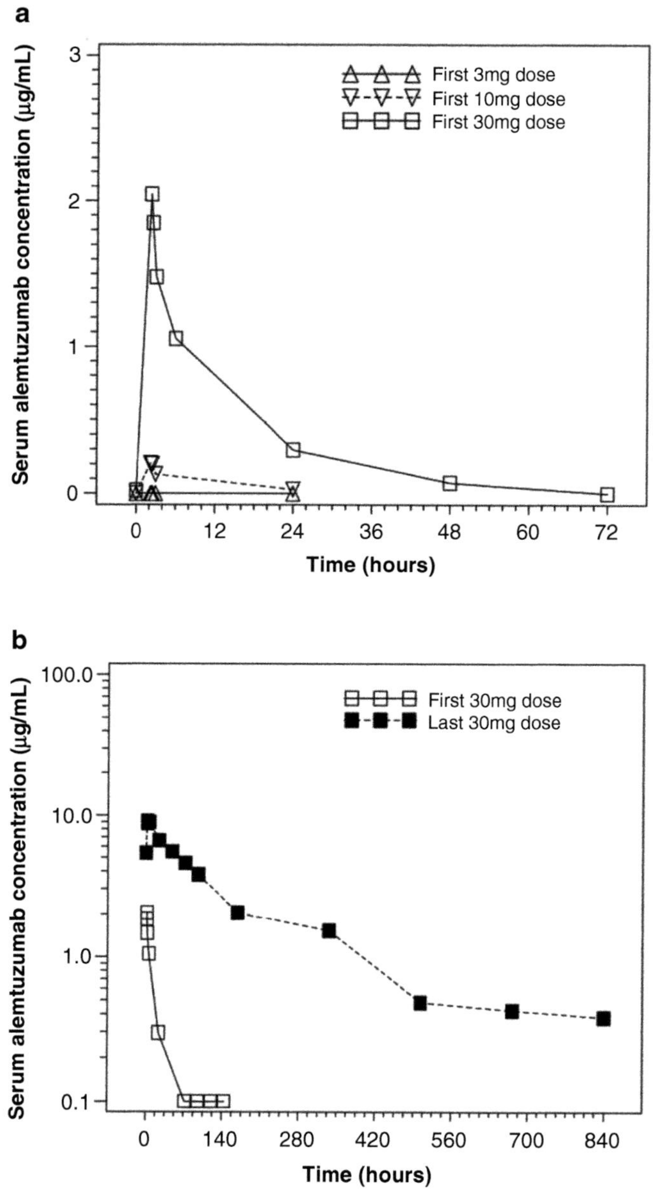

Fig. 5.4 Pharmacokinetics of alemtuzumab. Mean serum alemtuzumab concentrations as a function of time after infusion of the first 3, 10, and 30 mg dose (**a**) or the first and the last 30 mg dose (**b**). Dose and schedule of intravenous (IV) alemtuzumab comprised of a 2-h IV infusion at a starting dose of 3 mg on day 1, 10 mg on day 2, and 30 mg three times weekly for a total of 8–12 weeks. Alemtuzumab pharmacokinetics displayed nonlinear elimination kinetics and systemic clearance decreased with repeated administration

5.3.4.1 Distribution

It has been shown that alemtuzumab is widely distributed in body organs. By a quantitative radioimmunoprecipitation assay, radioactivity was detected in the blood, spleen, liver, lungs, kidneys, stomach, intestine, and bone of nude mice carrying subcutaneously implanted tumors that were injected with ^{35}S-methionine-labeled alemtuzumab. Tumor uptake increased over time, whereas uptake in normal tissues decreased, indicating evidence for specific antibody binding [64].

5.3.4.2 Metabolism

Little is known about the mechanisms of alemtuzumab metabolism. It is speculated that alemtuzumab is degraded by a nonspecific catabolism of proteins in the liver and other organs.

5.3.4.3 Excretion

Little is known about the mechanisms of alemtuzumab excretion.

5.3.5 Overcoming Alemtuzumab Resistance

The combined use of alemtuzumab and other agents with different mechanisms of action such as fludarabine, cyclophosphamide, or rituximab may be one of the optimal solutions for overcoming alemtuzumab resistance. It has been demonstrated that alemtuzumab combined with a purine analog or rituximab exerted a significantly higher proapoptotic effect than single agents in vitro, downregulating the antiapoptotic proteins FLIP and Bcl-2 (alemtuzumab plus purine analog) or significantly increasing expression of the apoptotic protein Bax (alemtuzumab plus rituximab). However, it is unclear if the combined use of alemtuzumab and a purine analog or rituximab is clinically beneficial for patients with CLL [65].

5.3.6 Characteristic Toxicities and Management

5.3.6.1 Infusion Reactions

Infusion reactions are one of the most commonly occurring adverse reactions with alemtuzumab. Infusion reactions are mediated by cytokine release, such as TNF-α, IFN-γ, or IL-6, likely derived from NK cells. When cytokines are released into the circulation, systemic symptoms including rigor, fever, nausea, vomiting, skin rash, dyspnea, hypotension, and bronchospasms can occur. Infusion reactions usually occur with the first infusion with significant variability in the severity of symptoms and tend to decrease in frequency and severity over the subsequent weeks of treatment. Initial dose escalation is recommended to reduce the risk of infusion reactions. Prophylactic administrations of histamine antagonists (diphenhydramine) and antipyretic analgesics (acetaminophen) are also recommended. Steroids (hydrocortisone) may be added in cases with prior severe infusion reactions [55, 56].

5.3.6.2 Opportunistic Infections

Reactivation of herpesvirus, including cytomegalovirus (CMV), herpes simplex, and varicella zoster, were the most common opportunistic infections observed in patients receiving alemtuzumab. Antiviral prophylaxis (acyclovir, famciclovir, valaciclovir) is recommended, and monitoring for CMV antigenemia or DNA is highly recommended in order to promptly start administration of ganciclovir or valganciclovir to prevent CMV reactivation. Sulfamethoxazole-trimethoprim prophylaxis against PCP is also recommended [55, 57, 66]. In addition, patients with resolved HBV receiving alemtuzumab should be closely monitored with HBV DNA so as to promptly start administration of nucleoside/nucleotide analogs to prevent HBV reactivation.

5.3.6.3 Cytopenia

Thrombocytopenia and prolonged neutropenia have been reported in patients receiving alemtuzumab. Thrombocytopenia is most common during the first 2 weeks of treatment, and neutropenia is most common during weeks 5 and 6 [66]. Hemolytic anemia, pure red cell aplasia, bone marrow aplasia, and hypoplasia have also been reported following alemtuzumab treatment, but the pathogenesis remains unclear.

5.4 Conclusions

Rituximab and alemtuzumab represent an important advance in the treatment of CLL. Although the mechanism of action of and resistance to these mAbs are being increasingly studied, the relative contribution of each mechanism in response to these mAbs has yet to be clarified. Further investigation on the mechanism of action of and resistance to these mAbs, as well as pharmacokinetics and managing toxicities of these mAbs, is needed to design more effective therapies, including combination therapy of these mAbs and other agents with different mechanisms of action. Moreover, since some of the causes of response variability for rituximab and alemtuzumab can be applied to other mAbs, a better understanding of rituximab and alemtuzumab may lead to the development of subsequent generations of mAbs.

References

1. von Mehren M, Adams GP, Weiner LM. Monoclonal antibody therapy for cancer. Annu Rev Med. 2003;54:343–69. doi:10.1146/annurev.med.54.101601.152442.
2. Structure of rituximab. In-house data. Zenyaku Kogyo Co., Ltd.
3. Reff ME, Carner K, Chambers KS, Chinn PC, Leonard JE, Raab R, et al. Depletion of B cells in vivo by a chimeric mouse human monoclonal antibody to CD20. Blood. 1994;83:435–45.
4. Smith MR. Rituximab (monoclonal anti-CD20 antibody): mechanisms of action and resistance. Oncogene. 2003;22:7359–68. doi:10.1038/sj.onc.1206939.

5. Keating GM, Rituximab A. Review of its use in chronic lymphocytic leukaemia, low-grade or follicular lymphoma and diffuse large B-cell lymphoma. Drugs. 2010;70:1445–76. doi:10.2165/11201110-000000000-00000.
6. Villamor N, Montserrat E, Colomer D. Mechanism of action and resistance to monoclonal antibody therapy. Semin Oncol. 2003;30:424–33. doi:10.1016/S0093-7754(03)00261-6.
7. Cragg MS, Morgan SM, Chan HT, Morgan BP, Filatov AV, Johnson PW, et al. Complement-mediated lysis by anti-CD20 mAb correlates with segregation into lipid rafts. Blood. 2003;101:1045–52. doi:10.1182/blood-200206-1761.
8. Byrd JC, Kitada S, Flinn IW, Aron JL, Pearson M, Lucas D, et al. The mechanism of tumor cell clearance by rituximab in vivo in patients with B-cell chronic lymphocytic leukemia: evidence of caspase activation and apoptosis induction. Blood. 2002;99:1038–43. doi:10.1182/blood.V99.3.1038.
9. Alas S, Emmanouilides C, Bonavida B. Inhibition of interleukin 10 by rituximab results in down-regulation of Bcl-2 and sensitization of B-cell non-Hodgkin's lymphoma to apoptosis. Clin Cancer Res. 2001;7:709–23.
10. Deans JP, Li H, Polyak MJ. CD20-mediated apoptosis: signalling through lipid rafts. Immunology. 2002;107:176–82. doi:10.1046/j.1365-2567.2002.01495.x.
11. Janas E, Priest R, Wilde JI, White JH, Malhotra R. Rituxan (anti-CD 20 antibody)-induced translocation of CD 20 into lipid rafts is crucial for calcium influx and apoptosis. Clin Exp Immunol. 2005;139:439–46. doi:10.1111/j.1365-2249.2005.02720.x.
12. Bellosillo B, Villamor N, López-Guillermo A, Marcé S, Esteve J, Campo E, et al. Complement-mediated cell death induced by rituximab in B-cell lymphoproliferative disorders is mediated in vitro by a caspase-independent mechanism involving the generation of reactive oxygen species. Blood. 2001;98:2771–7. doi:10.1182/blood.V98.9.2771.
13. Beum PV, Peek EM, Lindorfer MA, Beurskens FJ, Engelberts PJ, Parren PW, et al. Loss of CD20 and bound CD20 antibody from opsonized B cells occurs more rapidly because of trogocytosis mediated by Fc receptor-expressing effector cells than direct internalization by the B cells. J Immunol. 2011;187:3438–47. doi:10.4049/jimmunol.1101189.
14. Beers SA, French RR, Chan HT, Lim SH, Jarrett TC, Vidal RM, et al. Antigenic modulation limits the efficacy of anti-CD20 antibodies: implications for antibody selection. Blood. 2010;115:5191–201. doi:10.1182/blood-2010-01-263533.
15. Lim SH, Vaughan AT, Ashton-Key M, Williams EL, Dixon SV, Chan HT, et al. Fc gamma receptor IIb on target B cells promotes rituximab internalization and reduces clinical efficacy. Blood. 2011;118:2530–40. doi:10.1182/blood-2011-01-330357.
16. Manshouri T, Do K, Wang X, Giles FJ, O'Brien SM, Saffer H, et al. Circulating CD20 is detectable in the plasma of patients with chronic lymphocytic leukemia and is of prognostic significance. Blood. 2003;101:2507–13. doi:10.1182/blood-2002-06-1639.
17. O'Brien SM, Kantarjian H, Thomas DA, Giles FJ, Freireich EJ, Cortes J, et al. Rituximab dose-escalation trial in chronic lymphocytic leukemia. J Clin Oncol. 2001;19:2165–70.
18. Cartron G, Dacheux L, Salles G, Solal-Celigny P, Bardos P, Colombat P, et al. Therapeutic activity of humanized anti-CD20 monoclonal antibody and polymorphism in IgG Fc receptor FcγRIIIa gene. Blood. 2002;99:754–8. doi:10.1182/blood.V99.3.754.
19. Weng WK, Levy R. Two immunoglobulin G fragment C receptor polymorphisms independently predict response to rituximab in patients with follicular lymphoma. J Clin Oncol. 2003;21:3940–7. doi:10.1200/JCO.2003.05.013.
20. Cornec D, Tempescul A, Querellou S, Hutin P, Pers JO, Jamin C, et al. Identification of patients with indolent B cell lymphoma sensitive to rituximab monotherapy. Ann Hematol. 2012;91:715–21. doi:10.1007/s00277-011-1369-y.
21. Farag SS, Flinn IW, Modali R, Lehman TA, Young D, Byrd JC. FcγRIIIa and FcγRIIa polymorphisms do not predict response to rituximab in B-cell chronic lymphocytic leukemia. Blood. 2004;103:1472–4. doi:10.1182/blood-200307-2548.

22. Harjunpää A, Junnikkala S, Meri S. Rituximab (aanti-CD20) therapy of B-cell lymphomas: direct complement killing is superior to cellular effector mechanisms. Scand J Immunol. 2000;51:634–41. doi:10.1046/j.1365-3083.2000.00745.x.
23. Golay J, Zaffaroni L, Vaccari T, Lazzari M, Borleri GM, Bernasconi S, et al. Biologic response of B lymphoma cells to anti-CD20 monoclonal antibody rituximab in vitro: CD55 and CD59 regulate complement-mediated cell lysis. Blood. 2000;95:3900–8.
24. Golay J, Lazzari M, Facchinetti V, Bernasconi S, Borleri G, Barbui T, et al. CD20 levels determine the in vitro susceptibility to rituximab and complement of B-cell chronic lymphocytic leukemia: further regulation by CD55 and CD59. Blood. 2001;98:3383–9. doi:10.1182/blood.V98.12.3383.
25. Racila E, Link BK BK, Weng WK, Witzig TE, Ansell S, Maurer MJ, et al. A polymorphism in the complement component C1qA correlates with prolonged response following rituximab therapy of follicular lymphoma. Clin Cancer Res. 2008;14:6697–703. doi:10.1158/1078-0432.CCR-08-0745.
26. Pharmacokinetics of IDEC-C2B8 in patients with CD20 positive B-cell non-Hodgkin lymphoma. In-house data. Zenyaku Kogyo Co., Ltd.
27. Scheidhauer K, Wolf I, Baumgartl HJ, Von Schilling C, Schmidt B, Reidel G, et al. Biodistribution and kinetics of 131I-labelled anti-CD20 MAB IDEC-C2B8 (rituximab) in relapsed non-Hodgkin's lymphoma. Eur J Nucl Med. 2002;29:1276–82. doi:10.1007/s00259-002-0820-7.
28. Harjunpää A, Wiklund T, Collan J, Janes R, Rosenberg J, Lee D, et al. Complement activation in circulation and central nervous system after rituximab (Anti-CD20) treatment of B-cell lymphoma. Leuk Lymphoma. 2001;42:731–8. doi:10.3109/10428190109099335.
29. Gaetano ND, Xiao Y, Erba E, Bassan R, Rambaldi A, Golay J, et al. Synergism between fludarabine and rituximab revealed in a follicular lymphoma cell line resistant to the cytotoxic activity of either drug alone. Br J Haematol. 2001;114:800–9. doi:10.1046/j.1365-2141.2001.03014.x.
30. Chow KU, Sommerlad WD, Boehrer S, Schneider B, Seipelt G, Rummel MJ, et al. Anti-CD20 antibody (IDEC-C2B8, rituximab) enhances efficacy of cytotoxic drugs on neoplastic lymphocytes in vitro: role of cytokines, complement, and caspases. Haematologica. 2002;87:33–43.
31. Fischer K, Cramer P, Busch R, Böttcher S, Bahlo J, Schubert J, et al. Bendamustine in combination with rituximab for previously untreated patients with chronic lymphocytic leukemia: a multicenter phase II trial of the German Chronic Lymphocytic Leukemia Study Group. J Clin Oncol. 2012;30:3209–16. doi:10.1200/JCO.2011.39.2688.
32. Fischer K, Cramer P, Busch R, Stilgenbauer S, Bahlo J, Schweighofer CD, et al. Bendamustine combined with rituximab in patients with relapsed and/or refractory chronic lymphocytic leukemia: a multicenter phase II trial of the German Chronic Lymphocytic Leukemia Study Group. J Clin Oncol. 2011;29:3559–66. doi:10.1200/JCO.2010.33.806.
33. Wu L, Adams M, Carter T, Chen R, Muller G, Stirling D, et al. Lenalidomide enhances natural killer cell and monocyte-mediated antibody-dependent cellular cytotoxicity of rituximab-treated $CD20^+$ tumor cells. Clin Cancer Res. 2008;14:4650–7. doi:10.1158/1078-0432.CCR-07-4405.
34. Ramsay AG, Johnson AJ, Lee AM, Gorgün G, Dieu RL, Blum W, et al. Chronic lymphocytic leukemia T cells show impaired immunological synapse formation that can be reversed with an immunomodulating drug. J Clin Invest. 2008;118:2427–37. doi:10.1172/JCI35017.
35. Ramsay AG, Gribben JG. Immune dysfunction in chronic lymphocytic leukemia T cells and lenalidomide as an immunomodulatory drug. Haematologica. 2009;94:1198–202. doi:10.3324/haematol.2009.009274.
36. Lapalombella R, Yu B, Triantafillou G, Liu Q, Butchar JP, Lozanski G, et al. Lenalidomidedown-regulatestheCD20antigenandantagonizesdirectand antibody-dependentcellularcytotoxicityofrituximabonprimarychronic lymphocytic leukemia cells. Blood. 2008;112:5180–9. doi:10.1182/blood-200801-133108.

37. Badoux XC, Keating MJ, Wen S, Wierda WG, O'Brien SM, Faderl S, et al. Phase II study of lenalidomide and rituximab as salvage therapy for patients with relapsed or refractory chronic lymphocytic leukemia. J Clin Oncol. 2013;31:584–91. doi:10.1200/JCO.2012.42.862.
38. Shimizu R, Kikuchi J, Wada T, Ozawa K, Kano Y, Furukawa Y. HDAC inhibitors augment cytotoxic activity of rituximab by upregulating CD20 expression on lymphoma cells. Leukemia. 2010;24:1760–8. doi:10.1038/leu.2010.157.
39. Damm JK, Gordon S, Ehinger M, Jerkeman M, Gullberg U, Hultquist A, Drott K. Pharmacologically relevant doses of valproate upregulate CD20 expression in three diffuse large B-cell lymphoma patients in vivo. Exp Hematol Oncol. 2015;4:4. doi:10.1186/2162-3619-4-4.
40. Frys S, Simons Z, Hu Q, Barth MJ, Gu JJ, Mavis C, et al. Entinostat, a novel histone deacetylase inhibitor is active in B-cell lymphoma and enhances the anti-tumour activity of rituximab and chemotherapy agents. Br J Haematol. 2015;169:506–19. doi:10.1111/bjh.13318.
41. Winkler U, Jensen M, Manzke O, Schulz H, Diehl V, Engert A. Cytokine-release syndrome in patients with B-cell chronic lymphocytic leukemia and high lymphocyte counts after treatment with an anti-CD20 monoclonal antibody (rituximab, IDEC-C2B8). Blood. 1999;94:2217–22.
42. Byrd JC, Waselenko JK, Maneatis TJ, Murphy T, Ward FT, Monahan BP, et al. Rituximab therapy in hematologic malignancy patients with circulating blood tumor cells: association with increased infusion-related side effects and rapid blood tumor clearance. J Clin Oncol. 1999;17:791–5.
43. Nitta E, Izutsu K, Sato T, Ota Y, Takeuchi T, Kamijo A, et al. A high incidence of late-onset neutropenia following rituximab-containing chemotherapy as a primary treatment of CD20-positive B-cell lymphoma: a single-institution study. Ann Oncol. 2007;18:364–9. doi:10.1093/annonc/mdl393.
44. Dunleavy K, Hakim F, Kim HK, Janik JE, Grant N, Nakayama T, et al. B-cell recovery following rituximab-based therapy is associated with perturbations in stromal derived factor-1 and granulocyte homeostasis. Blood. 2005;106:795–802. doi:10.1182/blood-2004-08-3198.
45. Stallworth JR, Jerrell JM, Tripathi A. Cost-effectiveness of hydroxyurea in reducing the frequency of pain episodes and hospitalization in pediatric sickle cell disease. Ann Hematol. 2011;90:145–50. doi:10.1002/ajh.21772.
46. Hui CK, Cheung WW, Zhang HY, Au WY, Yueng YH, Leung AY, et al. Kinetics and risk of de novo hepatitis B infection in HBsAg-negative patients undergoing cytotoxic chemotherapy. Gastroenterology. 2006;131:59–68. doi:10.1053/j.gastro.2006.04.015.
47. Yeo W, Chan TC, Leung NW, Lam WY, Mo FK, Miu Ting Chu MT, et al. Hepatitis B virus reactivation in lymphoma patients with prior resolved hepatitis B undergoing anticancer therapy with or without rituximab. J Clin Oncol. 2009;27:605–11. doi:10.1200/JCO.2008.18.0182.
48. Evens AM, Jovanovic BD, Su YC, Raisch DW, Ganger D, Belknap SM, et al. Rituximab-associated hepatitis B virus (HBV) reactivation in lymphoproliferative diseases: meta-analysis and examination of FDA safety reports. Ann Oncol. 2011;22:1170–80. doi:10.1093/annonc/mdq583.
49. Tsutsumi Y, Yamamoto Y, Ito S, Ohigashi H, Shiratori S, Naruse H, et al. Hepatitis B virus reactivation with a rituximab-containing regimen. World J Hepatol. 2015;7:2344–51. doi:10.4254/wjh.v7.i21.2344.
50. Kusumoto S, Tanaka Y, Suzuki R, Watanabe T, Nakata M, Takasaki H, et al. Monitoring of hepatitis B virus (HBV) DNA and risk of HBV reactivation in B-cell lymphoma: a prospective observational study. Clin Infect Dis. 2015;61:719–29. doi:10.1093/cid/civ344.
51. Nissen JC, Hummel M, Brade J, Kruth J, Hofmann WK, Buchheidt D, et al. The risk of infections in hematologic patients treated with rituximab is not influenced by cumulative rituximab dosage – a single center experience. BMC Infect Dis. 2014;14:364. doi:10.1186/1471-2334-14-364.
52. Structure of alemtuzumab. In-house data. Sanofy Co., Ltd.
53. Dyer MJ, Hale G, Hayhoe FG, Waldmann H. Effects of CAMPATH-1 antibodies in vivo in patients with lymphoid malignancies: influence of antibody isotype. Blood. 1989;73:1431–9.

54. Hale G, Dyer MJ, Clark MR, Phillips JM, Marcus R, Riechmann L, et al. Remission induction in non-Hodgkin lymphoma with reshaped human monoclonal antibody CAMPATH-1H. Lancet. 1988;17(2):1394–9. doi:10.1016/S0140-6736(88)90588-0.
55. Alinari L, Lapalombella R, Andritsos L, Baiocchi RA, Lin TS, Byrd JC. Alemtuzumab (Campath-1H) in the treatment of chronic lymphocytic leukemia. Oncogene. 2007;26:3644–53. doi:10.1038/sj.onc.1210380.
56. Cheson BD. Monoclonal antibody therapy of chronic lymphocytic leukaemia. Best Pract Res Clin Haematol. 2010;23:133–43. doi:10.1016/j.beha.2010.01.006.
57. Jaglowski SM, Alinari L, Lapalombella R, Muthusamy N, Byrd JC. The clinical application of monoclonal antibodies in chronic lymphocytic leukemia. Blood. 2010;116:3705–14. doi:10.1182/blood-2010-04-001230.
58. Ginaldi L, De Martinis M, Matutes E, Farahat N, Morilla R, Dyer MJ, et al. Levels of expression of CD52 in normal and leukemic B and T cells: correlation with in vivo therapeutic responses to Campath-1H. Leuk Res. 1998;22:185–91. doi:10.1016/S0145-2126(97)00158-6.
59. Mone AP, Cheney C, Banks AL, Tridandapani S, Mehter N, Guster S, et al. Alemtuzumab induces caspase-independent cell death in human chronic lymphocytic leukemia cells through a lipid raft-dependent mechanism. Leukemia. 2006;20:272–9. doi:10.1038/sj.leu.2404014.
60. Albitar M, Do KA, Johnson MM, Giles FJ, Jilani I, O'Brien S, et al. Free circulating soluble CD52 as a tumor marker in chronic lymphocytic leukemia and its implication in therapy with anti-CD52 antibodies. Cancer. 2004;101:999–1008. doi:10.1002/cncr.20477.
61. Lin TS, Flinn IW, Modali R, Lehman TA, Webb J, Waymer S, et al. FCGR3A and FCGR2A polymorphisms may not correlate with response to alemtuzumab in chronic lymphocytic leukemia. Blood. 2005;105:289–91. doi:10.1182/blood-2004-02-0651.
62. Lozanski G, Heerema NA, Flinn IW, Smith L, Harbison J, Webb J, et al. Alemtuzumab is an effective therapy for chronic lymphocytic leukemia with p53 mutations and deletions. Blood. 2004;103:3278–81. doi:10.1182/blood-200310-3729.
63. A Phase II Study, including pharmacokinetics, of CAMPATH-1H in patients with B-cell chronic lymphocytic leukemia who have received treatment with a purine analogue (CAM213 study). In-house data. Sanofy Co., Ltd.
64. Hutchins JT, Kull Jr FC, Bynum J, Knick VC, Thurmond LM, Ray P. Improved biodistribution, tumor targeting, and reduced immunogenicity in mice with a gamma 4 variant of Campath-1H. Proc Natl Acad Sci U S A. 1995;19(92):11980–4.
65. Smolewski P, Szmigielska-Kaplon A, Cebula B, Jamroziak K, Rogalinska M, Kilianska Z, et al. Proapoptotic activity of alemtuzumab alone and in combination with rituximab or purine nucleoside analogues in chronic lymphocytic leukemia cells. Leuk Lymphoma. 2005;46:87–100. doi:10.1080/13693780400007151.
66. Elter T, Vehreschild JJ, Gribben J, Cornely OA, Engert A, Hallek M. Management of infections in patients with chronic lymphocytic leukemia treated with alemtuzumab. Ann Hematol. 2009;88:121–32. doi:10.1007/s00277-008-0566-9.

Rituximab and Alemtuzumab for Chronic Lymphocytic Leukemia: Clinical Pharmacology and Therapeutic Results

6

Suguru Fukuhara and Kensei Tobinai

Abstract

In the last decade, extensive investigation into the pathogenesis of B-cell chronic lymphocytic leukemia (B-CLL) has led to dramatic changes in the treatment strategy for B-CLL. The addition of anti-CD20 antibody to its management has remarkably improved the survival of B-CLL patients. Fludarabine, cyclophosphamide, and rituximab (FCR) is a standard treatment for physically fit patients without *p53* defects, while bendamustine and rituximab (BR) is considered as a treatment option for those older than 65 years. Chlorambucil with anti-CD20 antibody (obinutuzumab, rituximab, or ofatumumab) is recommended for unfit patients with relevant comorbidities without *p53* defects. Alemtuzumab has proven efficacy in patients with *p53* defects and has become a therapeutic option for these patients, but its role in the management of B-CLL patients is hampered by its substantial toxicity.

Keywords

Rituximab • Alemtuzumab • Chronic lymphocytic leukemia

6.1 Introduction

Chronic lymphocytic leukemia/small lymphocytic lymphoma (CLL/SLL) is the most commonly diagnosed type of lymphoid malignancy in Western countries and affects mainly elderly patients with a median age of 67–72 years at initial diagnosis

S. Fukuhara (✉) • K. Tobinai
Department of Hematology, National Cancer Center Hospital,
5-1-1 Tsukiji, Chuo-ku, Tokyo 104-0045, Japan
e-mail: sufukuha@ncc.go.jp

T. Ueda (ed.), *Chemotherapy for Leukemia*, DOI 10.1007/978-981-10-3332-2_6

[1–5]. Most cases of CLL arise from mature B lymphocytes (B-CLL) [6], with B-CLL patients exhibiting a highly variable clinical course. A considerable number of B-CLL patients have asymptomatic and indolent clinical courses, with the possibility of a normal life expectancy, although some have rapid disease progression. It has been considered that B-CLL treatment should be palliative without aiming for a cure, with no proven survival benefit from early intervention [7–10]. Therefore, the watch-and-wait approach remains the standard therapy for patients with early-stage, asymptomatic B-CLL. Treatment is recommended for B-CLL patients who have developed the following active diseases: advanced disease (Binet stage C or Rai stage III/IV), progressive disease (rapid enlargement of lymph nodes or spleen or a rapid lymphocyte doubling time), constitutional symptoms (weight loss, night sweating, or fever), or complications (autoimmune hemolytic anemia and/or thrombocytopenia poorly responsive to corticosteroid therapy or repeated episodes of infection) [6].

The Rai [11] and Binet [12] clinical staging systems have been used to define disease extent and prognosis. However, cytogenetic abnormalities also play an important role, including chromosomal aberrations, immunoglobulin heavy chain variable region genes (IGHV) hypermutation, and *p53* mutation status in particular [13–21]. The *p53* gene defects such as the deletion of the short arm of chromosome 17 (*del17p*) and/or *p53* mutation are associated with an adverse prognosis and with resistance to most chemotherapeutic agents used for B-CLL treatment. Therefore, treatment decisions have recently been based on these cytogenetic abnormalities (Fig. 6.1) [22]. In addition, treatment decisions have to take into consideration the patient's physical fitness, comorbidity burden, and concomitant medications. The German CLL Study Group (GCLLSG) established the cumulative illness rating scale (CIRS) score [23] to assess a patient's physical fitness, and patients are classified into three categories according the risk [24]. Physically fit patients without or

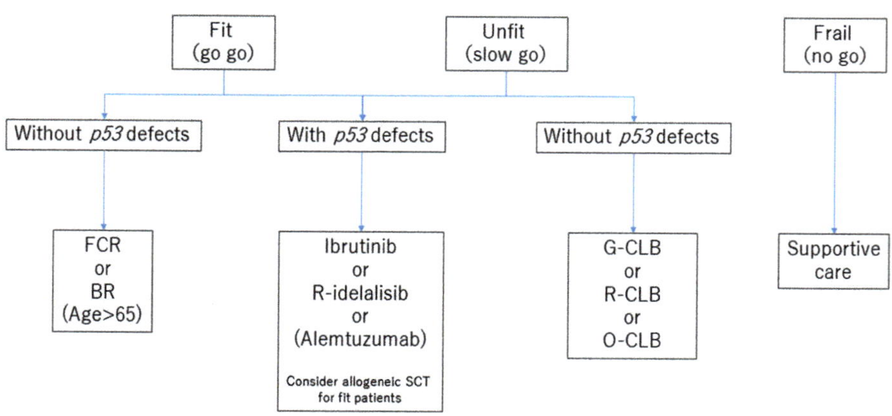

Fig. 6.1 Treatment strategy of B-CLL by the GCLLSG. *Abbreviations*: *FCR* fludarabine, cyclophosphamide, and rituximab, *BR* bendamustine and rituximab, *R-idelalisib* rituximab and idelalisib, *SCT* stem cell transplantation, *G-CLB* obinutuzumab and chlorambucil, *R-CLB* rituximab and chlorambucil, *O-CLB* ofatumumab and chlorambucil

only with mild comorbidities (go go) are recommended to receive the standard therapies aiming at long-term remissions and prolongation of survival. Physically unfit patients with relevant comorbidities (slow go) are recommended to receive less intensive therapies for disease control. Frail patients with multiple and/or severe comorbidities (no go) are recommended to receive supportive or palliative care. Treatment strategies based on GCLLSG are shown in Fig. 6.1 [22].

Several cytotoxic agents have been found to be active for B-CLL, and chlorambucil was regarded as the standard treatment for B-CLL for several decades [25]. In the mid-1990s, single-agent fludarabine therapy offered a higher response rate and comparable survival for B-CLL patients compared to anthracycline-based regimens [26, 27], and fludarabine or fludarabine-based chemotherapy such as fludarabine and cyclophosphamide (FC) was used widely, especially in younger patients [28–30]. Subsequently, the addition of rituximab to fludarabine-based chemotherapy (FR, FCR) achieved a first breakthrough for B-CLL treatment [31–35], and chemoimmunotherapy has become a new standard treatment for B-CLL. However, patients with high-risk cytogenetics, such as *p53* defects, still remain with poor prognosis primarily due to chemoimmunotherapy resistance [36, 37]. Alemtuzumab is active for such patients with these genomic abnormalities, and alemtuzumab administration has improved the survival rate of these patients [38–43].

In the present decade, progression in the understanding of B-CLL pathogenesis has facilitated the development of novel drugs targeting B-cell receptor signaling [44, 45]. Ibrutinib, which targets the Bruton's tyrosine kinase (BTK), and idelalisib, which targets the phosphatidylinositol 3-kinase (PI3K), have high efficacy for B-CLL patients, particularly those with *p53* defects, and are already approved in most Western countries for both relapsed B-CLL and for first-line treatment of B-CLL patients with *p53* defects [46–53]. Currently, many other novel agents are under investigation.

This review focuses mainly on rituximab and alemtuzumab and summarizes the available clinical data for B-CLL treatment.

6.2 Anti-CD20 Antibody for B-CLL Treatment

CD20 is a transmembrane protein expressed on the surface of mature B cells from the pre-B cell until plasma cell differentiation and plays a role in B-cell proliferation and differentiation [54–57]. Since CD20 is also present on most B-cell malignancies but not on hematopoietic stem cells and normal plasma cells, it was considered to be a suitable molecular target for B-cell malignancies.

6.2.1 Rituximab

Rituximab is a chimeric humanized monoclonal antibody that binds to the surface antigen CD20. Rituximab is considered to enhance an anticancer effect through antibody-dependent cell-mediated cytotoxicity (ADCC), complement-dependent cytotoxicity (CDC), and apoptosis [58, 59]. In early pivotal trials in patients with low-grade B-cell non-Hodgkin lymphoma (NHL), rituximab monotherapy at a dose of 375 mg/m^2 weekly for a total of four doses achieved an overall response rate (ORR) of 40–63% [60–64]. Importantly, rituximab has additional synergistic effects with various chemotherapeutic agents [65–68], and the addition of rituximab to chemotherapy was able to provide clinical benefit in most B-cell malignancies. [69–71]

6.2.1.1 Rituximab Monotherapy

One of the pivotal phase II trials described above [60] involved 30 patients with relapsed/refractory B-CLL, and the ORR was achieved in only 13% of patients. Another phase II trial of rituximab monotherapy (four infusions of 375 mg/m^2 once a week) for relapsed and/or refractory B-CLL patients demonstrated an ORR of 25%, while the complete response rate (CRR) was only 3%. Moreover, the duration of response was only 10 months [72]. Similarly, in a phase II trial for untreated B-CLL patients, rituximab monotherapy yielded a modest ORR of 51% and a CRR of 4% with a median progression-free survival (PFS) of 18.6 months [73].

It has been reported that the level of CD20 expression on B-CLL cells is significantly less compared to that found on normal B cells and other B-cell malignancies [74, 75]. Additionally, pharmacokinetic studies showed that the level of rituximab antibody in the serum of B-CLL patients was markedly lower than that of other indolent B-cell NHL [60]. These reasons may explain why standard dose rituximab has less activity as a single agent in B-CLL patients than in patients with low-grade B-cell NHL such as follicular lymphoma.

To overcome the reduced efficacy of rituximab in B-CLL, higher doses or denser dosing regimens were investigated, and these regimens showed a higher efficacy compared to standard doses [76]. In a dose-escalation trial of rituximab in B-CLL patients, 50 patients received four weekly infusions of rituximab with the dose escalated from 500 to 2250 mg/m^2. The response rate was correlated with dose: The ORR was 22% for patients treated at lower doses (500–825 mg/m^2), 43% at intermediate doses (1000–1500 mg/m^2), and 75% at the highest dose (2250 mg/m^2). In another study, rituximab was administered at doses ranging from 250 to 375 mg/m^2, three times a week for a total of 4 weeks, and an ORR and CRR of 45% and 3%, respectively, was obtained [77]. For asymptomatic untreated early-stage B-CLL, eight consecutive weekly infusions of rituximab at a dose of 375 mg/m^2 resulted in an ORR and CRR of 82% and 9%, respectively [78]. Based on the results as described above, rituximab monotherapy is currently less commonly used, and it is primary used in combination with chemotherapy.

6.2.1.2 Rituximab Maintenance Therapy

The use of rituximab as maintenance therapy has been explored and has prolonged the PFS in indolent B-cell NHL patients [79, 80]. There have been also several studies evaluating the efficacy of rituximab as maintenance therapy in B-CLL [80–82]. In these studies, patients who achieved at least a partial response (PR) at the completion of the induction therapy received maintenance therapy with rituximab for 6 months or longer. These studies demonstrated that maintenance with rituximab improved response and prolonged PFS, particularly in patients with detectable disease after induction therapy. Therefore, rituximab maintenance might have a potential survival benefit in B-CLL, although a randomized trial is needed for validation.

6.2.1.3 Combination with Chemotherapy

For Physically Fit Patients

Single-agent fludarabine therapy showed higher response and longer survival in B-CLL patients with untreated or relapsed disease, as compared with anthracycline-based regimens [26, 27]. Furthermore, fludarabine in combination with cyclophosphamide (FC) was the most effective regimen, although CR was achieved in only 23–38% of patients [28–30]. Since the combination of rituximab with fludarabine showed a synergistic effect in substantial preclinical studies [67], the addition of rituximab to a fludarabine-containing regimen (F or FC) was investigated.

Combination of Fludarabine and Rituximab (FR)

The treatment outcome of rituximab combined with fludarabine was evaluated in a phase II trial of GCLLSG [83]. Thirty-one previously untreated or relapsed B-CLL patients received fludarabine at standard doses (25 mg/m^2 per day, days 1–5, 29–33, 57–61, and 85–89) and rituximab (375 mg/m^2, days 57, 85, 113, and 151). ORR and CRR were 87% and 32%, respectively. Toxicity of FR regimen was manageable with grade 3 or 4 neutropenia in 42% and severe infections in 13% of patients. In a randomized phase II trial, the CALGB 9712 trial, fludarabine with concurrent rituximab was compared to sequential rituximab in previously untreated B-CLL patients [31]. Patients received six courses of fludarabine with or without rituximab, followed by four weekly administrations of rituximab. Among a total of 104 patients, those receiving concurrent regimen obtained a higher response rate (ORR and CRR; 90% and 47% in concurrent arm and 77% and 28% in sequential arm, respectively) with increased grade 3 or 4 neutropenia (74% vs. 41%). In a retrospective comparative analysis of CALGB 9712 and CALGB 9011 trial, 104 patients of the CALGB 9712 protocol treated with FR were compared to 178 patients of the CALGB 9011 protocol treated with single-agent fludarabine (F) [32]. The patients receiving FR had a significantly better PFS ($P < 0.0001$) and overall survival (OS) ($P = 0.0006$) than patients receiving fludarabine alone. The 2-year PFS was estimated at 67% in the FR arm and 45% in the F arm, and the 2-year OS was estimated at 93% and 81% in the FR and F arms, respectively. The incidence of infections was similar between the treatment arms. These results demonstrate that FR is a potent and feasible treatment option for B-CLL patients.

Combination of Fludarabine, Cyclophosphamide, and Rituximab (FCR)

Chemoimmunotherapy with FCR is currently recognized as the standard treatment for physically fit young patients with untreated B-CLL (Fig. 6.1). In a phase II trial conducted at the MD Anderson Cancer Center (MDACC), 300 patients with

Table 6.1 Phase III trial in previously untreated B-CLL

Study	Patient characteristics	Treatment	N	ORR (%)	CRR (%)	Median PFS (months)	Median OS
Hallek et al. (CLL-8) [33, 85]	Physically fit	FCR vs. FC	817				
		FCR	408	90	44	56.8	NR at 5.9 years
		FC	409	80	22	32.9	86 months
Eichhorst et al. (CLL-10) [103, 104]	Physically fit without *del17p*	BR vs. FCR	564				
		BR	280	97.8	31.5	43.2	
		FCR	284	97.8	40.7	53.7	
Goede et al. (CLL-11) [110, 111]	Physically unfit	G-CLB vs. R-CLB vs. CLB	781				NR
		G-CLB	238	77.3	22.3	29.9	
		R-CLB	233	31.4	0	16.3	
		CLB	118	65.7	7.3	11.1	
		G-CLB	333	78.4	20.7	29.2	
		R-CLB	330	65.1	7.0	15.4	
Hillmen et al. (COMPL-EMENT-1) [121]	Physically unfit	O-CLB vs. CLB	447				NR at 28.9 months
		O-CLB	221	82	12	22.4	
		CLB	223	69	1	13.1	
Hillmen et al. (CAM307) [42]		Alemtuzumab vs. CLB	297				NR at 24.6 months
		Alemtuzumab	149	83	24	14.6	
		CLB	148	55	2	11.7	

ORR overall response rate; *CRR* complete response rate; *PFS* progression-free survival; *OS* overall survival; *NR* not reached; *FCR* fludarabine, cyclophosphamide, and rituximab; *FC* fludarabine and cyclophosphamide; *BR* bendamustine and rituximab; *G-CLB* obinutuzumab and chlorambucil; *R-CLB* rituximab and chlorambucil; *CLB* chlorambucil; *O-CLB* ofatumumab and chlorambucil

previously untreated B-CLL were enrolled and received FCR [35, 84]. ORR was achieved in 95%, CR in 72%, nodular PR (nPR) in 10%, PR due to cytopenia in 7%, and PR due to residual disease in 6% of patients. With a median follow-up of 6 years, the 6-year overall and failure-free survivals were 77% and 51%, respectively. The median time to progression (TTP) was 80 months.

These results were superior to a historical control receiving previous generations of B-CLL therapy and led to the large randomized CLL8 trial by GCLLSG, which compared outcomes of FCR to those of FC as a first-line treatment for B-CLL patients (Table 6.1) [33, 85]. In CLL8, 817 physically fit patients with untreated B-CLL were randomly assigned to receive six courses of FC (intravenous fludarabine (25 mg/m^2 per day) and cyclophosphamide (250 mg/m^2 per day) for the first 3 days of each 28-day treatment course) with or without rituximab (375 mg/m^2 on day 0 of the first course and 500 mg/m^2 on day 1 of the second to sixth courses). The FCR arm obtained a significantly higher ORR than the FC arm (90% vs. 80%, $p < 0.001$) with a significantly higher CRR (44% vs. 22%, $p > 0.001$) and improved survival. With a median follow-up of 5.9 years, the median PFS were 56.8 and 32.9 months for the FCR and FC arms (HR = 0.59, 95% CI 0.50–0.69, $P < 0.001$), respectively, and the median OS was not reached for the FCR arm and was 86.0 months for the FC arm (HR = 0.68, 95% CI 0.54–0.89, $P = 0.001$). In the analysis of prognostic factors including molecular cytogenetics, the improved survival benefit with FCR was applied for most prognostic subgroups including *11q* deletion, although FCR did not improve the survival of patients with *del17p*. Furthermore, in a subgroup of patients with a mutated IGHV status, patients who were treated with FCR had a significant longer survival than those treated with FC. Median PFS was not reached for the FCR arm and was 41.9 months for the FC arm (HR 0.47, 95% CI 0.33–0.68, $P = 0.001$). The 5-year OS after FCR and FC were 86.3% and 79.8%, respectively. The Kaplan-Meier PFS curve appeared to plateau, and these findings might suggest a curative treatment with FCR for these particular B-CLL patients. In the safety analysis, neutropenia occurred more frequently in FCR arms (grades 3–4, FCR 34%, FC 21%), while other adverse events including infection, anemia, and thrombocytopenia were similar. Moreover, there was no significant difference in secondary malignancies including Richter's transformation between FCR arms (13.1%) and FC arms (17.4%) ($p = 0.1$).

Similar results were shown in a phase III trial comparing FCR with FC in patients with previously treated B-CLL [34]. Five hundred and fifty-two patients with no prior administration of rituximab were enrolled and randomly assigned to FCR or FC treatment arm. FCR significantly improved PFS (HR 0.65, $P < 0.001$; median, 30.6 months for FCR vs. 20.6 months for FC), ORR (69.9% vs. 58.0%, $p = 0.0034$), and CRR (24.3% vs. 14.0%, $P < 0.001$). The rate of grade 3 or 4 adverse events including neutropenia and serious adverse events was higher in the FCR arm compared to the FC arm, although the incidence of infections did not differ between the treatment arms, and FCR was well tolerated. These findings led to the establishment of rituximab in B-CLL treatment, and the FCR regimen was recognized as a standard regimen for physically fit patients with untreated B-CLL.

Consequently, the hypothesis that a more intensive chemotherapy might increase the therapeutic effect of FCR regimen was investigated. The addition of other agents to FCR regimen, such as mitoxantrone [37, 86], lenalidomide [87], or alemtuzumab [88], demonstrated encouraging clinical activity in previously untreated B-CLL, with an ORR of 92–100% and a CRR of 58–82%. While these more intensive chemotherapy regimens showed remarkable efficacy, there was a considerable increase in the incidence of adverse events, especially infections, in most of these trials. Despite showing substantial efficacy, these more intensive regimens have not been evaluated by a randomized comparison to the FCR regimen and thus have not become the standard regimen for untreated B-CLL patients.

Modified FCR Regimen

However, it is important to note that B-CLL patients are mostly elderly, and the FCR regimen was often too toxic and therefore not applicable to these patients. Therefore, modified FCR regimens of lower intensity were investigated to maintain the efficacy but reduce the adverse events, especially neutropenia and infections.

Two modified FCR regimens with reduced fludarabine and cyclophosphamide dosages and increased rituximab frequency were examined in phase II trials [89–91]. One trial demonstrated favorable outcome and reduced toxicity compared to the previous trials with FCR, although the median age of patients in this trial was only 58 years [89, 90]. Another trial focused on patients over 65 years old and demonstrated high efficacy, although myelosuppression was severe and frequent dose adjustments were required [91]. Therefore, these trial results could not be generalized to unfit or frail elderly B-CLL patients.

Another alternative attempt to reduce the toxicity of FCR regimen was to substitute fludarabine (and cyclophosphamide) with other purine analogs (cladribine, pentostatin, or bendamustine). The combination of cladribine [92] or pentostatin [93, 94] and rituximab with or without cyclophosphamide seemed to be inferior to FCR regimen or could not demonstrate a lower toxicity compared to FCR regimen. Therefore, these are not considered as a standard treatment for physically fit patients with B-CLL, and the value of these regimens remains to be elucidated.

Combination of Bendamustine and Rituximab (BR)

Bendamustine has structural similarities to both alkylating agents and purine analogs and had considerable activity for indolent B-cell malignancies including B-CLL [95–97]. Bendamustine produced significantly greater efficacy but more frequent neutropenia and infection than chlorambucil in previously untreated B-CLL patients and therefore did not show a benefit in OS [98, 99]. In a small phase I/II trial, single-agent bendamustine yielded an ORR of 56% in relapsed/refractory B-CLL patients [100]. Based on these results, BR regimen was conducted for relapsed/refractory and previously untreated B-CLL patients and showed promising outcomes.

In a phase II trial of 78 relapsed/refractory B-CLL patients where most had previously received a fludarabine-containing regimen, patients received bendamustine 70 mg/m^2 per day on days 1 and 2 and rituximab 375 mg/m^2 on day 0 for the first course and 500 mg/m^2 on day 1 for subsequent courses every 28 days for up to six courses [101]. Based on intent-to-treat analysis, ORR and CRR were achieved in 59.0% and 9.0% of patients, respectively. ORR was 45.5% in fludarabine-refractory patients and 60.5% in fludarabine-sensitive patients. With a median follow-up of 24 months, the median event-free survival (EFS) was 14.7 months. The incidence of grade 3 or 4 severe infections, neutropenia, thrombocytopenia, and anemia were 12.8%, 23.1%, 28.2%, and 16.6%, respectively. In genetic analyses, patients with *del17p* did not respond to BR regimen, similar to other purine analogs.

BR regimen was also investigated in previously untreated B-CLL patients [102]. The dose and schedule of BR regimen were essentially as described above, but the dose of bendamustine was increased to 90 mg/m^2 per day. Out of 117 patients, ORR and CRR were 88.0% and 23.1%, respectively. With a median follow-up time of 27.0 months, median EFS was 33.9 months, and 90.5% of patients were alive. Grade 3 or 4 infections, neutropenia, thrombocytopenia, and anemia were documented in 7.7%, 19.7%, 22.2%, and 19.7% of patients, respectively. In a genetic analysis, BR had modest activity for patients with *del17p*, as for relapsed/refractory patients. In comparison to FCR regimen, BR appeared to show similar efficacy, with a lower incidence of severe infections and neutropenia.

From promising results, a phase III trial, CLL10 trial of the GCLLSG, comparing the BR regimen with FCR regimen for previously untreated B-CLL in physically fit patients without *del17p* was conducted (Table 6.1) [103, 104]. A total of 564 patients with CIRS score ≤6 and creatinine clearance >70 ml/min and without *del17p* were enrolled, and these patients received up to six courses of BR or FCR. Patient background was well balanced between the two arms excluding age (22% in BR vs. 14% in FCR, aged >70 years, $p = 0.020$) and the proportion of unmutated IGHV status (68% in BR vs. 55% in FCR, $P = 0.003$). The ORR was 97.8% in both arms, although BR was inferior to FCR in CRR (31.5% vs. 40.7%, $P = 0.026$), in MRD negativity in peripheral blood (62.9% vs. 74.1%, $P = 0.0024$), in MRD negativity in the bone marrow (31.6% vs. 58.1%, $P < 0.001$), and in the median PFS (43.2 vs. 53.7 months, HR = 1.589, 95% CI 1.25–2.079, $P = 0.001$) with a median follow-up time of 35.9 months. In particular, physically fit patients (CIRS ≤3, only one CIRS item, age <65 years) benefited the most from FCR. However, there was no statistical difference in PFS between both arms in patients ≥65 years, CIRS 4–6 or >1 CIRS item. The 3-year OS was 92.2% in the BR arm and 90.6% in the FCR arm, with no significant difference (HR = 1.030, 95% CI 0.618–1.717, $p = 0.910$). In safety analysis, grade 3 or 4 severe neutropenia and infections were more frequently documented in the FCR arm (87.7% vs. 67.8%, $p < 0.001$, and 39.8% vs. 25.4%, $p = 0.001$), especially in elderly patients >70 years (48.4% vs. 26.8%, $p = 0.001$). The incidence of anemia and thrombocytopenia was not significantly different (14.2% vs. 12.0%, $p = 0.46$, and 22.4% vs. 16.5%, $p = 0.096$). Treatment-related mortality also did not differ significantly between both treatment arms (3.9% in FCR and 2.1% in BR). Based on these results, FCR regimen remains the standard therapy in physically fit young patients. The BR regimen can be an alternative regimen in elderly fit patients, as the FCR regimen more frequently causes severe neutropenia and infection in these patients (Fig. 6.1).

For Unfit Patients

Chlorambucil is a nitrogen mustard alkylating agent and has been considered the standard treatment of B-CLL for several decades, especially in elderly patients with relevant comorbidities, since chlorambucil offers a modest response rate, but low toxicity and the convenience of oral intake [25]. In the past, several more potent and promising agents, including fludarabine, bendamustine, and alemtuzumab, had not demonstrated any survival benefit compared to chlorambucil [42, 98, 99, 105–107]. The addition of rituximab to chemotherapy had increased the efficacy of B-CLL chemotherapy regimens under evaluation, and the addition of rituximab to chlorambucil (R-CLB) showed similarly encouraging results in some phase II trials [108,

109]. In these phase II trials, R-CLB was well tolerated and of benefit. These compared favorably with published results for chlorambucil monotherapy and subsequently led to the CLL11 phase III trial (Table 6.1) [110, 111]. The CLL11 trial by GCLLSG evaluated the efficacy of rituximab or obinutuzumab in combination with chlorambucil (R-CLB or G-CLB) in comparison to chlorambucil alone in patients with previously untreated B-CLL and relevant comorbidities. In this trial, R-CLB showed a survival benefit compared to chlorambucil monotherapy (the details are described below). Taken together, R-CLB has become one of the current standard treatments for physically unfit B-CLL patients.

6.2.2 Ofatumumab

Ofatumumab is a humanized novel type I CD20 antibody that binds to a CD20 epitope that is distinct from that recognized by rituximab [112, 113]. Ofatumumab demonstrates enhanced CDC activity and equivalent ADCC activity compared to rituximab and showed potent activity even in cells with low CD20 expression levels, including B-CLL cells, in preclinical studies [112–116].

6.2.2.1 Ofatumumab Monotherapy

In clinical trials, ofatumumab monotherapy has shown promising efficacy in B-CLL patients who were refractory to fludarabine and alemtuzumab (FA-ref) or refractory to fludarabine with bulky disease (BF-ref) [117]. In the Hx-CD20-406 trial, 138 patients, including 59 with FA-ref and 79 with BF-ref, received eight weekly infusions of ofatumumab followed by four monthly infusions at a dose of 300 mg for the first infusion and 2000 mg for the subsequent infusions. The ORR was 58% and 47% in FA-ref and BF-ref patients, respectively. Median PFS and OS were 5.7 and 13.7 months in FA-ref patients and 5.9 and 15.4 months in BF-ref patients, respectively. The incidence of grade 3 or 4 neutropenia and severe infections was 14% and 12% in FA-ref patients and 6% and 8% in BF-ref patients, respectively. Other adverse events were primarily grade 1 or 2 neutropenia, and ofatumumab monotherapy was well tolerated. Moreover, in ad hoc retrospective analysis, ofatumumab showed similar efficacy in patients with prior rituximab treatment, compared to rituximab-naïve patients [118]. Based on these results, ofatumumab was approved for B-CLL patients refractory to fludarabine and alemtuzumab.

Recently, two clinical trials have reported interesting results. One was a large retrospective, phase IV, observational study of ofatumumab monotherapy in heavily pretreated B-CLL patients with poor prognosis, and the ORR and CRR observed in this trial were 22% and 3%, respectively, which was lower than those previously reported [119]. Another was a randomized phase III trial (RENATE trial) comparing ofatumumab with ibrutinib in previously treated B-CLL patients [49]. In this study, ibrutinib significantly improved the response rate and PFS compared to ofatumumab. Taken together, the role of single ofatumumab monotherapy in relapsed/refractory B-CLL patients is still unclear.

6.2.2.2 Ofatumumab Maintenance

The efficacy of ofatumumab maintenance was evaluated in phase III (PROLONG trial) [120]. The enrolled B-CLL patients demonstrated CR or PR after the second- or third-line treatment and were randomly assigned to receive ofatumumab (300 mg followed by 1000 mg 1 week later and every 8 weeks for up to 2 years) or to undergo observation. Among 474 patients, PFS was improved in the ofatumumab arm compared with the observation arm (29•4 vs. 15.2 months, HR 0.50, 95% CI 0.38–0.66, $p < 0.0001$) with acceptable toxicities. Grade 3 or 4 neutropenia was observed in 24% and 10%, and severe infections in 13% and 8% of patients in the ofatumumab and observation arms, respectively. At the time of the interim analysis, no significant difference in OS had been observed. Based on this trial results, maintenance therapy of ofatumumab for patients with relapsed B-CLL might be applied in the near future.

6.2.2.3 Combination with Chemotherapy

Ofatumumab in combination with chlorambucil (O-CLB) has also been investigated in previously untreated B-CLL patients, as with obinutuzumab and rituximab (Table 6.1) [121]. In a phase III trial, the COMPLEMENT 1 trial, 447 patients who were not eligible for fludarabine-based treatment were enrolled and received chlorambucil at a dose of 10 mg/m^2 on days 1–7 every 28 days up to 12 courses with or without ofatumumab at a dose of 300 mg and 1000 mg on days 1 and 8 of the first course, respectively, and day 1 of the subsequent courses. The median age was 69 years, and 87% of patients were ≥65 years or had more than two comorbidities or a CCr <70 ml/min. With a median follow-up of 28.9 months, O-CLB significantly improved ORR (82% vs. 69%, $P < 0.001$) with superior CRR (12% vs. 1%) and PFS (22.4 vs. 13.1 months, $P < 0.001$). Grade 3 or 4 neutropenia occurred frequently in O-CLB arm (26% vs. 14%), but infections were of similar frequency in both treatment arms. The addition of ofatumumab to chlorambucil led to clinically significant improvements with a manageable toxicity in previously untreated B-CLL patients with relevant comorbidities and became a novel treatment option for these patients. Ofatumumab in combination with chlorambucil is approved by the US Food and Drug Administration (FDA) and European Medicines Agency (EMA) to treat previously untreated B-CLL patients for whom fludarabine-based therapy is considered inappropriate.

Ofatumumab in combination with bendamustine (BO) has also been assessed in several phase II trials [121–123]. In the phase II trial by Gruppo Italiano Malattie EMatologiche dell'Adulto (GIMEMA), 47 patients with relapsed/refractory B-CLL were enrolled and received bendamustine (70 mg/m^2 on day 1, 2 every 28 days) and ofatumumab (300 mg on day 1 and 1000 mg on day 8 at the first course and 1000 mg on day 1 at subsequent courses) up to six courses [122]. The ORR was 72.3%, with CR in 17% of patients. With a median follow-up of 24.2 months, the OS and PFS were achieved in 83.6% and 49.6% of patients, respectively. These results compared favorably with the efficacy of previously published treatments, such as BR and

FCR. Myelosuppression was the most common adverse event, and grade 3 or 4 neutropenia was observed in 61.7% of patients, although grade 3 or 4 infections were documented in only 6%. In another phase II trial, the efficacy of BO for patients with previously untreated and relapsed B-CLL was assessed [123]. In this trial, patients received the same dose and schedule as in the GIMEMA trial, although the dose of bendamustine was increased to 90 mg/m^2. Among 44 patients with previously untreated disease and 53 relapsed patients, respective ORR and CRR were 95% and 43% in the previously untreated subgroup and 74% and 11% in the relapsed subgroup. Grade 3 or 4 infections were documented in 11% and 15% of previously untreated and relapsed patients, respectively. In contrast, the phase II trial reported by Ujjani et al., which evaluated the efficacy of BO regimen in previously treated patients, was closed early due to unexpected adverse events including infusion-related reactions, infection, and neurotoxicity [124]. Based on these trials, BO regimen might be feasible and effective for both patients with relapsed B-CLL and those with previously untreated B-CLL who are physically unfit for fludarabine-based therapy. Ofatumumab in combination with bendamustine is also approved by EMA for the treatment of patients with previously untreated B-CLL who are not eligible for fludarabine-based therapy.

The combination of ofatumumab with fludarabine and cyclophosphamide (OFC) was evaluated in physically fit patients with previously untreated B-CLL [125, 126]. The phase III trial, COMPLEMENT 2, compared OFC with FC, and OFC improved ORR (84% vs. 68%, $P = 0.0003$) and PFS (28.9 vs. 18.8 months, $P = 0.0032$) among a total of 365 patients [126]. Grade 3 or 4 neutropenia was frequently observed in the OFC arm (58%) compared with the FC arm (41%), but the incidence rate of severe infections was similar between both treatment arms.

6.2.3 Obinutuzumab

Obinutuzumab is a humanized, glycoengineered anti-CD20 antibody that binds to a type II epitope of CD20 [127]. Obinutuzumab enhanced ADCC, induced direct cell death, and showed a lower degree of CDC, resulting in superior efficacy as compared with type I anti-CD20 antibody such as rituximab in preclinical studies [127–131].

In a phase II trial in patients with relapsed/refractory B-CLL, 20 patients received obinutuzumab at a fixed dose of 1000 mg (on days 1, 8, and 15 of course 1 and on day 1 of subsequent courses every 21 days for a total of eight courses) [132]. The ORR was 30% and the median PFS was 10.7 months. Grade 3 or 4 neutropenia was documented in 20% of patients. This trial showed that obinutuzumab monotherapy is active in patients with relapsed/refractory B-CLL, and the CLL11 trial was subsequently conducted.

In the CLL11 trial, 781 patients with previously untreated B-CLL and CIRS >6 and/or an estimated creatinine clearance (CCr) <70 ml/min were randomly assigned to chlorambucil alone (0.5 mg/kg on days 1 and 15 of each course every 28 days for a total of six courses), chlorambucil combined with obinutuzumab (1000 mg on days 1, 8, and 15 of cycle 1 and on day 1 of subsequent courses), or chlorambucil combined with rituximab (375 mg/m^2 on day 1 of the first course and 500 mg/m^2 on day 1 of subsequent courses) (Table 6.1) [110, 111]. Among 781 patients, the median age was 73 years, CCr was 62 ml/min, and the median CIRS score was 8 at baseline. G-CLB or R-CLB yielded higher response rates than chlorambucil monotherapy (ORR, 77.3% vs. 65.6% vs. 31.4%; CRR, 22.3% vs. 7.3% vs. 0%) and prolonged PFS (median PFS; 26.7 vs. 16.3 vs. 11.1 months, $P < 0.0001$). The OS was also longer with G-CLB or R-CLB compared with CLB monotherapy (G-CLB vs. CLB alone; HR 0.47, 95% CI 0.29–0.76, $P = 0.0014$, R-CLB vs. CLB alone; HR 0.60, 95% CI 0.38–0.94, $P = 0.0242$). The G-CLB treatment, as compared with R-CLB, prolonged the PFS (HR 0.40, 95% CI 0.33–0.50, $P = 0.001$) and CRR, but did not demonstrate benefit in OS (HR 0.70, 95% CI 0.47–1.02, $P = 0.0632$). However, this result might not be conclusive due to the small number of death events in both treatment arms. In the safety analysis, the incidence of grade 3 or 4 neutropenia was higher with G-CLB and R-CLB compared to CLB alone (33%, 28%, and 10%, respectively), although the incidences of severe infections were similar among the three treatment arms (12%, 14%, and 14%, respectively). Based on these results, obinutuzumab was approved for use in combination with chlorambucil to treat patients with previously untreated B-CLL. G-CLB and R-CLB are considered current standard treatments for patients with relevant comorbidities and previously untreated B-CLL.

6.3 Alemtuzumab for B-CLL

Alemtuzumab is a recombinant, humanized anti-CD52 monoclonal antibody [133]. CD52 is a cell surface protein and is expressed at high density on most normal and malignant lymphocytes including B-CLL, but not on hematopoietic stem cells [134]. The binding of alemtuzumab to CD52 induces cell death through CDC, ADCC, and induction of apoptosis [135–138]. Early pilot studies demonstrated that alemtuzumab could cause tumor regression in patients with advanced NHL with a higher response for tumor cells in the blood and bone marrow, but less response in the bulky lymph node [139]. These promising results encouraged pilot studies evaluating alemtuzumab efficacy for B-CLL, and several pilot phase II studies demonstrated that alemtuzumab was an effective salvage therapy for patients with relapsed/refractory B-CLL [140–143].

6.3.1 Monotherapy

In the pivotal CAM 211 trial, 93 patients with relapsed/refractory B-CLL, who received at least one alkylating agent-based regimen and in whom fludarabine treatment had failed, were enrolled and received alemtuzumab monotherapy [143]. Alemtuzumab was administered using a dose-escalation protocol followed by 30 mg three times weekly up to a total of 12 weeks. The ORR and CRR were 33% and 2%, respectively. The ORR in the peripheral blood, bone marrow, and lymph node were 86%, 45%, and 74%, respectively, and the respective CRRs were 83%, 26%, and 27%. A lower response rate was inversely correlated with larger lymph nodes. With a median follow-up of 29 months, median TTP was 4.7 months for all patients and 9.5 months for responders. Median OS was 16 months for all patients and 32 months for responders. Clinical benefit was observed not only in responders but in patients with stable disease. In a subgroup of patients with stable disease, the median chemotherapy-free time before alemtuzumab was 3.8 months and was extended to 7.6 months after alemtuzumab treatment. The most common adverse events were grade 1 or 2 infusion-related toxicity, cytopenia, and infections caused by profound cellular immunosuppression. Grade 3 or 4 infections were documented in 26.9% of patients, and the most common opportunistic infection observed was CMV reactivation.

Alemtuzumab has proven survival benefits in patients with previously untreated B-CLL. In a randomized CAM307 trial, 297 patients with previously untreated B-CLL were randomly assigned to receive either chlorambucil (40 mg/m2 every 28 days, for up to 12 months) or alemtuzumab (same dose and schedule for relapsed/refractory patients) (Table 6.1) [42]. Alemtuzumab improved ORR (83% vs. 55%, $P < 0.0001$) with superior CRR (24% vs. 2%, $P < 0.0001$) compared to chlorambucil. Elimination of minimal residual disease (MRD) occurred in 31% of complete responders to alemtuzumab, but none to chlorambucil. With a median follow-up of 24.6 months, the median PFS was 14.6 months in alemtuzumab arm and 11.7 months in chlorambucil arm, and alemtuzumab reduced the risk of progression or death by 42% (HR 0.58, $P = 0.0001$). Alemtuzumab also yielded a favorable median time to alternative treatment compared to chlorambucil (23.3 vs. 14.7 months, $P <$ 0.0001). Moreover, alemtuzumab was relatively active in patients with high-risk cytogenetics of *del17p* (ORR was 64%, and median PFS was 10.7 months). More infusion-related reaction, neutropenia, and CMV events were observed in alemtuzumab and more nausea and vomiting in chlorambucil, although other adverse event profiles were similar between treatment arms.

From these results, alemtuzumab was approved by the FDA and EMA for single-agent therapy for patients with previously untreated and relapsed/refractory B-CLL.

Subcutaneous alemtuzumab demonstrates similar efficacy and safety as compared to intravenous administration in fludarabine-refractory B-CLL patients. In a phase II CLL2H trial, alemtuzumab was administered subcutaneously at the same dose as intravenous administration [43]. Among 103 patients, after a median follow-up time of 37.9 months, ORR, CRR, PFS, and OS were 34%, 4%, 7.7 months, and 19.1 months, respectively. Grade 3 or 4 neutropenia, non-CMV infections, and CMV infections were observed in 56%, 29%, and 8% of patients, respectively. Skin reactions at the injection site were generally mild, and induction of anti-alemtuzumab antibody was rare. Taken together, subcutaneous administration is the preferred delivery route for alemtuzumab.

6.3.2 Combination with Chemotherapy

Since alemtuzumab has proven efficacy in patients with high-risk cytogenetics such as *del17p* and *p53* mutations [38–43], alemtuzumab was a therapeutic option for patients with these poor prognoses. However, in the CAM307 trial described above, alemtuzumab produced a median PFS of only 10.7 months in patients with *del17p*. In the patients with relapsed/refractory patients, alemtuzumab achieved ORR in only 33% to 55% with few CRR, and the median PFS of these patients was only 4.7–7.7 months.

Corticosteroids have efficacy in a p53-independent manner, and the addition of high-dose corticosteroids to alemtuzumab was therefore considered to improve the outcome of B-CLL patients with *p53* defects. Some phase II trials [144, 145] demonstrated an ORR, CRR, and median PFS of 88–97%, 21–65%, and 18.3–32.8 months, respectively. These results were highly favorable in comparison with the results observed in B-CLL patients with *del17p* receiving FCR in the GCLLSG CLL8 trial (median PFS and OS, 11 and 28.8 months, respectively) and with those who received alemtuzumab in the CAM307 trial (median PFS, 11 months).

Alemtuzumab in combination with other chemotherapy has been evaluated in several trials. A phase III trial by a French study group compared alemtuzumab in combination with FC (FCA) to FCR in patients with previously untreated B-CLL [146]. However, this trial was terminated early due to excess toxicity, which were mainly infections. Another phase III trial compared alemtuzumab in combination with fludarabine (FA) to fludarabine monotherapy in patients with relapsed/refractory B-CLL [147]. FA regimen resulted in better PFS (23.7 vs. 16.5 months, HR 0.61, 95% CI 0.47–0.80, $P = 0.0003$) and OS (median not reached vs. 52.9 months, HR 0.65, 95% CI 0.45–0.94, $p = 0.021$) compared to fludarabine monotherapy. The incidence of serious adverse events occurred more frequently in the FA arm (33% vs. 25%), such as grade 3 or 4 lymphopenia (94% vs. 33%), CMV events (14% vs. <1%), and grade 1 or 2 potentially alemtuzumab infusion-related reaction (62% vs. 13%). Taken together, FA regimen might be another treatment option for patients with previously treated B-CLL.

6.3.3 Adverse Effects

Alemtuzumab causes profound suppression of cell-mediated immunity through T-cell and neutrophil depletion and is associated with a high proportion of bacterial and viral infections, especially opportunistic infections. Reactivated herpes viruses such as CMV are the most frequently observed opportunistic infections. Symptomatic CMV reactivation occurred in 4–29% of B-CLL patients treated with alemtuzumab [148]. In the first-line CAM307 study, 16% and 52% of alemtuzumab-treated patients had symptomatic and asymptomatic CMV reactivation, respectively.

Infusion-related reaction is an established complication of alemtuzumab. Most of these are generally grade 1 or 2 reactions and were resolved by introducing subcutaneous administration.

6.3.4 Role of Alemtuzumab for B-CLL

Alemtuzumab has efficacy in patients with high-risk cytogenetics of *p53* defects, although alemtuzumab is associated with a high risk of toxicity, especially from infections due to T-cell depletion. In addition, the outcome of the novel agents, ibrutinib or idelalisib, has been superior to that previously reported with alemtuzumab. As a result of the inferior risk/benefit ratio of alemtuzumab compared to these novel agents, alemtuzumab currently has a limited role in the treatment strategy of B-CLL. Moreover, the alemtuzumab license has been withdrawn in 2012 by Sanofi, and alemtuzumab is now only available within a compassionate use program through the manufacturer.

6.4 Future Development

The treatment strategy of B-CLL has evolved with the addition of anti-CD20 antibody to chemotherapy. In addition, two novel agents targeting BCR signaling, ibrutinib and idelalisib, have shown high efficacy and favorable toxicity in B-CLL patients, especially those with *p53* defects. Ibrutinib or idelalisib with rituximab might be a current new standard treatment for B-CLL patients with this high-risk cytogenetics. At present, many other novel agents such as SYK inhibitor, BCL-2 inhibitor, CDK inhibitor, or anti-CD37 antibody are under investigation. In the future, the treatment strategies combining such novel agents may provide effective long-term disease control with curative potential.

References

1. Morton LM, Wang SS, Devesa SS, et al. Lymphoma incidence patterns by WHO subtype in the United States, 1992–2001. Blood. 2006;107:265–76.

2. Watson L, Wyld P, Catovsky D. Disease burden of chronic lymphocytic leukaemia within the European Union. Eur J Haematol. 2008;81:253–8.
3. National Cancer Institute [Website]. Surveillance epidemiology and end results cancer statistics review. http://seer.cancer.gov/statfacts/html/clyl.html. Last accessed 25 April 2016.
4. Diehl LF, Hynds-Karnell L, Menck HR. The national cancer data base report on age, gender, treatment and outcomes of patients with chronic lymphocytic leukemia. Cancer. 1999;86:2684–92.
5. Molica S, Levato D. What is changing in the natural history of chronic lymphocytic leukemia? Haematologica. 2001;86:8–12.
6. Hallek M, Cheson BD, Catovsky D, et al. Guidelines for the diagnosis and treatment of chronic lymphocytic leukemia: a report from the International Workshop on Chronic Lymphocytic Leukemia updating the National Cancer Institute-Working Group 1996 guidelines. Blood. 2008;111:5446–56.
7. Dighiero G, Maloum K, Desablens B, et al. Chlorambucil in indolent chronic lymphocytic leukemia. N Engl J Med. 1998;338:1506–14.
8. Shustik C, Mick R, Silver R, et al. Treatment of early chronic lymphocytic leukemia: intermittent chlorambucil versus observation. Hematol Oncol. 1988;6:7–12.
9. Montserrat E, Fontanillas M, Estape J, et al. Chronic lymphocytic leukemia treatment: an interim report of PETHEMA trials. Leuk Lymphoma. 1991;5:89–92.
10. CLL Trialists' Collaborative Group. Chemotherapeutic options in chronic lymphocytic leukemia. J Natl Cancer Inst. 1999;91:861–8.
11. Rai KR, Sawitsky A, Cronkite EP, et al. Clinical staging of chronic lymphocytic leukemia. Blood. 1975;46:219–34.
12. Binet JL, Auquier A, Dighiero G, et al. A new prognostic classification of chronic lymphocytic leukemia derived from a multivariate survival analysis. Cancer. 1981;48:198–204.
13. Döhner H, Stilgenbauer S, Benner A, et al. Genomic aberrations and survival in chronic lymphocytic leukemia. N Engl J Med. 2000;343:1910–6.
14. Damle RN, Wasil T, Fais F, et al. Ig V gene mutation status and CD38 expression as novel prognostic indicators in chronic lymphocytic leukemia. Blood. 1999;94:1840–7.
15. Hamblin TJ, Davis Z, Gardiner A, et al. Unmutated Ig V(H) genes are associated with a more aggressive form of chronic lymphocytic leukemia. Blood. 1999;94:1848–54.
16. el Rouby S, Thomas A, Costin D, et al. p53 gene mutation in B-cell chronic lymphocytic leukemia is associated with drug resistance and is independent of MDR1/MDR3 gene expression. Blood. 1993;82:3452–9.
17. Döhner H, Fischer K, Bentz M, et al. p53 gene deletion predicts for poor survival and nonresponse to therapy with purine analogs in chronic B-cell leukemias. Blood. 1995;85:1580–9.
18. Zenz T, Kröber A, Scherer K, et al. Monoallelic TP53 inactivation is associated with poor prognosis in chronic lymphocytic leukemia: results from a detailed genetic characterization with longterm follow-up. Blood. 2008;112:3322–9.
19. Rossi D, Cerri M, Deambrogi C, et al. The prognostic value of TP53 mutations in chronic lymphocytic leukemia is independent of Del17p13: implications for overall survival and chemorefractoriness. Clin Cancer Res. 2009;15:995–1004.
20. Zenz T, Eichhorst B, Busch R, et al. TP53 mutation and survival in chronic lymphocytic leukemia. J Clin Oncol. 2010;28:4473–9.
21. Trbusek M, Smardova J, Malcikova J, et al. Missense mutations located in structural p53 DNA-binding motifs are associated with extremely poor survival in chronic lymphocytic leukemia. J Clin Oncol. 2011;29:2703–8.
22. Stilgenbauer S, Furman RR, Zent CS. Management of chronic lymphocytic leukemia. Am Soc Clin Oncol Educ Book. 2015:164–75.
23. Linn BS, Linn MW, Gurel L. Cumulative illness rating scale. J Am Geriatr Soc. 1968;16:622–6.
24. Gribben JG. One step back but 2 steps forward. Blood. 2009;114:3359–60.

25. CLL Trialists' CollaborativeGroup. Chemotherapeutic options in chronic lymphocytic leukemia: a meta-analysis of the randomized trials. CLL Trialists' Collaborative Group. J Natl Cancer Inst. 1999;91:861–8.
26. Johnson S, Smith AG, Löffler H, et al. Multicentre prospective randomised trial of fludarabine versus cyclophosphamide, doxorubicin, and prednisone (CAP) for treatment of advanced-stage chronic lymphocytic leukaemia. The French Cooperative Group on CLL. Lancet. 1996;347:1432–8.
27. Leporrier M, Chevret S, Cazin B, et al. Randomized comparison of fludarabine, CAP, and ChOP in 938 previously untreated stage B and C chronic lymphocytic leukemia patients. Blood. 2001;98:2319–25.
28. Eichhorst BF, Busch R, Hopfinger G, et al. Fludarabine plus cyclophosphamide versus fludarabine alone in first line therapy of younger patients with chronic lymphocytic leukemia. Blood. 2006;107:885–91.
29. Flinn IW, Neuberg DS, Grever MR, et al. Phase III trial of fludarabine plus cyclophosphamide compared with fludarabine for patients with previously untreated chronic lymphocytic leukemia: US intergroup trial E2997. J Clin Oncol. 2007;25:793–8.
30. Catovsky D, Richards S, Matutes E, et al. Assessment of fludarabine plus cyclophosphamide for patients with chronic lymphocytic leukaemia (the LRF CLL4 trial): a randomised controlled trial. Lancet. 2007;370:230–9.
31. Byrd JC, Peterson BL, Morrison VA, et al. Randomized phase 2 study of fludarabine with concurrent versus sequential treatment with rituximab in symptomatic, untreated patients with B-cell chronic lymphocytic leukemia: results from cancer and leukemia group B 9712 (CALGB 9712). Blood. 2003;101:6–14.
32. Byrd JC, Rai K, Peterson BL, et al. Addition of rituximab to fludarabine may prolong progression-free survival and overall survival in patients with previously untreated chronic lymphocytic leukemia: an updated retrospective comparative analysis of CALGB 9712 and CALGB 9011. Blood. 2005;105:49–53.
33. Hallek M, Fischer K, Fingerle-Rowson G, et al. Addition of rituximab to fludarabine and cyclophosphamide in patients with chronic lymphocytic leukaemia: a randomised, open-label, phase 3 trial. Lancet. 2010;376:1164–74.
34. Robak T, Dmoszynska A, Solal-Céligny P, et al. Rituximab plus fludarabine and cyclophosphamide prolongs progression-free survival compared with fludarabine and cyclophosphamide alone in previously treated chronic lymphocytic leukemia. J Clin Oncol. 2010;28:1756–65.
35. Keating MJ, O'Brien S, Albitar M, et al. Early results of a chemoimmunotherapy regimen of fludarabine, cyclophosphamide, and rituximab as initial therapy for chronic lymphocytic leukemia. J Clin Oncol. 2005;23:4079–88.
36. Stilgenbauer S, Schnaiter A, Paschka P, et al. Gene mutations and treatment outcome in chronic lymphocytic leukemia: results from the CLL8 trial. Blood. 2014;123:3247–54.
37. Bosch F, Abrisqueta P, Villamor N, et al. Rituximab, fludarabine, cyclophosphamide, and mitoxantrone: a new, highly active chemoimmunotherapy regimen for chronic lymphocytic leukemia. J Clin Oncol. 2009;27:4578–84.
38. Stilgenbauer S, Döhner H. Campath-1H-induced complete remission of chronic lymphocytic leukemia despite p53 gene mutation and resistance to chemotherapy. N Engl J Med. 2002;347:452–3.
39. Lozanski G, Heerema NA, Flinn IW, et al. Alemtuzumab is an effective therapy for chronic lymphocytic leukemia with p53 mutations and deletions. Blood. 2004;103:3278–81.
40. Osuji NC, Del Giudice I, Matutes E, et al. The efficacy of alemtuzumab for refractory chronic lymphocytic leukemia in relation to cytogenetic abnormalities of p53. Haematologica. 2005;90:1435–6.
41. Zenz T, Häbe S, Denzel T, et al. Detailed analysis of p53 pathway defects in fludarabine-refractory chronic lymphocytic leukemia (CLL): dissecting the contribution of 17p deletion, TP53 mutation, p53-p21 dysfunction, and miR34a in a prospective clinical trial. Blood. 2009;114:2589–97.

42. Hillmen P, Skotnicki AB, Robak T, et al. Alemtuzumab compared with chlorambucil as first-line therapy for chronic lymphocytic leukemia. J Clin Oncol. 2007;25:5616–23.
43. Stilgenbauer S, Zenz T, Winkler D, et al. Subcutaneous alemtuzumab in fludarabine-refractory chronic lymphocytic leukemia: clinical results and prognostic marker analyses from the CLL2H study of the German Chronic Lymphocytic Leukemia Study Group. J Clin Oncol. 2009;27:3994–4001.
44. Jones JA, Byrd JC. How will B-cell-receptor-targeted therapies change future CLL therapy? Blood. 2014;123:1455–60.
45. Stevenson FK, Krysov S, Davies AJ, et al. B-cell receptor signaling in chronic lymphocytic leukemia. Blood. 2011;118:4313–20.
46. Herman SE, Gordon AL, Hertlein E, et al. Bruton tyrosine kinase represents a promising therapeutic target for treatment of chronic lymphocytic leukemia and is effectively targeted by PCI-32765. Blood. 2011;117:6287–96.
47. Advani RH, Buggy JJ, Sharman JP, et al. Bruton tyrosine kinase inhibitor ibrutinib (PCI-32765) has significant activity in patients with relapsed/refractory B-cell malignancies. J Clin Oncol. 2013;31:88–94.
48. Byrd JC, Furman RR, Coutre SE, et al. Targeting BTK with ibrutinib in relapsed chronic lymphocytic leukemia. N Engl J Med. 2013;369:32–42.
49. Byrd JC, Brown JR, O'Brien S, et al. Ibrutinib versus ofatumumab in previously treated chronic lymphoid leukemia. N Engl J Med. 2014;371:213–23.
50. Burger JA, Tedeschi A, Barr PM, et al. Ibrutinib as initial therapy for patients with chronic lymphocytic leukemia. N Engl J Med. 2015;373:2425–37.
51. Hoellenriegel J, Meadows SA, Sivina M, et al. The phosphoinositide 3′-kinase delta inhibitor, CAL-101, inhibits B-cell receptor signaling and chemokine networks in chronic lymphocytic leukemia. Blood. 2011;118:3603–12.
52. Brown JR, Byrd JC, Coutre SE, et al. Idelalisib, an inhibitor of phosphatidylinositol 3-kinase p110δ, for relapsed/refractory chronic lymphocytic leukemia. Blood. 2014;123:3390–7.
53. Furman RR, Sharman JP, Coutre SE, et al. Idelalisib and rituximab in relapsed chronic lymphocytic leukemia. N Engl J Med. 2014;370:997–1007.
54. Stashenko P, Nadler LM, Hardy R, et al. Characterization of a human B lymphocyte-specific antigen. J Immunol. 1980;125:1678–85.
55. Tedder TF, Boyd AW, Freedman AS, et al. The B cell surface molecule B1 is functionally linked with B cell activation and differentiation. J Immunol. 1985;135:973–9.
56. Tedder TF, Klejman G, Schlossman SF, et al. Structure of the gene encoding the human B lymphocyte differentiation antigen CD20 (B1). J Immunol. 1989;142:2560–8.
57. Nadler LM, Korsmeyer SJ, Anderson KC, et al. B cell origin of non-T cell acute lymphoblastic leukemia. A model for discrete stages of neoplastic and normal pre-B cell differentiation. J Clin Invest. 1984;74:332–40.
58. Glennie MJ, French RR, Cragg MS, et al. Mechanisms of killing by anti-CD20 monoclonal antibodies. Mol Immunol. 2007;44:3823–37.
59. Maloney DG. Anti-CD20 antibody therapy for B-cell lymphomas. N Engl J Med. 2012;366:2008–16.
60. McLaughlin P, Grillo-López AJ, Link BK, et al. Rituximab chimeric anti-CD20 monoclonal antibody therapy for relapsed indolent lymphoma: half of patients respond to a four-dose treatment program. J Clin Oncol. 1998;16:2825–33.
61. Maloney DG, Grillo-López AJ, Bodkin DJ, et al. IDEC-C2B8: results of a phase I multiple-dose trial in patients with relapsed non-Hodgkin's lymphoma. J Clin Oncol. 1997;15:3266–74.
62. Maloney DG, Grillo-López AJ, White CA, et al. IDEC-C2B8 (rituximab) anti-CD20 monoclonal antibody therapy in patients with relapsed low-grade non-Hodgkin's lymphoma. Blood. 1997;90:2188–95.
63. Igarashi T, et al. Factors affecting toxicity, response and progression-free survival in relapsed patients with indolent B-cell lymphoma and mantle cell lymphoma treated with rituximab: a Japanese phase II study. Ann Oncol. 2002;13:928–43.

64. Tobinai K, Kobayashi Y, Narabayashi M, et al. Feasibility and pharmacokinetic study of a chimeric anti-CD20 monoclonal antibody (IDEC-C2B8, rituximab) in relapsed B-cell lymphoma. The IDEC-C2B8 Study Group. Ann Oncol. 1998;9:527–34.
65. Alas S, Bonavida B. Rituximab inactivates signal transducer and activation of transcription 3 (STAT3) activity in B-non-Hodgkin's lymphoma through inhibition of the interleukin 10 autocrine/paracrine loop and results in down-regulation of Bcl-2 and sensitization to cytotoxic drugs. Cancer Res. 2001;61:5137–44.
66. Alas S, Emmanouilides C, Bonavida B. Inhibition of interleukin 10 by rituximab results in down-regulation of bcl-2 and sensitization of B-cell non-Hodgkin's lymphoma to apoptosis. Clin Cancer Res. 2001;7(3):709–23.
67. Di Gaetano N, Xiao Y, Erba E, et al. Synergism between fludarabine and rituximab revealed in a follicular lymphoma cell line resistant to the cytotoxic activity of either drug alone. Br J Haematol. 2001;114:800–9.
68. Chow KU, Sommerlad WD, Boehrer S, et al. Anti-CD20 antibody (IDEC-C2B8, rituximab) enhances efficacy of cytotoxic drugs on neoplastic lymphocytes in vitro: role of cytokines, complement, and caspases. Haematologica. 2002;87:33–43.
69. Hiddemann W, Buske C, Dreyling M, et al. Treatment strategies in follicular lymphomas: current status and future perspectives. J Clin Oncol. 2005;23:6394–9.
70. Coiffier B, Lepage E, Briere J, et al. CHOP chemotherapy plus rituximab compared with CHOP alone in elderly patients with diffuse large-B-cell lymphoma. N Engl J Med. 2002;346:235–42.
71. Pfreundschuh M, Trümper L, Osterborg A, et al. CHOP-like chemotherapy plus rituximab versus CHOP-like chemotherapy alone in young patients with good-prognosis diffuse large-B-cell lymphoma: a randomised controlled trial by the MabThera International Trial (MInT) Group. Lancet Oncol. 2006;7:379–91.
72. Huhn D, von Schilling C, Wilhelm M, et al. Rituximab therapy of patients with B-cell chronic lymphocytic leukemia. Blood. 2001;98:1326–31.
73. Hainsworth JD, Litchy S, Barton JH, et al. Single-agent rituximab as first-line and maintenance treatment for patients with chronic lymphocytic leukemia or small lymphocytic lymphoma: a phase II trial of the Minnie Pearl Cancer Research Network. J Clin Oncol. 2003;21:1746–51.
74. Almasri NM, Duque RE, Iturraspe J, et al. Reduced expression of CD20 antigen as a characteristic marker for chronic lymphocytic leukemia. Am J Hematol. 1992;40:259–63.
75. Prevodnik VK, Lavrenčak J, Horvat M, et al. The predictive significance of CD20 expression in B-cell lymphomas. Diagn Pathol. 2011;6:33.
76. O'brien SM, Kantarjian H, Thomas DA, et al. Rituximab dose-escalation trial in chronic lymphocytic leukemia. J Clin Oncol. 2001;19:2165–70.
77. Byrd JC, Murphy T, Howard RS, et al. Rituximab using a thrice weekly dosing schedule in B-cell chronic lymphocytic leukemia and small lymphocytic lymphoma demonstrates clinical activity and acceptable toxicity. J Clin Oncol. 2001;19:2153–64.
78. Ferrajoli A, Keating MJ, O'Brien S, Cortes J, Thomas DA. Experience with rituximab immunotherapy as an early intervention in patients with Rai stage 0 to II chronic lymphocytic leukemia. Cancer. 2011;117:3182–6.
79. Salles G, Seymour JF, Offner F, et al. Rituximab maintenance for 2 years in patients with high tumour burden follicular lymphoma responding to rituximab plus chemotherapy (PRIMA): a phase 3, randomised controlled trial. Lancet. 2011;377:42–51.
80. Luin-Nelemans HC, Hoster E, Hermine O, et al. Treatment of older patients with mantle-cell lymphoma. N Engl J Med. 2012;367:520–31.
81. Del Poeta G, Del Principe MI, Buccisano F, et al. Consolidation and maintenance immunotherapy with rituximab improve clinical outcome in patients with B-cell chronic lymphocytic leukemia. Cancer. 2008;112:119–28.
82. Wiernik PH, Adiga GU. Single-agent rituximab in treatment-refractory or poor prognosis patients with chronic lymphocytic leukemia. Curr Med Res Opin. 2011;27:1987–93.

83. Schulz H, Klein SH, Rehwald U, et al. Phase II study of a combined immunochemotherapy using rituximab and fludarabine in patients with chronic lymphocytic leukemia. Blood. 2002;100:3115–20.
84. Tam CS, O'Brien S, Wierda W, et al. Long-term results of the fludarabine, cyclophosphamide, and rituximab regimen as initial therapy of chronic lymphocytic leukemia. Blood. 2008;112:975–80.
85. Fischer K, Bahlo J, Fink AM, et al. Long-term remissions after FCR chemoimmunotherapy in previously untreated patients with CLL: updated results of the CLL8 trial. Blood. 2016;127:208–15.
86. Faderl S, Wierda W, O'Brien S, et al. Fludarabine, cyclophosphamide, mitoxantrone plus rituximab (FCM-R) in frontline CLL <70 years. Leuk Res. 2010;34:284–8.
87. Mato AR, Foon KA, Feldman T, et al. Reduced-dose fludarabine, cyclophosphamide, and rituximab (FCR-Lite) plus lenalidomide, followed by lenalidomide consolidation/maintenance, in previously untreated chronic lymphocytic leukemia. Am J Hematol. 2015;90:487–92.
88. Parikh SA, Keating MJ, O'Brien S, et al. Frontline chemoimmunotherapy with fludarabine, cyclophosphamide, alemtuzumab, and rituximab for high-risk chronic lymphocytic leukemia. Blood. 2011;118:2062–8.
89. Foon KA, Boyiadzis M, Land SR, et al. Chemoimmunotherapy with low-dose fludarabine and cyclophosphamide and high dose rituximab in previously untreated patients with chronic lymphocytic leukemia. J Clin Oncol. 2009;27:498–503.
90. Foon KA, Mehta D, Lentzsch S, et al. Long-term results of chemoimmunotherapy with low-dose fludarabine, cyclophosphamide and high-dose rituximab as initial treatment for patients with chronic lymphocytic leukemia. Blood. 2012;119:3184–5.
91. Dartigeas C, Van Den Neste E, Berthou C, et al. Evaluating abbreviated induction with fludarabine, cyclophosphamide, and dose-dense rituximab in elderly patients with chronic lymphocytic leukemia. Leuk Lymphoma. 2015 Sep 28;1–7 [Epub ahead of print].
92. Robak T, Smolewski P, Cebula B, et al. Rituximab plus cladribine with or without cyclophosphamide in patients with relapsed or refractory chronic lymphocytic leukemia. Eur J Haematol. 2007;79:107–13.
93. Kay NE, Geyer SM, Call TG, et al. Combination chemoimmunotherapy with pentostatin, cyclophosphamide, and rituximab shows significant clinical activity with low accompanying toxicity in previously untreated B chronic lymphocytic leukemia. Blood. 2007;109:405–11.
94. Reynolds C, Di Bella N, Lyons RM, et al. A phase III trial of fludarabine, cyclophosphamide, and rituximab vs. pentostatin, cyclophosphamide, and rituximab in B-cell chronic lymphocytic leukemia. Investig New Drugs. 2012;30:1232–40.
95. Leoni LM, Bailey B, Reifert J, et al. Bendamustine (Treanda) displays a distinct pattern of cytotoxicity and unique mechanistic features compared with other alkylating agents. Clin Cancer Res. 2008;14:309–17.
96. Rummel MJ, Al-Batran SE, Kim SZ, et al. Bendamustine plus rituximab is effective and has a favorable toxicity profile in the treatment of mantle cell and low-grade non-Hodgkin's lymphoma. J Clin Oncol. 2005;23:3383–9.
97. Robinson KS, Williams ME, van der Jagt RH, et al. Phase II multicenter study of bendamustine plus rituximab in patients with relapsed indolent B-cell and mantle cell non-Hodgkin's lymphoma. J Clin Oncol. 2008;26:4473–9.
98. Knauf WU, Lissichkov T, Aldaoud A, et al. Phase III randomized study of bendamustine compared with chlorambucil in previously untreated patients with chronic lymphocytic leukemia. J Clin Oncol. 2009;27:4378–84.
99. Knauf WU, Lissitchkov T, Aldaoud A, et al. Bendamustine compared with chlorambucil in previously untreated patients with chronic lymphocytic leukaemia: updated results of a randomized phase III trial. Br J Haematol. 2012;159:67–77.
100. Bergmann MA, Goebeler ME, Herold M, et al. Efficacy of bendamustine in patients with relapsed or refractory chronic lymphocytic leukemia: results of a phase I/II study of the German CLL Study Group. Haematologica. 2005;90:1357–64.

101. Fischer K, Cramer P, Busch R, et al. Bendamustine combined with rituximab in patients with relapsed and/or refractory chronic lymphocytic leukemia: a multicenter phase II trial of the German Chronic Lymphocytic Leukemia Study Group. J Clin Oncol. 2011;29:3559–66.
102. Fischer K, Cramer P, Busch R, et al. Bendamustine in combination with rituximab for previously untreated patients with chronic lymphocytic leukemia: a multicenter phase II trial of the German Chronic Lymphocytic Leukemia Study Group. J Clin Oncol. 2012;30:3209–16.
103. Eichhorst B, Fink AM, Busch R, et al. Frontline chemoimmunotherapy with fludarabine (F), cyclophosphamide (C), and rituximab (R) (FCR) shows superior efficacy in comparison to bendamustine (B) and rituximab (BR) in previously untreated and physically fit patients (pts) with advanced chronic lymphocytic leukemia (CLL): final analysis of an international, randomized study of the German CLL study group (GCLLSG) (CLL10 study). Blood. 2014;124:abst19.
104. Cramer P, Langerbeins P, Eichhorst B, et al. Advances in first-line treatment of chronic lymphocytic leukemia: current recommendations on management and first-line treatment by the German CLL Study Group (GCLLSG). Eur J Haematol. 2016;96:9–18.
105. Rai KR, Peterson BL, Appelbaum FR, et al. Fludarabine compared with chlorambucil as primary therapy for chronic lymphocytic leukemia. N Engl J Med. 2000;343:1750–7.
106. Eichhorst BF, Bahlo J, Busch R, et al. First line therapy of elderly patients with chronic lymphocytic leukemia (CLL) – long term follow-up results of a randomized phase III study of the German CLL study group (CLL5 study of the GCLLSG). Hematol Oncol. 2013;31(Suppl.1):151–200. Abst107
107. Eichhorst BF, Busch R, Stilgenbauer S, et al. First-line therapy with fludarabine compared with chlorambucil does not result in a major benefit for elderly patients with advanced chronic lymphocytic leukemia. Blood. 2009;114:3382–91.
108. Hillmen P, Gribben JG, Follows GA, et al. Rituximab plus chlorambucil as first-line treatment for chronic lymphocytic leukemia: final analysis of an open-label phase II study. J Clin Oncol. 2014;32:1236–41.
109. Foà R, Del Giudice I, Cuneo A, et al. Chlorambucil plus rituximab with or without maintenance rituximab as first-line treatment for elderly chronic lymphocytic leukemia patients. Am J Hematol. 2014;89:480–6.
110. Goede V, Fischer K, Busch R, et al. Obinutuzumab plus chlorambucil in patients with CLL and coexisting conditions. N Engl J Med. 2014;370:1101–10.
111. Goede V, Fischer K, Engelke A, et al. Obinutuzumab as frontline treatment of chronic lymphocytic leukemia: updated results of the CLL11 study. Leukemia. 2015;29:1602–4.
112. Teeling JL, French RR, Cragg MS, et al. Characterization of new human CD20 monoclonal antibodies with potent cytolytic activity against non-Hodgkin lymphomas. Blood. 2004;104:1793–800.
113. Teeling JL, Mackus WJ, Wiegman LJ, et al. The biological activity of human CD20 monoclonal antibodies is linked to unique epitopes on CD20. J Immunol. 2006;177:362–71.
114. Beum PV, Lindorfer MA, Beurskens F, et al. Complement activation on B lymphocytes opsonized with rituximab or ofatumumab produces substantial changes in membrane structure preceding cell lysis. J Immunol. 2008;181:822–32.
115. Pawluczkowycz AW, Beurskens FJ, Beum PV, et al. Binding of submaximal C1q promotes complement-dependent cytotoxicity (CDC) of B cells opsonized with anti-CD20 mAbs ofatumumab (OFA) or rituximab (RTX): considerably higher levels of CDC are induced by OFA than by RTX. J Immunol. 2009;183:749–58.
116. Beum PV, Lindorfer MA, Peek EM, et al. Penetration of antibody-opsonized cells by the membrane attack complex of complement promotes Ca(2+) influx and induces streamers. Eur J Immunol. 2011;41:2436–46.
117. Wierda WG, Kipps TJ, Mayer J, et al. Ofatumumab as single-agent CD20 immunotherapy in fludarabine-refractory chronic lymphocytic leukemia. J Clin Oncol. 2010;28:1749–55.
118. Wierda WG, Padmanabhan S, Chan GW, et al. Ofatumumab is active in patients with fludarabine-refractory CLL irrespective of prior rituximab: results from the phase 2 international study. Blood. 2011;118:5126–9.

119. Moreno C, Montillo M, Panayotidis P, et al. Ofatumumab in poor-prognosis chronic lymphocytic leukemia: a phase IV, non-interventional, observational study from the European Research Initiative on Chronic Lymphocytic Leukemia. Haematologica. 2015;100:511–6.
120. van Oers MH, Kuliczkowski K, Smolej L, et al. Ofatumumab maintenance versus observation in relapsed chronic lymphocytic leukaemia (PROLONG): an open-label, multicentre, randomised phase 3 study. Lancet Oncol. 2015;16:1370–9.
121. Hillmen P, Robak T, Janssens A, et al. Chlorambucil plus ofatumumab versus chlorambucil alone in previously untreated patients with chronic lymphocytic leukaemia (COMPLEMENT 1): a randomised, multicentre, open-label phase 3 trial. Lancet. 2015;385:1873–83.
122. Cortelezzi A, Sciumè M, Liberati AM, et al. Bendamustine in combination with ofatumumab in relapsed or refractory chronic lymphocytic leukemia: a GIMEMA multicenter phase II trial. Leukemia. 2014;28:642–8.
123. Offner F, Panagiotidis P, Afanasyev B, et al. Ofatumumab and bendamustine combination therapy in patients with untreated and relapsed chronic lymphocytic leukemia: initial results of the phase II study OMB115991. 2014. Available from: http://www.newevidence.com/oncology/ofatumumab-and-bendamustine-combination-therapy-in-patients-with-untreated-and-relapsed-chronic-lymphocytic-leukemia-initial-results-of-the-phase-ii-study-omb115991. Accessed 25 Apr 2016.
124. Ujjani C, Ramzi P, Gehan E, et al. Ofatumumab and bendamustine in previously treated chronic lymphocytic leukemia and small lymphocytic lymphoma. Leuk Lymphoma. 2015;56:915–20.
125. Wierda WG, Kipps TJ, Dürig J, et al. Chemoimmunotherapy with O-FC in previously untreated patients with chronic lymphocytic leukemia. Blood. 2011;117:6450–8.
126. Robak T, Grosicki S, Warzocha K, et al. Ofatumumab (O) in combination with fludarabine (F) and cyclophosphamide (C) (OFC) vs FC in patients with relapsed chronic lymphocytic leukemia (CLL): results of the phase III study COMPLEMENT 2. In: 20th Congress of European Hematology Association, LB219, 11–14 June 2015, Vienna, Austria.
127. Mössner E, Brünker P, Moser S, et al. Increasing the efficacy of CD20 antibody therapy through the engineering of a new type II anti-CD20 antibody with enhanced direct and immune effector cell mediated B-cell cytotoxicity. Blood. 2010;115:4393–402.
128. Dalle S, Reslan L, Besseyre de Horts T, et al. Preclinical studies on the mechanism of action and the anti-lymphoma activity of the novel anti-CD20 antibody GA101. Mol Cancer Ther. 2011;10:178–85.
129. Patz M, Isaeva P, Forcob N, et al. Comparison of the in vitro effects of the anti-CD20 antibodies rituximab and GA101 on chronic lymphocytic leukaemia cells. Br J Haematol. 2011;152:295–306.
130. Bologna L, Gotti E, Manganini M, et al. Mechanism of action of type II, glycoengineered, anti-CD20 monoclonal antibody GA101 in B-chronic lymphocytic leukemia whole blood assays in comparison with rituximab and alemtuzumab. J Immunol. 2011;186:3762–9.
131. Herter S, Herting F, Mundigl O, et al. Preclinical activity of the type II CD20 antibody GA101 (obinutuzumab) compared with rituximab and ofatumumab in vitro and in xenograft models. Mol Cancer Ther. 2013;12:2031–42.
132. Cartron G, de Guibert S, Dilhuydy MS, et al. Obinutuzumab (GA101) in relapsed/refractory chronic lymphocytic leukemia: final data from the phase 1/2 GAUGUIN study. Blood. 2014;124:2196–202.
133. Riechmann L, Clark M, Waldmann H, Winter G. Reshaping human antibodies for therapy. Nature. 1988;332:323–7.
134. Rossmann ED, Lundin J, Lenkei R, et al. Variability in B-cell antigen expression: implications for the treatment of B-cell lymphomas and leukemias with monoclonal antibodies. Hematol J. 2001;2:300–6.
135. Hale C, Bartholomew M, Taylor V, et al. Recognition of CD52 allelic gene products by CAMPATH-1H antibodies. Immunology. 1996;88:183–90.

136. Bindon CI, Hale G, Waldmann H. Importance of antigen specificity for complement-mediated lysis by monoclonal antibodies. Eur J Immunol. 1988;18:1507–14.
137. Xia MQ, Hale G, Waldmann H. Efficient complement-mediated lysis of cells containing the CAMPATH-1 (CDw52) antigen. Mol Immunol. 1993;30:1089–96.
138. Mone AP, Cheney C, Banks AL, et al. Alemtuzumab induces caspase-independent cell death in human chronic lymphocytic leukemia cells through a lipid raft-dependent mechanism. Leukemia. 2006;20:272–9.
139. Dyer MJS, Hale G, Marcus R, et al. Remission induction in patients with lymphoid malignancies using unconjugated CAMPATH-1 monoclonal antibodies. Leuk Lymphoma. 1990;2:179–93.
140. Osterborg A, Dyer MJ, Bunjes D, et al. Phase II multicenter study of human CD52 antibody in previously treated chronic lymphocytic leukemia. European Study Group of CAMPATH-1H Treatment in Chronic Lymphocytic Leukemia. J Clin Oncol. 1997;15:1567–74.
141. Rai KR, Freter CE, Mercier RJ, et al. Alemtuzumab in previously treated chronic lymphocytic leukemia patients who also had received fludarabine. J Clin Oncol. 2002;20:3891–7.
142. Ferrajoli A, O'Brien SM, Cortes JE, et al. Phase II study of alemtuzumab in chronic lymphoproliferative disorders. Cancer. 2003;98:773–8.
143. Keating MJ, Flinn I, Jain V, et al. Therapeutic role of alemtuzumab (Campath-1H) in patients who have failed fludarabine: results of a large international study. Blood. 2002;99:3554–61.
144. Pettitt AR, Jackson R, Carruthers S, et al. Alemtuzumab in combination with methylprednisolone is a highly effective induction regimen for patients with chronic lymphocytic leukemia and deletion of TP53: final results of the national cancer research institute CLL206 trial. J Clin Oncol. 2012;30:1647–55.
145. Stilgenbauer S, Cymbalista F, Leblond V, et al. Alemtuzumab combined with dexamethasone followed by alemtuzumab maintenance or allo-SCT in "ultra High-risk" CLL: final results from the CLL2O phase II study. Blood. 2014;124 suppl; abst.1991.
146. Lepretre S, Aurran T, Mahe B, et al. Excess mortality after treatment with fludarabine and cyclophosphamide in combination with alemtuzumab in previously untreated patients with chronic lymphocytic leukemia in a randomized phase 3 trial. Blood. 2012;119:5104–10.
147. Elter T, Gercheva-Kyuchukova L, Pylylpenko H, et al. Fludarabine plus alemtuzumab versus fludarabine alone in patients with previously treated chronic lymphocytic leukaemia: a randomised phase 3 trial. Lancet Oncol. 2011;12:1204–13.
148. O'Brien SM, Keating MJ, Mocarski ES. Updated guidelines on the management of cytomegalovirus reactivation in patients with chronic lymphocytic leukemia treated with alemtuzumab. Clin Lymphoma Myeloma. 2006;7:125–30.

Inotuzumab Ozogamicin for Acute Lymphoblastic Leukemia: Clinical Pharmacology and Therapeutic Results

7

Noriko Usui

Abstract

CD22 antigen is a B-cell lineage-restricted type I transmembrane protein, a member of Siglec family of cell surface receptors. Expression of CD22 is found in almost all the B cells and most B-lymphoid malignancies including non-Hodgkin lymphoma (NHL) and acute lymphoblastic leukemia (ALL).

Inotuzumab ozogamicin (INO) is one of the antibody-drug conjugates (ADCs) that consists of a cytotoxic drug, calicheamicin, attached to a humanized monoclonal anti-CD22 antibody. Based upon clinical trials, INO was shown to be effective for relapsed/refractory ALL as well as B-cell NHL. Single-agent treatment of INO (1.8 mg/m^2 once every 3–4 weeks or fractionated weekly, 0.8 mg/m^2 on day 1, and 0.5 mg/m2 on day 8 and 15 every 3–4 weeks) provided an objective response rate of 60% in the treatment of relapsed/refractory CD22-positive ALL patients. Combination of INO with rituximab and low-intensive conventional chemotherapy for patients with relapsed/refractory ALL showed better objective response. This review summarizes the clinical efficacy and safety of INO in the treatment of relapsed/refractory ALL, based on currently available data in the literature.

Keywords

Acute lymphoblastic leukemia • Inotuzumab ozogamicin • Relapsed/refractory • Allogeneic stem cell transplantation • Veno-occlusive disease

N. Usui (✉)
Division of Clinical Oncology and Hematology, Department of Internal Medicine, The Jikei University Daisan Hospital, 4-11-1 Izumi-Honcho, Komae, Tokyo 201-8601, Japan
e-mail: usuin@jikei.ac.jp

T. Ueda (ed.), *Chemotherapy for Leukemia*, DOI 10.1007/978-981-10-3332-2_7

7.1 Introduction

Inotuzumab ozogamicin (INO) is one of the antibody-drug conjugates (ADCs) developed for contribution to the treatment of B-cell lymphoid malignancies [1]. The antibody part is made of humanized monoclonal IgG4 antibody directed against the CD22 antigen present on B cells. And its conjugated drug is calicheamicin.

CD22 antigen is a B-cell lineage-restricted type I transmembrane protein, a member of Siglec family of cell surface receptors [2]. CD22 interacts with sialic acid-bearing molecules present on various blood cell types including lymphocytes (B and T cells), monocytes, and neutrophils [3]. CD22 is thought to regulate signal transduction of surface immunoglobulin (Ig) receptors on B cells, B-cell migration, and maintenance of peripheral B-cell tolerance [4]. CD22 is rapidly internalized by endocytosis with a half-life of less than 1 h upon ligand- or anti-CD22 monoclonal antibody (mAb) binding and is not shed in the extracellular environment [5–8].

Expression of CD22 is found in almost all the B cells and most B-lymphoid malignancies including non-Hodgkin lymphoma (NHL), chronic lymphocytic leukemia (CLL), acute lymphoblastic leukemia (ALL), and hairy cell leukemia (HCL) [9]. In ALL, up to 90–100% of mature B-ALL patients showed CD22 expression [4, 8], while 60–100% of patients with B-cell precursor ALL expressed CD22 [9].

Calicheamicin is a member of potent DNA-damaging cytotoxic products chemically modified by conversion to a more stable disulfide derivative of *N*-acetyl gamma-calicheamicin 1, 2-dimethyl hydrazine dichloride (NAc gamma-calicheamicin DMH) [10] that is many times potent in vitro than conventional anticancer drugs such as vincristine, mitomycin C, cisplatin, or doxorubicin [11]. Calicheamicin is used for conjugation to several monoclonal antibodies (mAbs) such as anti-CD33 mAb expressed on acute myeloid leukemia (AML), via linkers attached to the lysine residues of the mAbs [12, 13]. After internalization of antigen-antibody complex, ADC is routed through the endosomes and lysosomes in the cells, where calicheamicin is activated to attack DNA of the nucleus to kill the cells [2].

Anti-CD22 mAb without conjugated cytotoxic drug has shown to have no antitumor activity in preclinical models; however, conjugation with calicheamicin provided potent dose-depending cellular damage [1]. As several clinical studies of INO against relapse or refractory B-cell NHL indicated that this ADC is promising [14–17], INO is expected to be promising in the treatment for relapse or refractory B-cell ALL.

7.2 Clinical Pharmacology Based upon Studies for B-Cell NHL

7.2.1 Single-Agent Treatment of INO

First-in-human phase I study of single-agent INO was conducted as open-label in US and EU dose-escalation study of safety, tolerability, and pharmacokinetics (PK) against patients with CD22-positive B-cell NHL [14]. Doses ranged from 0.4 to 2.4 mg/m^2 administered once every 3 weeks to 36 patients in the maximum tolerated dose (MTD) lead-in cohort (as part 1). At 2.4 mg/m^2, criteria for escalation stop were met since two patients within this six-patient cohort had dose-limiting toxicities (DLTs) (one had grade 4 of thrombocytopenia, and another had grade 4 neutropenia). Therefore, 1.8 mg/m^2 was decided as the MTD. In addition, reversible thrombocytopenia is major toxicity of INO and became the cause of delay of treatment. Since no DLTs occurred in the six-patient cohort of 1.8 mg/m^2 once every 4 weeks, this dose and schedule (1.8 mg/m^2 q-4 weeks) was declared MTD and was selected for the part 2 of this study to evaluate its efficacy. Among the 49 patients in the part 2, there were 22 patients with follicular lymphoma (FL) and 26 patients with diffuse large B-cell lymphoma (DLBCL), and overall response was 41% including 68% in FL and 15% in DLBCL (Table 7.1).

Pharmacokinetic samples in this phase I study were available for INO, anti-CD22 antibody, and free and total calicheamicin derivatives. The data indicated that disposition was nonlinear with the number of dose or increasing dose. Nonlinearity is seen commonly with other antibodies as well [18]. It is due to target-mediated drug disposition, in which elimination and distribution are affected by the antibody and target cell interaction [19]. Mean end of infusion peak concentrations for 2.4 mg/m^2 once every 3 weeks and 1.8 mg/m^2 once every 3 weeks could not be distinguished from each other. For the INO and total calicheamicin, increases in area under the curve extrapolated over dosing interval (AUCT) with period and increases in AUCT with dose were observed. Anti-CD22 mAb and total calicheamicin exhibited similar trends of elimination but with a longer half-life than that of INO, suggesting that the acetyl butyrate linker is noticeably stable in plasma [14].

Phase I study of INO in Japan was conducted for patients with follicular lymphoma pretreated with rituximab-based therapy [15]. Based upon this study, safety and efficacy of INO 1.8 mg/m^2 q-4weeks for 13 Japanese patients were similar to phase I study in the USA/EU, but efficacy was better (Table 7.1).

Table 7.1 Inotuzumab ozogamicin against relapse or refractory non-Hodgkin lymphoma

Author	Year	IO	Dose	No. of patients	Response (%)
Advani A	2010	Single	1.8 mg/m^2	FL: 22	FL: 68
				DLBCL:26	DLBCL: 15
Ogura M	2010	Single	1.8 mg/m^2	FL: 10	FL: 80
Ogura M	2012	W RIT	1.8 mg/m^2	FL: 6	FL: 100
				MCL:2	MCL: 50
				MALT: 1	MALT: 100
				DLBCL:1	DLBCL: 0
Fayad L	2013	W RIT	1.8 mg/m^2	FL: 39	FL: 87
				DLBCL: 67	DLBCL: 74

FL follicular lymphoma, *DLBCL* diffuse large B-cell lymphoma, *MCL* mantle cell lymphoma, *MALT* mucosa-associated lymphoma, *W RIT* combination with rituximab

Table 7.2 Adverse events of inotuzumab ozogamicin monotherapy (1.8 mg/m² once every 4 weeks)

Events	EU/US pts (*N* = 49)		JPN pts (*N* = 10)	
	All grades (%)	Grade 3/4 (%)	All grades (%)	Grade 3/4 (%)
Thrombocytopenia	89.8	63.3	100	50
Asthenia	67.3	8.2	40	0
Nausea	51	2	70	0
Neutropenia	51	34.7	80	40
AST increased	40.8	0	80	0
Abdominal pain	30.6	0	N/A	N/A
Anorexia	30.6	2	80	0
ALP increased	26.5	4.1	60	0
Anemia	26.5	6.1	60	0
Leukopenia	26.5	18.4	90	20
Lymphopenia	N/A	N/A	80	40
Vomiting	26.5	4.1	N/A	N/A
Constipation	24.5	4.1	40	0
Hyperbilirubinemia	22.4	2	40	0
Headache	20.4	0	40	0
ALT increased	18.4	4.1	60	0
Epistaxis	18.4	0	40	0

EU/US pts European/US patients, *JPN pts* Japanese patients, *AST* aspartate aminotransferase, *ALP* alkaline phosphatase, *ALT* alanine aminotransferase, *N/A* not available

Adverse events of INO 1.8 mg/m² q-4 weeks for patients with relapsed/refractory B-cell NHL observed in phase I studies of both the EU/USA and Japan are listed in Table 7.2 [14, 15]. The most common adverse events were thrombocytopenia, neutropenia, asthenia, and increase of aspartate transaminase (AST)/alanine aminotransferase (ALT). Thrombocytopenia and neutropenia were the most common reason for dose modification.

7.2.2 Combination of INO with Rituximab

Based upon the phase I results and data demonstrating synergy between INO and rituximab in animal models [1, 20], phase I/II study was conducted to evaluate the safety and efficacy of the combination of rituximab and INO (R-INO) in patients with relapsed/refractory NHL [17].

R-INO was administered once every 4 weeks: rituximab on day 1 and INO on day 2 of each cycle. The study was performed in two parts: dose escalation (DE) to define the MTD (part 1) and an expanded cohort to further evaluate efficacy and safety of the MTD (part 2). Rituximab was administered at a fixed dose of 375 mg/m² on day 1, and INO was administered as DE from 0.8 to 1.3 to 1.8 mg/m² on day 2. For part 1, 15 patients received R-INO during DE, and no DLTs were observed at the 0.8 or 1.3 mg/m² dose levels, while only one of seven patients had a DLT (delayed dosing was the result of low neutrophils and platelets) at the highest planned INO dose (1.8 mg/m^2). MTD for the regimen was declared to be 375 mg/m^2 of rituximab on day 1 and 1.8 mg/m^2 of INO on day 2 once every 4 weeks.

For part 2, 104 patients were enrolled with 103 dosed in the expanded MTD cohort, and ORR was 87% and 74%, for patients with relapsed FL and relapsed/refractory DLBCL (Table 7.1).

The safety and efficacy of INO combined with rituximab were also investigated in the phase I study for Japanese patients with relapsed/refractory B-cell NHL [16]. A total of ten patients (FL 6, DLBCL 1, mantle cell lymphoma (MCL) 2, mucosa-associated lymphoid tissue lymphoma (MALT) 1) were treated by R-INO regimen that was 375 mg/m^2 of rituximab on day 1 and 1.8 mg/m^2 of INO on day 2 once every 4 weeks and repeated up to eight cycles, or until occurrence of disease progression or intolerable toxicity. Drug exposure increased with successive doses, similar to the pharmacokinetic profiles observed in the phase I study of INO monotherapy [15]. Although the number of patients is small, the efficacy of combination treatment indicates to be promising (Table 7.1).

7.3 Therapeutic Results of INO

7.3.1 Clinical Efficacy for B-Cell Acute Lymphoblastic Leukemia

7.3.1.1 Single-Agent Treatment

Single-Dose Schedule

The first phase II study of single-agent INO 1.3–1.8 mg/m^2 once every 3–4 weeks was conducted for 49 patients with relapsed/refractory ALL [21]. Patients received a median of two (range 1–5) INO courses. A total of 82% of the patients received more than two cycles, and 47% received more than three cycles of INO. In all patients, CD22 was expressed in more than 50% of blasts and for 28 patients (57%) with more than 90% of blasts.

The overall response rate (ORR) was 57% (28 of 49 patients) including nine patients (18%) who had complete remission (CR) and 19 patients (39%) who had CR with incomplete recovery of peripheral blood cells (CRi) (Table 7.3). The treatment was well tolerated, with only two patients (4%) dying within 4 weeks of start of therapy from nondrug-related complications.

Among the 28 patients obtaining CR, 18 had chromosomal abnormalities at the start of therapy, and 16 (89%; 43% of all patients) achieved a complete cytogenetic response (CCyR). Multiparameter flow cytometry for MRD was performed in 27 patients achieving CR, and reversal to MRD-negative status was observed in 17 patients (63% in CR). Most responses occurred early in the course of treatment, and among nine patients who achieved CR, eight of these did so after one cycle and one patient after two cycles.

The median overall survival (OS) time was 5.1 and 7.9 months in all patients and 28 responders, respectively [22, 23]. Twenty-two patients (45%) received allo-SCT

Table 7.3 Inotuzumab ozogamicin for patients with relapsed/refractory acute lymphoblastic leukemia

Patient characteristics	Single dose ($N = 49$)	Weekly dose ($N = 41$)
Prior therapy (regimen)		
One, two, three, or more (%)	27, 49, 24	39, 24, 37
Prior allo-SCT (%)	14	7
Karyotype		
Diploid t(9;22), t(4;11), others (%)	24, 14, 10, 51	22, 20, 7, 51
Response (%)	57	59
CR, CRp, CRi (%)	18, 29, 10	20, 30, 9
Early death (%)	4	5
MRD negativity in CR (%)	63	70
Allo-SCT as post-therapy (%)	45	34
Overall survival (median) (months)	5.1	7.3
Toxicity		
Hyperbilirubinemia (%)	29	5
Elevated transaminase (%)	57	27
Veno-occlusive disease (%)	10	2

Allo-SCT allogeneic stem cell transplantation, *CR* complete remission, *CRp* complete remission with incomplete platelet recovery, *CRi* complete remission with incomplete peripheral blood cell count recovery, *MRD* minimal residual disease

after treatment of INO, and five patients (23%) had clinical evidence for veno-occlusive disease (VOD). Drug-related fever and hypotension were commonly observed during the first 1–2 days of infusion. Fever was reported in 29 (59%) patients and was grade 3/4 in nine (31%) of these patients. Grade 1/2 hypotension was reported in 12 (24%) patients, and grade 3/4 hypotension was observed in only one (2%) patient. Another commonly seen adverse event was elevated liver transaminase (grade 1/2 elevations were observed in 27 of 49 (55%) patients, one grade 3/4) (Table 7.4).

Weekly Dose Schedule

Preclinical studies suggested that lower-dose more frequent schedules of INO might improve anti-ALL efficacy and reduce toxicities. This resulted in amending the study abovementioned [21] to change the dose schedule of INO to weekly, 0.8 mg/m^2 on day 1 and 0.5 mg/m^2 on day 8 and 15 every 3–4 weeks, for the same total dose of INO 1.8 mg/m^2 per course [22].

A total of 41 patients were enrolled. Overall, 24 (59%) patients responded to weekly dose INO; 8 (20%) patients had CR, 13 (32%) patients had CRp (3%), and 3 (7%) had CRi. These response rates are found to be similar to INO single-dose schedule which is given every 3–4 weeks (Table 7.3) [21]. Since receiving INO

Table 7.4 Non-hematologic adverse events during the first cycle of inotuzumab ozogamicin therapy for relapsed/refractory acute lymphoblastic leukemia

	Single dose ($N = 49$)		Weekly ($N = 41$)	
Events	Grade 1–2	Grade 3–4	Grade 1–2	Grade 3–4
Fever on day 1–2	20 (41%)	9 (18%)	3 (7%)	6 (15%)
Hypotension	12 (24%)	1 (2%)	6 (15%)	0
Hyperbilirubinemia	12 (24%)	2 (4%)	2 (5%)	0
Increase transaminase	27 (55%)	1 (2%)	9 (22%)	2 (5%)
Increase amylase	0	1 (2%)	1 (2%)	0
Nausea	6 (12%)	0	5 (12%)	0
Vomiting	3 (6%)	0	0	0
Diarrhea	3 (6%)	0	1 (2%)	0
Mucositis	0	1 (2%)	0	0
Anorexia	1 (2%)	0	0	0
Headache	1 (2%)	0	1 (2%)	0
Constipation	1 (2%)	0	0	0
Hypokalemia	0	1 (2%)	0	1 (2%)
Hypoalbuminemia	1 (2%)	0	0	0

earlier led to better outcomes, median OS for patients who received INO as salvage 1, 2, or 3 were 9.2, 4.3, and 6.6 months, respectively ($p = 0.002$). MRD-negative was achieved in 17 of 24 (70%) patients who had responded to INO. A total of 14 (34%) patients were able to undergo allo-SCT, and nine of 14 (65%) were reported to be alive [23].

Fever and hypotension were less common with weekly INO. Drug-related fever within 1–2 days of infusion was seen in nine of 41 (21%) patients treated with weekly dose compared with 29 of 49 (59%) patients with the single-dose INO. Liver toxicity was also less common with weekly dose INO. Only 11 of 41 (27%) patients had elevated liver transaminases (elevation of AST/ALT) with weekly INO compared with 28 of 49 (57%) with single-dose INO. VOD was observed in only one (2%) patient among those who underwent allo-SCT (Table 7.4).

The preliminary report of another phase II study for weekly dose schedule of INO (total dose of 1.8 mg/m^2 per course) in patients with relapsed/refractory ALL indicated similar results [24]. A total of 35 patients enrolled in this study, and ORR (CR, CRi, CRp) was 66%, and 78% (18 of 23) of patients with response achieved MRD-negative status. Overall, the median time to attain remission and MRD negativity was 25 days. A total of 34% (12 of 35) of patients were able to undergo allo-SCT, and six of them were reported to be alive. INO was discontinued in five patients due to adverse events, and the elevated AST/ALT was the most common reason (grade 3/4 in two patients, 6%). The incidence of grade 3 or more transaminitis with weekly INO appears to be comparable with single-dose INO schedule (2%) [22]. However, grade 1/2 transaminitis is much less common with weekly dose schedule. Other relevant INO-related grade 3/4 adverse events were observed

Table 7.5 Factors related to response of inotuzumab ozogamicin for relapsed/refractory acute lymphoblastic leukemia

Characteristic	Category	No.	No of response (%)	*P* value
Age (years)	<60	65	37 (57)	0.79
	≧60	25	15 (65)	
PS (ECOG)	0–1	81	48 (59)	0.39
	≧2	9	4 (44)	
Salvage regimen	S1	29	22 (76)	
Prior therapy	S1, CRD1 <12M	15	11 (73)	
	S1, CRD1≧12M	9	7 (78)	0.056
	S2	34	17 (50)	
	≧S3	27	13 (48)	
Karyotype	Diploid	21	17 (81)	
	Ph positive/t(9;22)	15	6 (40)	
	t (4;11)	8	3 (38)	0.047
	Other	46	26 (57)	
% CD22 positive	>90	59	33 (56)	
	70–89	22	13 (59)	0.823
	50–69	9	6 (67)	
Prior allo-SCT	Yes	10	5 (50)	

S1 1 salvage regimen, *CRD1* first complete remission duration, *12M* 12 months, *S2* two salvage regimens, *S3* three salvage regimens, *Ph* Philadelphia, *allo-SCT* allogeneic stem cell transplantation

including thrombocytopenia (31%), neutropenia (26%), and neutropenic fever (20%).

Factors Related to Response in Single-Agent Treatment of INO
In the total study groups combining single-dose schedule and weekly dose schedule, lower response rates were observed among patients with Philadelphia chromosome (*BCR-ABL1*)-positive ALL and those with translocation (4, 11) (38–40% versus 57–81% for others; *p* value 0.047). Response rate was also lower in patients treated in salvage 2 or later (48–50% versus 76% in salvage 1; $p = 0.056$) (Table 7.5). In addition, baseline or pretreatment high peripheral blood absolute blast count [PBABC ($\geqq 1.0 \times 10^9$/L)] and thrombocytopenia ($<100 \times 10^9$/L) were also associated with lower probability of marrow CR achievement by univariate analysis [25].

By univariate and multivariate analysis, patients with complex karyotype including t(4;11), t(9;22), or chromosome 17 abnormality, number of previous therapies (regimens), baseline thrombocytopenia, and high PBABC were associated with worse survival.

7.3.1.2 Combination of INO with Conventional Chemotherapy (Table 7.6)

The preliminary results of clinical trials of combining INO with chemotherapy have been reported in December 2015 [26, 27]. A total of 48 patients with relapsed/

Table 7.6 Response of inotuzumab ozogamicin combining with mini-hyper-CVD for acute lymphoblastic leukemia

	Relapse/refractory ALL	Newly ALL(elderly)
	(*N* = 48) *N* (%)	(*N* = 34) *N* (%)
Age median (range)	35 (9–87)	69 (60–79)
CR	24 (52)	25/31[a] (81)
CRp	8 (17)	5/31[a] (31)
CRi	2 (4)	
Cytogenetic CR		19/19 (100)
Negative MRD on D21		20/25 (80)
Negative MRD overall		33/33 (100)
ORR	37 (74)	30/31[a] (97)
No response	5 (11)	1/31[a] (3)
Early death	7 (15)	0
Too early for evaluation	2 (4)	

CR complete remission, *CRp* complete remission with incomplete platelet recovery, *CRi* complete remission with incomplete peripheral blood cell count recovery, *MRD* minimal residual disease, *D21* day 21

[a]Since 3 among 34 patients started therapy in CR, 31 patients were evaluated for response

refractory B-cell ALL have been enrolled and received lower intensity chemotherapy, which was referred to as mini-hyper-CVD (cyclophosphamide and dexamethasone at 50% dose reduction, no anthracycline, methotrexate at 75% dose reduction, cytarabine at 0.5 $g/m^2 \times 4$ doses). Rituximab and intrathecal chemotherapy were given for the first four courses. INO was given on day 3 of each of the first four courses. Patients received INO at 1.8 mg/m^2 for cycle 1 followed by 1.3 mg/m^2 for subsequent cycles. Early death was encountered in seven (15%) patients. The ORR was 74% (24 (52%) CR, 8 (17%) CRp, 2 (4%) marrow CR). Nineteen (41%) patients proceeded to receive allo-SCT. The 1-year PFS and OS rates were 60% and 46%, respectively. Median survival for patients with CR/CRp/marrow CR(CRi) was 18 versus 1 month in patients with refractory disease ($p < 0.001$). As it was observed in monotherapy of INO, median survival was 17 months in patients treated as the first salvage therapy (ST), 6 months in patients treated as the second ST, and 7 months in patients treated as the third or more ST. Grade 3/4 non-hematological toxicities included infections, mucositis, hypertransaminasemia, and VOD (n = 6; 1 in a patient who had prior allo-SCT, 1 at D35 of CAR T cell, and 3 post-allo-SCT following INO therapy). INO with mini-hyper-CVD chemotherapy is considered to be effective for patients with relapsed/refractory ALL.

INO and mini-hyper-CVD combination has also been tested in the frontline setting in elderly B-ALL patients (≧60 years of age) [27]. Rituximab and intrathecal chemotherapy were given for the first four courses. INO was given on day 3 of each of the first four courses. The first six patients received 1.3 mg/m^2 for cycle 1 followed by 0.8 mg/m^2 for subsequent cycles, and patients seven onward received 1.8 mg/m^2 for cycle 1 followed by 1.3 mg/m^2 for subsequent cycles. A total of 34 patients with a median age of 69 years old (range 60–79) were treated, and median follow-up was 19 months. Of the 31 patients evaluable for response (three started in CR), 30 (97%) achieved CR/CRp (25 CR, 5 CRp). All patients achieving CR have also achieved flow cytometry MRD-negative status, in 80% at the time of CR achievement. Median time to platelet and neutrophil recovery was 23 days (18–91) and 16 days (12–49) after induction and was 22 days (14–64) and 17 days (13–49) after subsequent cycles. Grade 3/4 toxicities ≥10% included prolonged thrombocytopenia (n = 27; 79%), infections during consolidation (n = 25; 73%) or during induction (n = 18; 52%), hyperglycemia (n = 17; 50%), hypokalemia (n = 12; 35%), hyperbilirubinemia (n = 8; 24%), increased ALT/AST (n = 7, 21%), and hemorrhage (n = 6; 18%). VOD was observed in four patients (11%). Two patients (6%) received allogeneic stem cell transplantation. The 2-year progression-free survival (PFS) and OS rates were 87% and 70%, respectively. Since these results appear to be better than those achieved with a conventional chemotherapy-only approach, the authors indicated that INO plus mini-hyper-CVD may become the new standard of care for frontline treatment of older patients with ALL.

7.3.1.3 Role of Allogeneic Stem Cell Transplant After INO Treatment

Currently, allo-SCT is the most effective therapeutic approach for durable disease control in relapsed/refractory ALL patients [28]. In several clinical trials, single-agent treatment INO allowed large number (20–45%) of refractory B-ALL patients to proceed with allo-SCT.

The outcomes of heavily pretreated 26 patients (median age of 33 years ranged 5–70 years) who received allo-SCT after single-dose or weekly INO have been reported [29]. INO was administered intravenously at the first three adults, and three children received a dose of 1.3 mg/m^2. A total of 23 patients who achieved at least marrow CR underwent allo-SCT directly, whereas three patients who did not respond to INO received chemotherapy before starting the allo-SCT conditioning regimen. The majority of the patients received a matched related or unrelated donor transplant with myeloablative conditioning regimens (85%). A total of 15 (58%) patients had no MRD at the time of allo-SCT. Median follow-up duration was 13 months, and OS survival at 1 year was reported as 20%. Patients without MRD at the time of SCT had a markedly better 1-year OS of 42%. The cumulative incidence of non-relapse mortality (NRM) at 6 months and 1 year was 40% and 60%, respectively, with five deaths attributed to VOD at a median of 23 days posttransplant.

Observed regimen-related toxicities appear within an expected range of transplant-related complications (Table 7.7) [29]. However, there were marked hepatic toxicity, hypertransaminasemia, hyperbilirubinemia, and VOD. As it was mentioned above, five patients had fatal VOD that occurred in a median of two courses of INO (range 1–5 courses) administered at a median of 40 days (range 27–68 days) before the start of the conditioning regimen for allo-SCT, including two patients who had received previous allo-SCT. Diffuse alveolar hemorrhage (DAH) developed in four patients including one patient who also had VOD.

Allo-SCT as post-remission therapy after re-induction with INO for relapsed/refractory ALL is seemed promising when the patients can attain CR and continue

Table 7.7 Regimen-related toxicities in patients with relapsed/refractory ALL who received allogeneic stem cell transplantation after treatment with inotuzumab ozogamicin (*N* = 26)

	Grade, *N* (%)	
Toxicity	All grades	Grade 3/4
Liver		
Transaminases	24 (92%)	7 (27%)
Hyperbilirubinemia	17 (65%)	10 (38%)
Veno-occlusive disease		5 (19%)
Gastrointestinal tract		
Diarrhea	12 (47%)	2 (8%)
Mucositis	24 (92%)	5 (19%)
Nausea/vomiting	21 (82%)	1 (4%)
Urinary tract/kidney		
Creatinine rise	15 (58%)	9 (35%)
Hemorrhage cystitis	6 (23%)	4 (15%)
Lung		
Diffuse alveolar hemorrhage		4 (15%)

MRD negativity just before starting conditioning therapy for allo-SCT. However, appropriate management of VOD is required to obtain better outcome by allo-SCT.

7.3.1.4 Toxicity of INO in the Treatment for ALL

INO is based on an antibody conjugation platform that is similar to gemtuzumab ozogamicin (GO), a humanized anti-CD33 mAb conjugated to calicheamicin for the treatment of CD33-positive acute myeloid leukemia [14, 30]. INO and GO have the same cytotoxic component, calicheamicin; however, the toxicity profile is different since the antigen targets, dosing regimens, and pharmacokinetics are different [31]. Major toxicities of GO have been associated with thrombocytopenia, increase of liver enzymes, and VOD, especially among patients who received allo-SCT [30]. Thrombocytopenia was also a notable in the treatment of INO for patients with ALL; because of the nature of the disease in these patients, treatment with INO was usually continued. Transient abnormalities in liver function were also often found, but VOD development was rare (0.03%) in INO as a single-agent treatment [21] (Table 7.4). Five of 26 patients (19%) who underwent allo-SCT developed VOD (Table 7.7), but the cause of VOD might not be only INO. INO does attack CD22 antigen but not CD33 antigen (target of GO) expressed in liver sinusoids [32], and it has been hypothesized to sensitize the liver to VOD associated with allo-SCT. Historically, regimens containing total body irradiation (TBI) plus thiotepa combined with other alkylating agents have been associated with high VOD rates [33]. Therefore, VOD post-remission with INO might be a result from synergistic toxic effects with conditioning regimen of allo-SCT.

7.3.2 Future Prospective of INO in the Treatment of ALL

In phase I/II studies, single-agent treatment of INO for patients with relapsed/refractory ALL has been shown to provide approximately 60% of the patients. In spite of quite high response rates and MRD negativity, response duration was not long and OS was limited. Therefore, about 30–40% of patients are required to undergo allo-SCT as post-remission therapy. In order to reduce risk of VOD or severe drug-related toxicity, appropriate adjustment of conditioning regimens will be required.

Currently, an international randomized phase III clinical trial comparing single-agent INO with investigator choice of chemotherapy (FLAG (fludarabine, cytarabine, and G-CSF), HIDAC (high-dose cytarabine), or cytarabine and mitoxantrone) in patients with relapsed/refractory ALL is ongoing, and Japanese patients have been enrolled. Results of this phase III study will provide true efficacy of INO including optimal dose and schedule.

Combination of INO with rituximab and low-intensive conventional chemotherapy for patients with relapsed/refractory ALL provided better outcomes than single-agent INO. Although appropriate management of VOD in post-remission therapy is required, the use of INO in combination therapy will be one of the best salvage induction therapies and will be a frontline therapy for elderly patients with ALL.

Future studies will be planned to investigate the role of INO not only as single agent but also as combination to cure rates in newly diagnosed patients with adult ALL.

Conflict of Interest Disclosure Dr. Usui has received research grants and honoraria from CIMIC, Takeda, Eli Lilly Japan, Pfizer, Nippon Boehringer-Ingelheim, Sysmex, Janssen Pharmaceutical, Zenyaku Kogyo, Kyowa Hakko Kirin, Astellas Pharma, Otsuka Pharmaceutical, Celgene, SymBio Pharmaceuticals, Huya Bioscience International, Chugai Pharmaceutical, Bristol-Myers Squibb, and Solasia Pharma.

References

1. Dijoseph J, Armellino D, Boghaert E, Khandke K, Dougher M, Sridharan L, et al. Antibody-targeted chemotherapy with CMC-544: a CD22-targeted immunoconjugate of calicheamicin for the treatment of B-lymphoid malignancies. Blood. 2004;103:1807–14.
2. Shor B, Gerber H-P, Sapra P. Preclinical and clinical development of inotuzumab-ozogamicin in hematological malignancies. Mol Immunol. 2015;67(2 Pt A):107–16.
3. Nitschke L. CD22 and Siglec-G: B-cell inhibitory receptors with distinct functions. Immunol Rev. 2009;230:128–43.
4. Piccaluga PP, Arpinati M, Candoni A, Laterza C, Paolini S, Gazzola A, et al. Surface antigens analysis reveals significant expression of candidate targets for immunotherapy in adult acute lymphoid leukemia. Leuk Lymphoma. 2011;52:325–7.
5. de Vries JF, Zwaan CM, De Bie M, Voerman JS, den Boer ML, van Dongen JJ, et al. The novel calicheamicin-conjugated CD22 antibody inotuzumab ozogamicin (CMC-544) effectively kills primary pediatric acute lymphoblastic leukemia cells. Leukemia. 2012;26:255–64.

6. Gerber HP, Koehn FE, Abraham RT. The antibody-drug conjugate: an enabling modality for natural product-based cancer therapeutics. Nat Prod Rep. 2013;30:625–39.
7. John B, Herrin BR, Raman C, Wang YN, Bobbitt KR, Brody BA, et al. The B cell coreceptor CD22 associates with AP50, a clathrin-coated pit adapter protein, via tyrosine-dependent interaction. J Immunol. 2003;170:3534–43.
8. Raponi S, De Propris MS, Intoppa S, Milani ML, Vitale A, Elia L, et al. Flow cytometric study of potential target antigens (CD19, CD20, CD22, CD33) for antibody-based immunotherapy in acute lymphoblastic leukemia: analysis of 552 cases. Leuk Lymphoma. 2011;52:1098–107.
9. Olejniczak SH, Stewart CC, Donohue K, Czuczman MS. A quantitative exploration of surface antigen expression in common B-cell malignancies using flow cytometry. Immunol Investig. 2006;35:93–114.
10. Lee MD, Manning JK, Williams DR, Kuck NA, Testa RT, Borders DB. Calicheamicins, a novel family of antitumor antibiotics, 3. Isolation, purification and characterization of calicheamicins beta 1Br, gamma 1Br, alpha 2I, alpha 3I, beta 1I, gamma 1I and delta 1I. J Antibiot. 1989;42:1070–87.
11. DiJoseph JF, Dougher MM, Evans DY, Zhou BB, Damle NK. Preclinical anti-tumor activity of antibody-targeted chemotherapy with CMC-544 (inotuzumab ozogamicin), a CD22-specific immunoconjugate of calicheamicin, compared with non-targeted combination chemotherapy with CVP or CHOP. Cancer Chemother Pharmacol. 2011;67:741–9.
12. Hamann PR, Hinman LM, Hollander I, Beyer CF, Lindh D, Holcomb R, et al. Gemtuzumab ozogamicin, a potent and selective anti-CD33 antibody-calicheamicin conjugate for treatment of acute myeloid leukemia. Bioconjug Chem. 2002;13:47–58.
13. Hamann PR, Hinman LM, Beyer CF, Lindh D, Upeslacis J, Flowers DA, Bernstein I. An anti-CD33 antibody-calicheamicin conjugate for treatment of acute myeloid leukemia. Choice Linker Bioconjug Chem. 2002;13:40–6.
14. Advani A, Coiffier B, Czuczman M, Dreyling M, Foran J, Gine E, et al. Safety, pharmacokinetics, and preliminary clinical activity of inotuzumab ozogamicin, a novel immunoconjugate for the treatment of B-cell non-Hodgkin's lymphoma: results of a phase I study. J Clin Oncol. 2010;28:2085–93.
15. Ogura M, Tobinai K, Hatake K, Uchida T, Kasai M, Oyama T, et al. Phase I study of inotuzumab ozogamicin (CMC-544) in Japanese patients with follicular lymphoma pretreated with rituximab-based therapy. Cancer Sci. 2010;101:1840–5.
16. Ogura M, Hatake K, Ando K, Tobinai K, Tokushige K, Ono C, et al. Phase I study of anti-CD22 immunoconjugate inotuzumab ozogamicin plus rituximab in relapsed/refractory B-cell non-Hodgkin lymphoma. Cancer Sci. 2012;103:933–8.
17. Fayad L, Offner F, Smith MR, Verhoef G, Johnson P, Kaufman JL, et al. Safety and clinical activity of a combination therapy comprising two antibody-based targeting agents for the treatment of non-Hodgkin lymphoma: results of a phase I/II study evaluating the immunoconjugate inotuzumab ozogamicin with rituximab. J Clin Oncol. 2013;31:573–83.
18. Lobo E, Hansen R, Balthasar J. Antibody pharmacokinetics and pharmacodynamics. J Pharm Sci. 2004;93:2645–68.
19. Cao Y, Jusko W. Incorporating target-mediated drug disposition in a minimal physiologically-based pharmacokinetic model for monoclonal antibodies. J Pharmacokinet Pharmacodyn. 2014;41:375–87.
20. DiJoseph JF, Dougher MM, Kalyandrug LB, Armellino DC, Boghaert ER, Hamann PR, et al. Antitumor efficacy of a combination of CMC-544 (inotuzumab ozogamicin), a CD22-targeted cytotoxic immunoconjugate of calicheamicin, and rituximab against non-Hodgkin's B-cell lymphoma. Clin Cancer Res. 2006;12:242–9.
21. Kantarjian H, Thomas D, Jorgensen J, Jabbour E, Kebriaei P, Rytting M, et al. Inotuzumab ozogamicin, an anti-CD22-calecheamicin conjugate, for refractory and relapsed acute lymphocytic leukaemia: a phase 2 study. Lancet Oncol. 2012;13:403–11.

22. Kantarjian H, Thomas D, Jorgensen J, Kebriaei P, Jabbour E, Rytting M, et al. Results of inotuzumab ozogamicin, a CD22 monoclonal antibody, in refractory and relapsed acute lymphocytic leukemia. Cancer. 2013;119:2728–36.
23. Yilmaz M, Richard S, Jabbour E. The clinical potential of inotuzumab ozogamicin in relapsed and refractory acute lymphocytic leukemia. Ther Adv Hematol. 2015;6:253–61.
24. Advani A., Stein A., Kantarjian H. A phase II study of weekly inotuzumab ozogamicin (INO) in adult patients with CD22-positive acute lymphoblastic leukemia (ALL) in second or later salvage. In: 56th ASH annual meeting and exposition, 6–9 December, San Francisco, 2014; Abstract 2255.
25. Jabbour E, O'Brien S, Huang X, Thomas D, Rytting M, Sasaki K, et al. Prognostic factors for outcome in patients with refractory and relapsed acute lymphocytic leukemia treated with inotuzumab ozogamicin, a CD22 monoclonal antibody. Am J Hematol. 2015;90:193–6.
26. Sasaki K, Kantarjian HM, O'Brien S, Thomas DA, Ravandi F, Guillermo Garcia-Manero G, et al. Salvage chemotherapy with inotuzumab ozogamicin (INO) combined with mini-Hyper-CVD for adult patients with relapsed/refractory (R/R) acute lymphoblastic leukemia (ALL). Blood. 2015;126:3721.
27. Jabbour E, O'Brien S, Sasaki K, DeThomas DA, Garcia-Manero G, Ravandi F, et al. Frontline inotuzumab ozogamicin in combination with low-intensity chemotherapy (mini-hyper-CVD) for older patients with acute lymphoblastic leukemia (ALL). Blood. 2015;126:83.
28. Fielding AK, Richards SM, Chopra R, Lazarus HM, Litzow MR, Buck G, et al. Outcome of 609 adults after relapse of acute lymphoblastic leukemia (ALL); an MRC UKALL12/ECOG 2993 study. Blood. 2007;109:944–50.
29. Kebriaei P, Wilhelm K, Ravandi F, Brandt M, De Lima M, Ciurea S, et al. Feasibility of allografting in patients with advanced acute lymphoblastic leukemia after salvage therapy with inotuzumab ozogamicin. Clin Lymphoma Myeloma Leuk. 2013;13:296–301.
30. Larson R, Sievers E, Stadtmauer E, Lowenberg B, Estey E, Dombret H, et al. Final report of the efficacy and safety of gemtuzumab ozogamicin (mylotarg) in patients with CD33-positive acute myeloid leukemia in first recurrence. Cancer. 2005;104:1442–52.
31. Dowell J, Korth-Bradley J, Liu H, King SP, Berger MS. Pharmacokinetics of gemtuzumab ozogamicin, an antibody-targeted chemotherapy agent for the treatment of patients with acute myeloid leukemia in first relapse. J Clin Pharmacol. 2001;41:1206–14.
32. Rajvanshi P, Shulman HM, Sievers EL, McDonald GB. Hepatic sinusoidal obstruction after gemtuzumab ozogamicin (Mylotarg) therapy. Blood. 2002;99:2310–4.
33. Lee J, Gooley T, Bensinger W, Schiffman K, Mcdonald G. Veno-occlusive disease of the liver after busulfan, melphalan, and thiotepa conditioning therapy: incidence, risk factors, and outcome. Biol Blood Marrow Transplant. 1999;5:306–15.

Blinatumomab for Acute Lymphoblastic Leukemia: Clinical Pharmacology and Therapeutic Results

8

Satoru Takada

Abstract

Blinatumomab, a bispecific CD19/CD3 T-cell engager (BiTE), is a genetically engineered single-stranded bispecific monoclonal antibody. It consists of mouse monoclonal variant chains that bind to CD19 at the N-terminus and to CD3 at the C-terminus. Since many cases of B-lineage acute lymphoblastic leukemia (B-ALL) express CD19 on the leukemic cells, blinatumomab can associate B-ALL leukemic cells with T cells and form immune synapses between them, which result in T-cell activation and proliferation. Thereafter, the leukemic cells are killed by perforin-mediated cell lysis.

Blinatumomab can induce complete remission (CR) in 40–60% of cases of relapsed/refractory B-cell precursor (B-precursor) ALL, and 40–60% of CR patients become minimal residual disease (MRD) negative. Blinatumomab is effective for patients who have recurred after chemotherapy and after allogeneic hematopoietic stem cell transplantation (allo-HSCT). The characteristic adverse effects of this drug are central nervous system disorders (tremor, dizziness, confusion, encephalopathy, ataxia, aphasia) and cytokine releasing syndromes (flu-like symptoms, hypotension pulmonary edema, multi-organ failure). The efficacy of blinatumomab for de novo B-precursor ALL patients and in combination therapies with other anticancer drugs has not been investigated.

Keywords

Blinatumomab • CD19/CD3 bispecific T-cell engager • B-precursor ALL

S. Takada (✉)
Leukemia Research Center, Saiseikai Maebashi Hospital,
564-1 Kamishindenmachi, Maebashi, Gunma 371-0821, Japan
e-mail: s-takada@maebashi.saiseikai.or.jp

T. Ueda (ed.), *Chemotherapy for Leukemia*, DOI 10.1007/978-981-10-3332-2_8

8.1 Introduction

Acute lymphoblastic leukemia (ALL) is classified as B-cell precursor acute lymphoblastic leukemia (B-precursor ALL), T-cell precursor acute lymphoblastic leukemia (T-precursor ALL), or Burkitt's leukemia according to its cell origin. Furthermore, B-precursor ALL is subclassified in some types of leukemia by its genetic abnormality, one of which is Philadelphia chromosome-positive acute lymphoblastic leukemia (Ph-ALL) [1]. In adult ALL, more than 80% of patients achieve complete remission (CR) [2, 3]. Unfortunately, many of these patients will relapse, and the results of treatment for relapsed patients are dismal even if they receive allogeneic hematopoietic stem cell transplantation (allo-HSCT) [4]. Molecular targeted therapies for ALL are currently being developed, and some such drugs are already in use in clinical practice. They are roughly categorized into two types of drugs. One category is that of an inhibitor of an intracellular signaling pathway that is important for the survival and/or proliferation of leukemic cells. For example, Abl tyrosine kinase inhibitors, such as imatinib, nilotinib, and dasatinib, have dramatically improved the treatment of Ph-ALL [5]. Another type of molecular targeted drug is a monoclonal antibody that binds to a protein on the leukemic cell surface and induces antigen-dependent cellular cytotoxicity (ADCC) and complement-dependent cytotoxicity (CDC). For example, the anti-CD20 monoclonal antibody, rituximab, has improved the treatment of Burkitt's leukemia [6]. Recent innovations in antibody engineering have improved traditional monoclonal antibody killing of target cells, making their killing more potent and more efficient by conjugating toxins [7]. A more sophisticated approach of antibody engineering is the induction of highly effective cell lysis by T cells. One such approach involves the ectopic expression of a chimeric antigen receptor (CAR) construct in transfected autologous T cells of patients. The efficacy of a CD19 CAR T cell has already been reported [8]. Another approach is the generation of a bispecific antibody that transiently engages the T cell with target cells. In this chapter, we review the pharmacological profiles, the mechanism of its antileukemic effect, and the clinical results of the bispecific CD19/CD3 antibody, blinatumomab.

8.2 Structure and Chemical Characteristics of Blinatumomab

Blinatumomab is an artificial bispecific mouse monoclonal antibody that has an anti-CD19 single-chain Fv (scFv) fragment at the N-terminus and an anti-CD3 scFv fragment at the C-terminus (Fig. 8.1). The DNA fragment encoding the bispecific single-chain antibody CD19 × CD3 domain arrangement of anti-CD19 V light-chain (VL)-anti-CD19 V heavy-chain (VH)-anti-CD3VH-anti-CD3VL is transfected into DHFR-deficient Chinese hamster ovary cells. These cells produce an anti-CD19 scFv fragment at the N-terminus and an anti-CD3 scFv fragment at the C-terminus [9]. These fragments are connected by a non-glycosylated, five-amino-acid, non-immunogenic linker. This linker is so flexible that it enables blinatumomab to

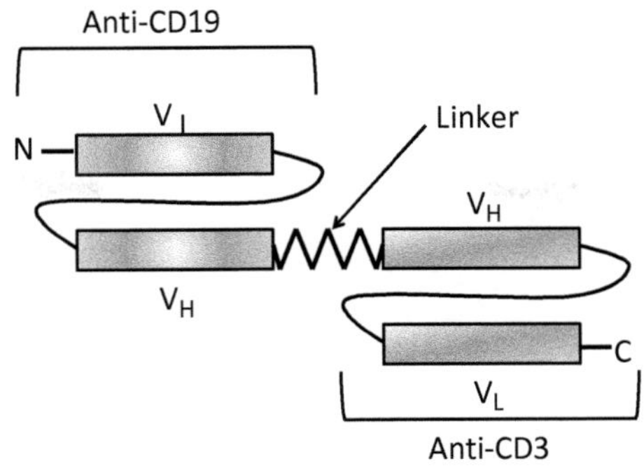

Fig. 8.1 Blinatumomab has anti-CD19 single-chain Fv (scFv) fragment at N-terminal and anti-CD3 scFv fragment at C-terminal. Each scFv is composed of V light chain and V heavy chain. Each scFv is connected by a flexible linker, which enables blinatumomab to bind a leukemic cell and a T cell

effectively bind both a leukemic cell and a T cell. Blinatumomab does not have a constant region. The molecular weight of blinatumomab is 54.1 kD, which is one third that of traditional monoclonal antibodies [10]. Blinatumomab binds more strongly to CD19 than to CD3, and the dissociation constants for CD19 and CD3 are 1.49×10^{-9} and 2.67×10^{-7} mol/L, respectively [11].

8.3 Mechanisms of Cytotoxicity of Blinatumomab

More than 95% of B-precursor ALL cells express CD19 on the leukemic cell surface [12]. Blinatumomab binds to both CD19 on the leukemic cell and to CD3 on T cells, thereby engaging T cells with CD19+ target leukemic cells and inducing cell toxicity. Blinatumomab can bind and activate both CD3 + CD4+ T cells and CD3 + CD8+ T cells. Because the activity of blinatumomab does not depend on the specificity of the T-cell receptor and does not require antigen presentation by major histocompatibility complex, leukemic cells are killed by polyclonal T cells [13]. Blinatumomab has two major effects on the T cell that is connected with the CD19+ leukemic cell through blinatumomab. The first effect is direct activation of the connected T cell, resulting in upregulation of the T-cell activation markers CD25, CD69, CD2, interferon (IFN)-γ, tumor necrosis factor (TNT)-α, interleukin (IL)-2, IL-6, and IL-10. The activated T cell then induces perforin-mediated cytotoxicity via granzyme entry into the CD19-positive leukemic cell. This leads to caspase activation and apoptosis of the CD19-positive leukemic cell. This effect is stronger in CD8-positive T cells than in CD4-positive T cells. The second effect is marked T-cell proliferation, leading to a supply of blinatumomab-activated T cells and serial killing of the CD19-positive target leukemic cells [14] (Fig. 8.2). This proliferation and serial killing of leukemic cells may be the reason why blinatumomab is effective for fully relapsed B-precursor ALL patients, who have so many target CD19-positive leukemic cells compared to the number of T cells. T-cell killing of CD19-positive leukemic cells

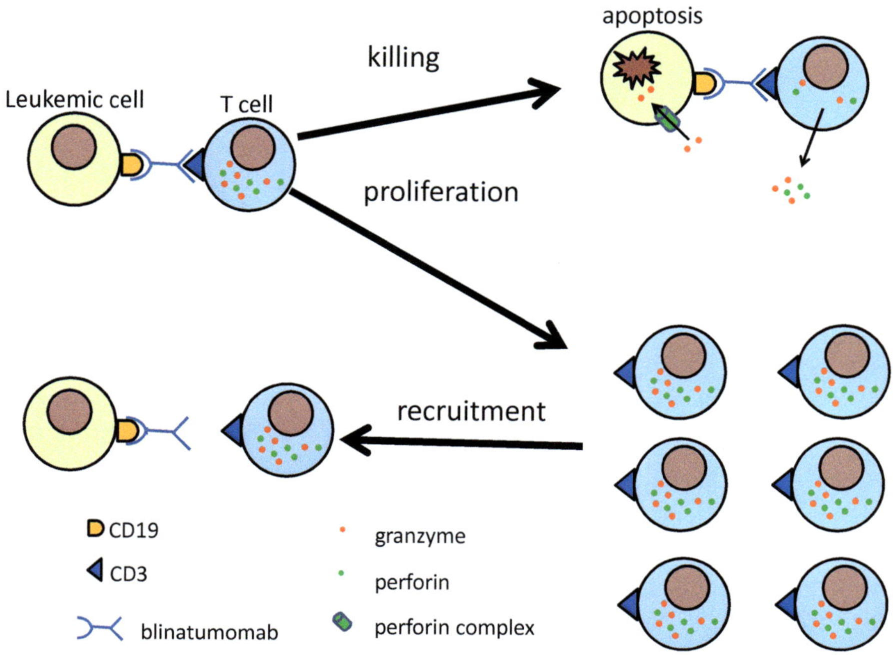

Fig. 8.2 Blinatumomab has two major effects to T cell, which is connected with CD19+ leukemic cell by blinatumomab. First effect is direct T-cell activation which results in killing of CD19+ leukemic cell with perforin-mediated cell cytotoxicity via granzyme entry. Second effect is T-cell proliferation. The proliferated T cells are recruited for serial killing of the CD19-positive target leukemic cell. Blinatumomab can bind to and activate both CD3 + CD4+ T cells and CD3 + CD8+ T cells. The activity of blinatumomab does not depend on the specificity of the T-cell receptor and not require antigen presentation by major histocompatibility complex

and activated T-cell proliferation continue for as long as the T cell can make an immune synapse with a CD19-positive leukemic cell via blinatumomab, and they expire following elimination of the CD19-positive leukemic cell. By redirecting unstimulated human T cells to CD19-positive target cells, blinatumomab shows significant cytotoxicity at concentrations of 10–100 pg/ml [9]. This concentration is about 100 times lower than that of rituximab, which shows cytotoxicity at a concentration of 2 μg/ml [15]. In the presence of blinatumomab, the effecter-to-target ratio of the blinatumomab-activated T cell and the CD19-positive target cell is as low as 2:1, which is very low compared with other immunotherapies [9].

8.4 Pharmacokinetics of Blinatumomab

The serum half-life (t1/2) of blinatumomab is very short compared with that of a traditional monoclonal antibody such as rituximab, because blinatumomab lacks the Fc region of an antibody. The average t1/2 of blinatumomab and rituximab is 1.25 h and 76.3 h, respectively [14, 16]. This short t1/2 is the reason why continuous intravenous (CIV) administration of blinatumomab is needed, whereas traditional monoclonal antibodies are administered intermittently. The systemic clearance is not affected by creatinine clearance, age, gender, weight, or body surface area [14]. A phase 1 trial of blinatumomab was carried out for 38 patients with relapsed/refractory non-Hodgkin lymphoma. In this trial, blinatumomab was given as CIV administration, using doses ranging from 5 to 60 μg/m^2 over a period of 4–6 weeks. This trial indicated that the maximum tolerated dose was 60 μg/m^2 and that the majority of tumor responses were seen during the first 4 weeks [17]. In the cases of patients who received 15 μg/m^2 of blinatumomab given as CIV administration, its serum concentration reached steady state within a day, and the steady-state concentration was 731 ± 163 pg/ml (mean ± SD; range: 492–1050 pg/ml) [14]. In vitro analysis, a cytolytic effect of blinatumomab was observed at concentrations between 10 and 100 pg/ml [9]. In this phase 1 study, tumor regression was observed in patients who were treated with 5 μg/m^2 of blinatumomab given as CIV administration [17]. Based on these results, it was recommended that blinatumomab should be given by CIV administration at a dose greater than 15 μg/m^2 for 4 weeks, with a 2-week rest between cycles.

8.5 Immunological Responses of Blinatumomab Infusion

8.5.1 Peripheral B-Cell Kinetics Induced by Blinatumomab Infusion

The number of B cells in peripheral blood that expressed CD19 on their surface rapidly decreased to a very low level with CIV administration of blinatumomab. The mean time to reach nadir was 2.18 ± 3.80 days (mean ± SD; range 0.003–13.94 days). The number of B cells in peripheral blood remained consistently very low during the treatment with blinatumomab, including the 2-week rest periods between cycles [14].

8.5.2 Peripheral T-Cell Kinetics Induced by Blinatumomab Infusion

In the setting of CIV administration of blinatumomab for MRD-positive ALL patients in CR, the number of peripheral T cell began to decrease within 1 h in response to the start of blinatumomab infusion. The nadir was reached within 0.36±0.24 days (mean±SD; range 0.06–1.09 days), and the number of peripheral T cells at nadir was as low as 10% of that at baseline. After the nadir had been reached, the number of peripheral T cells gradually began to increase and had recovered to 50% of the baseline number after 3.13 ± 1.85 days (mean ± SD; range 0.82–9.10 days). The number of peripheral T cells had recovered to baseline on days 8–9 and continued to increase up to day 17, when the number of expanded peripheral T cells had increased to double the number that was present before the start of blinatumomab. Although the number of peripheral T cell decreased after 17 days, their number was maintained above the baseline during CIV administration of blinatumomab [14].

8.5.3 Profile of Expanded T Cells Induced by Blinatumomab Infusion

Analysis of the expanded peripheral T-cell subsets showed three types of patterns: greater expansion of CD4+ T cells than CD8+ T cells, greater expansion of CD8+ T cells than CD4+ T cells, and approximately similar expansion of CD4+ and CD8+ T cells. Except for a very few cases, expansion of regulatory T cells in peripheral blood was not induced by administration of blinatumomab. The majority of expanded CD8+ T cells in peripheral blood were effecter memory T cells of CD45RA−/CD197 phenotype [14].

8.5.4 Cytokine Profiles Induced by Blinatumomab Infusion

Engagement of T cells with leukemic cells through blinatumomab activates T cells, and activated T cells produce inflammatory cytokines including IL-2, IL-6, IL-10, IFN-γ, and TNF-α. The levels of these cytokines in peripheral blood reached a maximum within 1 day after the start of blinatumomab administration and dropped to undetectable levels within 3 days after the start of blinatumomab administration. The elevation of inflammatory cytokines is not observed in patients with a low tumor burden because T-cell activation occurs when an immune synapse is made between a T cell and a CD19+ leukemic cell via blinatumomab [14].

8.6 Safety and Adverse Effects

8.6.1 Adverse CNS Events

The most common adverse CNS events are tremor (17%), dizziness (14%), confusion (7%), encephalopathy (5%), ataxia (5%), and somnolence. In many cases, these adverse CNS events are reversible with temporal interruption of blinatumomab, dexamethasone, and anticonvulsant, but they force the discontinuation of administration of blinatumomab. For the patients whose neurological adverse events are less than grade 4, blinatumomab can be reintroduced starting at the lowest dose (5 $\mu g/m^2$) after these events have resolved [18]. CNS events tend to occur in patients with CNS infiltration of leukemic cells or in those with underlying CNS diseases. These data suggest that blinatumomab should not be given to such patients. The mechanism of blinatumomab-induced CNS toxicity could involve direct T-cell-mediated toxicity and/or cytokine-mediated toxicity such as the CNS toxicity that is induced by CAR T-cell therapy [19]. These are the reasons why adverse CNS events tend to occur in patients who have a high tumor burden or in those who were given blinatumomab for the first time.

8.6.2 Cytokine Releasing Syndromes

Cytokine releasing syndromes (CRS) develop as the result of systemic inflammation that is caused by inflammatory cytokines such as IL-2, IL-6, IL-10, IFN-γ, and TNF-α, which are produced by blinatumomab-activated T cells. In most CRS cases, symptoms are flu-like such as pyrexia and myalgia. In severe CRS cases, inflammatory cytokines induce capillary leak and result in hypotension, pulmonary edema, coagulopathy, and multi-organ failure. The preventive administration of dexamethasone (10 $mg/m^2/day$) during the first 5 days of blinatumomab infusion and dose reduction of blinatumomab to 5 $\mu g/m^2/day$ (or 9 μg/day) during the first 7 days of blinatumomab effectively prevent development of CRS and do not affect the result of blinatumomab treatment. CRS usually develops in the first cycle of blinatumomab treatment, because T-cell activation and inflammatory cytokine release occur due to immune synapse formation between T cells and CD19-positive leukemic cells via blinatumomab [18, 20].

8.6.3 Hypogammaglobulinemia

Because B cells differentiate into plasma cells that produce immunoglobulins, B-cell elimination by blinatumomab results in hypogammaglobulinemia. Since CD19, but not CD20, expression is maintained on plasma blast cells, the period of hypogammaglobulinemia resulting from blinatumomab administration is prolonged compared to that resulting from an anti-CD20 antibody such as rituximab. Although the levels of all immunoglobulin classes in serum are decreased by treatment with blinatumomab, the greatest decrease is seen in the level of serum IgA. The serum levels of IgG, IgM, and IgA fall to 29%, 12%, and 6% of their respective baseline values. The level of each immunoglobulin class begins to recover in the order of IgM, IgG, and IgA after completion of blinatumomab treatment. It takes a long time to recover the level of serum immunoglobulins after completion of blinatumomab treatment because plasma cells have to be differentiated from naïve and memory B cells, which are regenerated by CD19-negative B-cell progenitors. Within 2 years, the levels of serum IgG and IgM, but not the levels of serum IgA, recover to more than 50% of the level of the pretreatment baseline. Because immunoglobulin is an important humoral factor for the eradication of foreign pathogens, it might be necessary to regularly monitor the level of serum immunoglobulin and to replenish it to the minimum level to prevent infection [21].

8.6.4 Other Adverse Effects

Cytopenias are frequently observed during blinatumomab treatment. It is difficult to determine whether these cytopenias are related to the effects of blinatumomab or to ALL itself. Neutropenia and febrile neutropenia (FN) more than grade 3 were developed in 25% and 16%, respectively, of ALL patients treated with blinatumomab [18]. It is necessary to pay attention to infectious disease both during and after treatment with blinatumomab, because hypogammaglobulinemia induced by blinatumomab results in patients with a compromised immune status.

8.7 Results of Clinical Trials of Blinatumomab (Table 8.1)

8.7.1 Clinical Results of Adult Patients with Relapsed or Refractory B-Precursor ALL Treated with Blinatumomab

Two results of phase 2 clinical trials of blinatumomab have been published to date. The first report included 36 relapsed or refractory B-precursor ALL patients with or without Philadelphia chromosome, including 21 patients who had received allo-HSCT before the treatment with blinatumomab. The median age was 32 years (range: 18–77 years of age). At the beginning of this trial, blinatumomab was administered at a dose of 15 μg/m^2 as CIV administration for 4 weeks with a 2-week rest between cycles. Because grade 4 CRS was observed, prophylactic treatment with dexamethasone at a dose of up to 24 mg for up to 5 days and/or 200 mg/m^2 of cyclophosphamide for up to 4 days was permitted, and the initial dose of

Table 8.1 Results of clinical trials of blinatumomab

Disease status	Age No. of patients	Results	Grade3–4 AEs	No. of TRM	References
R/R	32 years (18–77) *N* = 36	69% CR or CRh 88% MCR in CR and CRh	Leukopenia, thrombocytopenia, CNS disorder	6 (17%)	[20]
R/R	39 years (18–79) *N* = 168	43% CR or CRh 82% MCR in CR and CRh	FN, neutropenia, anemia, pyrexia Neurologic events, hepatic disorder	28 (17%)	[18]
R/R	10.4 years (4.3–18.5) *N* = 9	67% CR 67% MCR in CR and CRh	FN, anemia, CRS, anemia, thrombocytopenia, hepatic disorder	0 (0%)	[23]
CR with MRD	45 years (18–76) *N* = 116	80% MCR	Pyrexia, tremor, aphasia, encephalopathy	2 (2%)	[22]

R/R relapsed/refractory, *MRD* minimal residual disease, *CR* complete response, *CRh* CR with incomplete hematologic recovery, *MCR* molecular CR, *CNS* central nervous system blinatumomab in the first week of treatment was lowered to 5 μg/m^2 and was later increased to 15 μg/m^2. Sixty-nine percent of patients achieved a CR or CR with partial hematologic recovery (CRh), with 88% of responders achieving an MRD response. Forty-two percent of patients who achieved CR or CRh underwent subsequent allo-HSCT. The median overall survival (OS) and relapse-free survival (RFS) were 9.8 and 7.6 months, respectively. Frequent adverse events (AEs) during the treatment were pyrexia (81%), fatigue (50%), headache (47%), tremor (36%), and leukopenia (19%). The most frequent AEs of grade 3 or 4 were transient leukopenia and thrombocytopenia. Infectious diseases developed in 12 patients, including 5 deaths. None of the patients that died from infectious disease had achieved a CR or CRh. CNS events were observed in 22% of the patients. Two patients developed grade 4 CRS, and none of the nonresponders to blinatumomab treatment developed CRS [20].

The second report included 189 relapsed or refractory B-precursor ALL patients without Philadelphia chromosome, including 64 patients who had received allo-HSCT before the treatment with blinatumomab. The median age was 39 years (range: 18–79 years of age). In the first cycle, blinatumomab was administered as CIV administration at a dose of 9 μg/day for the first week and 28 μg/day for the next 3 weeks. After two cycles, blinatumomab was administered at a dose of 28 μg/day for 4 weeks with a 2-week rest between cycles. Within two cycles of blinatumomab treatments, 43% of patients achieved a CR or CRh, with 82% of responders achieving an MRD response. Forty percent of patients who achieved CR or CRh underwent subsequent allo-HSCT. The median OS and RFS times were 6.1 and 5.9 months, respectively. Allo-HSCT before the treatment of blinatumomab had no impact on the result of its treatment. Frequent AEs of grade 3 or 4 during the treatment were febrile FN (25%), neutropenia (16%), anemia (14%), neurological event (13%), and CRS (2%). Three deaths due to infectious disease were thought by the investigator to be treatment related [18].

8.7.2 Results of Blinatumomab Treatment of MRD-Positive Adult B-Precursor ALL Patients in Hematological CR

One hundred and sixteen patients in hematological CR with MRD after three or more intensive chemotherapies were treated with 15 μg/m^2/day of blinatumomab for 4 weeks with a 2-week rest between cycles. Seventy-eight percent of these patients achieved a complete MRD response after one cycle of treatment. Two fatal adverse events occurred, one of which was a subdural hemorrhage and the other was atypical pneumonia [22].

8.7.3 Clinical Results of Pediatric Patients with Relapsed or Refractory B-Precursor ALL Treated with Blinatumomab

The results of a phase 2 trial of blinatumomab for pediatric patients with relapsed or refractory B-precursor ALL have been reported. Thirty-nine patients, including patients who relapsed after allo-HSCT, were treated with blinatumomab. The median age was 9 years (range: 2–16 years of age). They received blinatumomab at a dose of 5 μg/m^2/day during the first week and at a dose of 15 μg/m^2/day during the next 3 weeks. The treatment was repeated with intervals of 2 weeks. Similar to adult patients with relapsed or refractory pre-B-ALL, 36% of the pediatric patients achieved CR or CRh within two cycles of treatment, and 42% of the patients who achieved CR or CRh were MRD negative. Frequently observed AEs were pyrexia (74%), anemia (33%), nausea (31%), headache (28%), and hypotension (21%). AEs of more than grade 3 were anemia (26%), pyrexia (21%), increased alanine aminotransferase (18%), increased aspartate aminotransferase (18%), FN (15%), and CRS (5%) [23].

8.8 Problems and Future Direction

As described here, about 40–60% of relapsed or refractory B-precursor ALL patients can obtain CR or CRh with blinatumomab treatment, and about 40–60% of these patients become MRD negative. However, it is not possible to identify the patients for whom blinatumomab is effective. It is currently thought that patients who achieve CR or CRh with blinatumomab should receive allo-HSCT to cure the leukemia if allo-HSCT is not a contraindication for them. However, according to a long-term follow-up of a German phase 2 study, 2 of 12 patients who became MRD negative and did not receive allo-HSCT as consolidation therapy maintained a long-term relapse-free status (more than 30 months). It is very interesting that they experienced severe adverse effects that were characteristic of blinatumomab treatment. One patient had a reversible grade 4 CRS, and the other had a reversible grade 3 neurological event [24].

Blinatumomab has been approved only for relapsed or refractory B-precursor ALL by the US Food and Drug Administration and the European Commission. The next step is to investigate how to use blinatumomab for de novo B-precursor ALL patients. Because about 80% of B-precursor ALL patients can achieve CR with conventional combination chemotherapy, it is impossible to compare the efficacy of blinatumomab as monotherapy with that of conventional combination chemotherapy [2, 3]. It is uncertain whether the combination of blinatumomab with cytotoxic anticancer drugs will improve treatment outcome because blinatumomab depends on T-cell cytotoxicity to exert its antileukemic effect, and this may be hindered by cytotoxic agents. From this point of view, as many cases of Ph-ALL express CD 19 [25] and TKIs do not affect T-cell function, combination therapies with TKIs and blinatumomab are very attractive for the treatment of Ph-ALL with CD 19 expression. Investigations regarding how to use blinatumomab more effectively should be continued.

References

1. Swerdlow S, Campo E, Harris N. World Health Organization classification of tumours of haematopoietic and lymphoid tissues. Lyon: IARC Press; 2008.
2. Gökbuget N, Hoelzer D. Treatment of adult acute lymphoblastic leukemia. Semin Hematol. 2009;46(1):64–75.
3. Couban S, Savoie L, Mourad YA, Leber B, Minden M, Turner R, Palada V, Shehata N, Christofides A, Lachance S. Evidence-based guidelines for the use of tyrosine kinase inhibitors in adults with Philadelphia chromosome-positive or BCR-ABL-positive acute lymphoblastic leukemia: a Canadian consensus. Curr Oncol. 2014;21(2):e265–309. doi:10.3747/co.21.1834.
4. Fielding AK, Richards SM, Chopra R, Lazarus HM, Litzow MR, Buck G, Durrant IJ, Luger SM, Marks DI, Couban S, Savoie L, Mourad YA, Leber B, Minden M, Turner R, Palada V, Franklin IM, McMillan AK, Tallman MS, Rowe JM, Goldstone AH, Medical Research Council of the United Kingdom Adult ALL Working Party, Eastern Cooperative Oncology Group. Outcome of 609 adults after relapse of acute lymphoblastic leukemia (ALL); an MRCUKALL12/ECOG 2993 study. Blood. 2007;109(3):944–50. Epub 2006 Oct 10
5. Chiaretti S, Foà R. Management of adult Ph-positive acute lymphoblastic leukemia. Hematol Am Soc Hematol Educ Program. 2015;2015(1):406–13. doi:10.1182/asheducation-2015.1.406.
6. Hoelzer D, Walewski J, Döhner H, Viardot A, Hiddemann W, Spiekermann K, Serve H, Dührsen U, Hüttmann A, Thiel E, Dengler J, Kneba M, Schaich M, Schmidt-Wolf IG, Beck J, Hertenstein B, Reichle A, Domanska-Czyz K, Fietkau R, Horst HA, Rieder H, Schwartz S, Burmeister T, Gökbuget N, German Multicenter Study Group for Adult Acute Lymphoblastic Leukemia. Improved outcome of adult Burkitt lymphoma/leukemia with rituximab and chemotherapy: report of a large prospective multicenter trial. Blood. 2014;124(26):3870–9. doi:10.1182/blood-2014-03-563627. Epub 2014 Oct 30
7. Kantarjian H, Thomas D, Jorgensen J, Jabbour E, Kebriaei P, Rytting M, York S, Ravandi F, Kwari M, Faderl S, Rios MB, Cortes J, Fayad L, Tarnai R, Wang SA, Champlin R, Advani A, O'Brien S. Inotuzumab ozogamicin, an anti-CD22-calecheamicin conjugate, for refractory and relapsed acute lymphocytic leukaemia: a phase 2 study. Lancet Oncol. 2012;13(4):403–11. doi:10.1016/S1470-2045(11)70386-2. Epub 2012 Feb 21
8. Maude SL, Teachey DT, Porter DL, Grupp SA. CD19-targeted chimeric antigen receptor T cell therapy for acute lymphoblastic leukemia. Blood. 2015;125(26):4017–23. doi:10.1182/blood-2014-12-580068. Epub 2015 May 21
9. Löffler A, Kufer P, Lutterbüse R, Zettl F, Daniel PT, Schwenkenbecher JM, Riethmüller G, Dörken B, Bargou RC. A recombinant bispecific single-chain antibody, CD19 x CD3, induces rapid and high lymphoma-directed cytotoxicity by unstimulated T lymphocytes. Blood. 2000;95(6):2098–103.
10. Wu J, Fu J, Zhang M, Liu D. Blinatumomab: a bispecific T cell engager (BiTE) antibody against CD19/CD3 for refractory acute lymphoid leukemia. J Hematol Oncol. 2015;8:104. doi:10.1186/s13045-015-0195-4.
11. Moore PA, Zhang W, Rainey GJ, Burke S, Li H, Huang L, Gorlatov S, Veri MC, Aggarwal S, Yang Y, Shah K, Jin L, Zhang S, He L, Zhang T, Ciccarone V, Koenig S, Bonvini E, Johnson S. Application of dual affinity retargeting molecules to achieve optimal redirected T cell killing of B cell lymphoma. Blood. 2011;117(17):4542–51. doi:10.1182/blood-2010-09-306449. Epub 2011 Feb 7

12. Raponi S, De Propris MS, Intoppa S, Milani ML, Vitale A, Elia L, Perbellini O, Pizzolo G, Foá R, Guarini A. Flow cytometric study of potential target antigens (CD19, CD20, CD22, CD33) for antibody-based immunotherapy in acute lymphoblastic leukemia: analysis of 552 cases. Leuk Lymphoma. 2011;52(6):1098–107. doi:10.3109/10428194.2011.559668. Epub 2011 Feb 24
13. Zimmerman Z, Maniar T, Nagorsen D. Unleashing the clinical power of T cells: CD19/CD3 bi-specific T cell engager (BiTE®) antibody construct blinatumomab as a potential therapy. Int Immunol. 2015;27(1):31–7. doi:10.1093/intimm/dxu089. Epub 2014 Sep 19
14. Klinger M, Brandl C, Zugmaier G, Hijazi Y, Bargou RC, Topp MS, Gökbuget N, Neumann S, Goebeler M, Viardot A, Stelljes M, Brüggemann M, Hoelzer D, Degenhard E, Nagorsen D, Baeuerle PA, Wolf A, Kufer P. Immunopharmacologic response of patients with B-lineage acute lymphoblastic leukemia to continuous infusion of T cell-engaging CD19/CD3-bispecific BiTE antibody blinatumomab. Blood. 2012;119(26):6226–33. doi:10.1182/blood-2012-01-400515. Epub 2012 May 16
15. Reff ME, Carner K, Chambers KS, Chinn PC, Leonard JE, Raab R, Newman RA, Hanna N, Anderson DR. Depletion of B cells in vivo by a chimeric mouse human monoclonal antibody to CD20. Blood. 1994;83(2):435–45.
16. Berinstein NL, Grillo-López AJ, White CA, Bence-Bruckler I, Maloney D, Czuczman M, Green D, Rosenberg J, McLaughlin P, Shen D. Association of serum Rituximab (IDEC-C2B8) concentration and anti-tumor response in the treatment of recurrent low-grade or follicular non-Hodgkin's lymphoma. Ann Oncol. 1998;9(9):995–1001.
17. Bargou R, Leo E, Zugmaier G, Klinger M, Goebeler M, Knop S, Noppeney R, Viardot A, Hess G, Schuler M, Einsele H, Brandl C, Wolf A, Kirchinger P, Klappers P, Schmidt M, Riethmüller G, Reinhardt C, Baeuerle PA, Kufer P. Tumor regression in cancer patients by very low doses of a T cell-engaging antibody. Science. 2008;321(5891):974–7. doi:10.1126/science.1158545.
18. Topp MS, Gökbuget N, Stein AS, Zugmaier G, O'Brien S, Bargou RC, Dombret H, Fielding AK, Heffner L, Larson RA, Neumann S, Foà R, Litzow M, Ribera JM, Rambaldi A, Schiller G, Brüggemann M, Horst HA, Holland C, Jia C, Maniar T, Huber B, Nagorsen D, Forman SJ, Kantarjian HM. Safety and activity of blinatumomab for adult patients with relapsed or refractory B-precursor acute lymphoblastic leukaemia: a multicentre, single-arm, phase 2 study. Lancet Oncol. 2015;16(1):57–66. doi:10.1016/S1470-2045(14)71170-2. Epub 2014 Dec 16
19. Maude SL, Frey N, Shaw PA, Aplenc R, Barrett DM, Bunin NJ, Chew A, Gonzalez VE, Zheng Z, Lacey SF, Mahnke YD, Melenhorst JJ, Rheingold SR, Shen A, Teachey DT, Levine BL, June CH, Porter DL, Grupp SA. Chimeric antigen receptor T cells for sustained remissions in leukemia. N Engl J Med. 2014;371(16):1507–17. doi:10.1056/NEJMoa1407222.
20. Topp MS, Gökbuget N, Zugmaier G, Klappers P, Stelljes M, Neumann S, Viardot A, Marks R, Diedrich H, Faul C, Reichle A, Horst HA, Brüggemann M, Wessiepe D, Holland C, Alekar S, Mergen N, Einsele H, Hoelzer D, Bargou RC. Phase II trial of the anti-CD19 bispecific T cell-engager blinatumomab shows hematologic and molecular remissions in patients with relapsed or refractory B-precursor acute lymphoblastic leukemia. J Clin Oncol. 2014;32(36):4134–40. doi:10.1200/JCO.2014.56.3247. Epub 2014 Nov 10
21. Zugmaier G, Topp MS, Alekar S, Viardot A, Horst HA, Neumann S, Stelljes M, Bargou RC, Goebeler M, Wessiepe D, Degenhard E, Gökbuget N, Klinger M. Long-term follow-up of serum immunoglobulin levels in blinatumomab-treated patients with minimal residual disease-positive B-precursor acute lymphoblastic leukemia. Blood Cancer J. 2014;4:244. doi:10.1038/bcj.2014.64.
22. Goekbuget N, Dombret H, Bonifacio M, Reichle A, Graux C, Havelange V, Buss EC, Faul C, Bruggemann M, Ganser A, Stieglmaier J, Wessels H, Haddad V, Zugmaier G, Nagorsen D, Bargou RC. BLAST: a confirmatory, single-arm, phase 2 study of Blinatumomab, a Bispecific T cell Engager (BiTE®) antibody construct, in patients with minimal residual disease B-precursor Acute Lymphoblastic Leukemia (ALL). Blood. 2014;124:379. Epub 2014 Dec 5

23. Schlegel P, Lang P, Zugmaier G, Ebinger M, Kreyenberg H, Witte KE, Feucht J, Pfeiffer M, Teltschik HM, Kyzirakos C, Feuchtinger T, Handgretinger R. Pediatric posttransplant relapsed/refractory B-precursor acute lymphoblastic leukemia shows durable remission by therapy with the T cell engaging bispecific antibody blinatumomab. Haematologica. 2014;99(7):1212–9. doi:10.3324/haematol.2013.100073. Epub 2014 Apr 11
24. Zugmaier G, Gökbuget N, Klinger M, Viardot A, Stelljes M, Neumann S, Horst HA, Marks R, Faul C, Diedrich H, Reichle A, Brüggemann M, Holland C, Schmidt M, Einsele H, Bargou RC, Topp MS. Long-term survival and T cell kinetics in relapsed/refractory ALL patients who achieved MRD response after blinatumomab treatment. Blood. 2015;126(24):2578–84. doi:10.1182/blood-2015-06-649111. Epub 2015 Oct 19
25. Westbrook CA, Hooberman AL, Spino C, Dodge RK, Larson RA, Davey F, Wurster-Hill DH, Sobol RE, Schiffer C, Bloomfield CD. Clinical significance of the BCR-ABL fusion gene in adult acute lymphoblastic leukemia: a Cancer and Leukemia Group B Study (8762). Blood. 1992;80(12):2983–90.

Mogamulizumab in Adult T-Cell Leukemia/Lymphoma

9

Michinori Ogura

Abstract

KW-0761, mogamulizumab, is a next-generation humanized anti-CC chemokine receptor 4 (CCR4) immunoglobulin G1 (IgG1) monoclonal antibody with a defucosylated Fc region, which markedly enhanced antibody-dependent cellular cytotoxicity. Because CCR4 is expressed on tumor cells from most patients with adult T-cell leukemia/lymphoma (ATL), CCR4 might represent a novel molecular target for immunotherapy by mogamulizumab. Phase I and II studies showed that mogamulizumab is active in patients with relapsed ATL with acceptable toxicity. A randomized phase II study demonstrated that the combination strategy of mogamulizumab with polychemotherapy showed a potentially less favorable safety profile and a higher complete response rate was achieved, providing the basis for further investigation of this novel treatment for newly diagnosed aggressive ATL. Based on these clinical studies, mogamulizumab was approved in patients with both newly diagnosed and relapsed/refractory CCR4+ ATL in Japan. Mogamulizumab is expected to become a core agent combined with other molecular targeting drugs and chemotherapeutic drugs in ATL and CCR4+ T-cell lymphoma.

Keywords

Mogamulizumab • CCR4 • ADCC • ATL

M. Ogura (✉)
The Department of Hematology, and the Department of Clinical Trial Center, Tokai Central Hospital, 4-6-2 Higashijimacho, Sohara, Kakamigahara, Gifu 504-8601, Japan
e-mail: mi-ogura@naa.att.ne.jp

T. Ueda (ed.), *Chemotherapy for Leukemia*, DOI 10.1007/978-981-10-3332-2_9

9.1 Introduction

Adult T-cell leukemia-lymphoma (ATL) is an aggressive peripheral T-cell neoplasm caused by human T-cell lymphotropic virus type I. The disease is resistant to conventional chemotherapeutic agents, and there currently exist limited treatment options; thus, it has a poor prognosis [1–4]. A phase III trial for previously untreated patients with aggressive ATL (acute, lymphoma, or unfavorable chronic type) age 33–69 years demonstrated that a dose-intensified multidrug regimen, VCAP-AMP-VECP (vincristine, cyclophosphamide, doxorubicin, and prednisone; doxorubicin, ranimustine, and prednisone; and vindesine, etoposide, carboplatin, and prednisone), resulted in median progression-free survival (PFS) and overall survival (OS) of 7.0 and 12.7 months, respectively [5]. This remains unsatisfactory compared with responses in other hematologic malignancies. Allogeneic hematopoietic stem cell transplantation has evolved into a potential approach to treating patients with ATL over the last decade. However, only a small fraction of patients with ATL have the opportunity to benefit from transplantation, such as those who are younger, have achieved sufficient disease control, and have an appropriate stem cell source [6, 7]. Therefore, the development of alternative treatment strategies for patients with ATL is an urgent issue.

Because CC chemokine receptor 4 (CCR4) is expressed on tumor cells from most patients with ATL [8, 9], CCR4 might represent a novel molecular target for immunotherapy. Accordingly, mogamulizumab, a next-generation humanized anti-CCR4 immunoglobulin G1 (IgG1) monoclonal antibody (mAb) with a defucosylated Fc region, which markedly enhances antibody-dependent cellular cytotoxicity (ADCC), was developed [10, 11].

In this chapter, mechanism of action and clinical data of phase I and phase II studies in relapsed ATL and randomized phase II study in newly diagnosed ATL will be described.

9.2 Mechanism of Action (Fig. 9.1)

Chemokines act as signaling molecules in the migration and tissue homing of various leukocytes. Among them, thymus and activation-regulated chemokine (TARC) and monocyte-derived chemokine (MDC) induce the selective recruitment of distinct subsets of T cells through triggering of a chemokine receptor, CCR4. The CCR4 gene is located on chromosome 3p24. CCR4 is a seven-domain transmembrane G protein-coupled receptor, and TARC/CCL17 and MDC/CCL22 are ligands of CCR4. The anti-CCR4 monoclonal antibody recognizes the N-terminal portion of the CCR4 molecule. KW-0761, mogamulizumab, is a next-generation humanized anti-CCR4 immunoglobulin G1 (IgG1) monoclonal antibody with a defucosylated Fc region, which markedly enhanced ADCC. Ishida et al. reported that the therapeutic defucosylated anti-CCR4 mAb induced a robust ADCC activity against not only CCR4-positive human ATL cells but also against other types of CCR4-positive human leukemia/lymphoma lines in the presence of PBMC from healthy

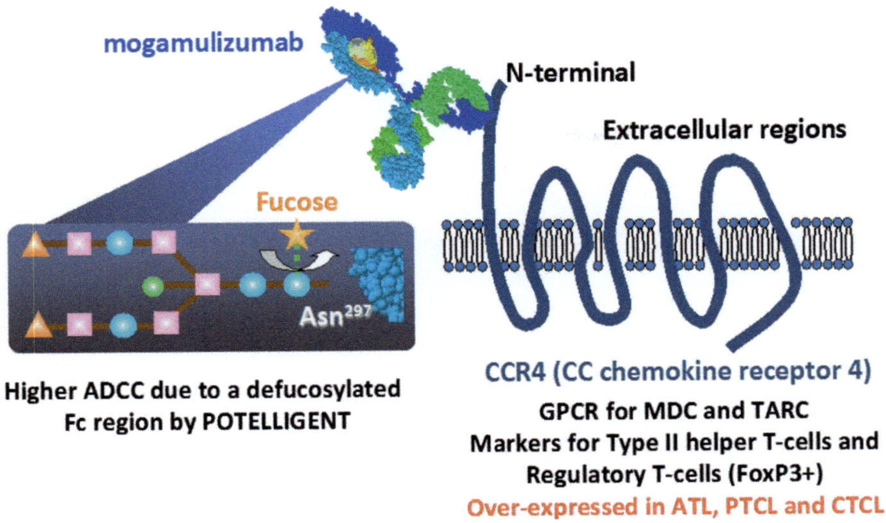

Fig. 9.1 CC chemokine receptor 4 (*CCR4*) and humanized anti-CCR4 monoclonal antibody, KW-0761. The CCR4 gene is located on chromosome 3p24. CCR4 is a seven-domain transmembrane G protein-coupled receptor, and TARC/CCL17 and MDC/CCL22 are ligands of CCR4. The anti-CCR4 monoclonal antibody recognizes the N-terminal portion of the CCR4 molecule

individuals in a dose-dependent manner in vitro. In addition, a robust ADCC of the therapeutic defucosylated anti-CCR4 mAb mediated by autologous effector cells was triggered in some ATL cells as well as cells from other types of PTCL patients in vitro [11, 12]. Highly enhanced ADCC activity without complement-dependent cytotoxicity or direct antitumor activities was also reported [11, 13]. Ishida et al. analyzed 103 patients with ATL and found that tumor cells from about 90% of patients showed CCR4 expression [14]. They also found that patients with CCR4-positive ATL were more likely to have skin infiltration and had a worse outcome than those with CCR4-negative ATL, indicating that CCR4 played an important pathogenetic role in ATL [14].

9.3 Phase I Study in Relapsed ATL

This phase I study assessed the safety, pharmacokinetics, and recommended phase II dose and efficacy of KW-0761 (mogamulizumab) in patients with relapsed CCR4-positive adult T-cell leukemia-lymphoma (ATL) or peripheral T-cell lymphoma (PTCL) [15]. In this study, 16 patients received KW-0761 once a week for 4 weeks by intravenous infusion (Table 9.1). Doses were escalated, starting at 0.01, 0.1, 0.5, and finally 1.0 mg/kg by a 3+3 design (Fig. 9.2). Fifteen patients completed the protocol treatment. Only one patient, at the 1.0 mg/kg dose, developed grade 3 dose-limiting toxicities, skin rash, and febrile neutropenia and grade 4 neutropenia. Other treatment-related grade 3–4 toxicities were lymphopenia (n = 10),

Table 9.1 Patient demographic and clinical characteristics by cohort in phase I study in relapsed ATL (Ref. [15])

Characteristic	Cohort and Dosage 1: 0.01 mg/kg	2: 0.1 mg/kg	3: 0.5 mg/kg	4: 1.0 mg/kg	Expanded: 1.0 mg/kg	Total
No. of patients	3	4[a]	3	3	3	16
Median age, years						62
Range	46-68	55-66	60-69	62-64	55-62	46-69
Sex						
Male	2	2	2	0	2	8
Female	1	2	1	3	1	8
Diagnosis						
ATL	2	4	3	2	2	13
PTCL	1(MF)	0	0	1(PTCL-NOS)	1(PTCL-NOS)	3
No. of prior chemotherapy regimens						
1	2	2	2	1	2	9
2	0	0	0	2	0	2
≥3	1	2	1	0	1	5

ATL **adult T-cell leukemia-lymphoma,** ***PTCL*** **peripheral T-cell lymphoma,** ***NOS*** **not otherwise specified,** ***MF*** **mycosis fungoides**

[a]One patient enrolled at 0.1 mg/kg was withdrawn due to early progressive disease

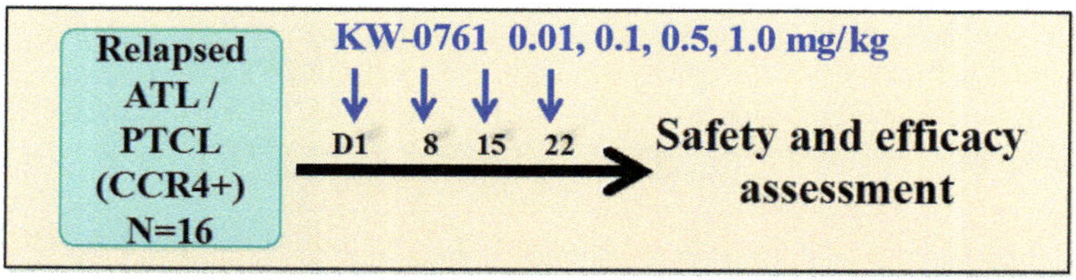

Fig. 9.2 Study design of phase I study of mogamulizumab in relapsed ATL and PTCL. This was a multicenter dose-escalation study with three to six patients at each dose level to determine the maximum-tolerated dose (*MTD*) and estimate the recommended phase II dose. Cohorts of patients received KW-0761 at 0.01, 0.1, 0.5, and 1.0 mg/kg, weekly for 4 weeks by intravenous infusion. Premedications (antihistamine and antipyretic) were administered before each KW-0761 (mogamulizumab) treatment

neutropenia (n = 3), leukopenia (n = 2), herpes zoster (n = 1), and acute infusion reaction/cytokine release syndrome (n = 1). Neither the frequency nor severity of toxicities increased with dose escalation. The maximum tolerated dose was not reached. Therefore, the recommended phase II dose was determined to be 1.0 mg/kg. No patients had detectable levels of anti-KW-0761 antibody. The plasma maximum and trough, and the area under the curve of 0–7 days of KW-0761, tended to increase dose and frequency dependently. Five patients (31%; 95% CI, 11–59%) achieved objective responses: two complete (0.1; 1.0 mg/kg) and three partial (0.01; 2 at 1.0 mg/kg) responses (Table 9.2). KW-0761 was tolerated at all the dose levels tested, demonstrating potential efficacy against relapsed CCR4-positive ATL or PTCL. Subsequent phase II studies at the 1.0 mg/kg dose are thus warranted.

Table 9.2 Summary of clinical response of each patient in phase I study in relapsed ATL (Ref. [15])

Patient No. by Cohort		Sex	Age(years)	Disease	No. of Infusions	Response				PFS(days)
						PB	Skin	LN[a]	OR	
1										
	101	M	46	MF tumor stage	4	-	PD	SD	PD	29
	102	M	60	ATL acute	4	-	SD	-	SD→CR[b]	617+
	103	F	68	ATL acute	4	CR	-	CR	PR[c]	85
2										
	201	M	55	ATL acute	4	CR	PR	SD	SD	50
	202	F	66	ATL acute	4	PR	-	SD	SD	36
	203	M	66	ATL acute	1	-	-	SD	PD[c]	8
	204	F	57	ATL acute	4	CR	CR	-	CR	379+
3										
	301	M	60	ATL acute	4	-	PD	-	PD	36
	302	M	64	ATL acute	4	-	-	PD	PD	29
	303	F	69	ATL lymphoma	4	-	-	SD	PD[c]	29
4										
	401	F	64	PTCL-NOS	4	CR	CR	PR	PR	198+
	402	F	62	ATL acute	4	CR	CR	PR	PR	64
	403	F	64	ATL lymphoma	4	-	-	SD	SD	43
Expanded										
	411	M	55	ATL acute	4	-	PD	-	PD	28
	412	M	62	ATL acute	4	CR	-	-	CR	107+
	413	F	58	PTCL-NOS	4	-	-	SD	SD	110+

PB **peripheral blood,** *LN* **lymph node,** *PFS* **progression-free survival,** *OR* **overall response,** *M* **male,** *MF* **mycosis fungoides,** *PD* **progressive disease,** *SD* **stable disease,** *F* **female,** *ATL* **adult T-cell leukemia-lymphoma,** *CR* **complete response,** *PR* **partial response,** *PTCL-NOS* **peripheral T-cell lymphoma, not otherwise specified**

[a]Target lesions among measurable enlarged lymph nodes and tumor nodules in extranodal organs

[b]The diseases had disappeared by 1 year after treatment and 102 was categorized as showing CR

[c]Patients had nontarget lesions (nonincrease on 103, increase on 203) and new tumor legions (303)

9.4 Phase II Study in Relapsed ATL

A multicenter phase II study of KW-0761 for patients with relapsed, aggressive CCR4-positive ATL was conducted to evaluate efficacy, pharmacokinetic profile, and safety [16]. The primary end point was overall response rate, and secondary end points included progression-free survival and overall survival from the first dose of KW-0761. Patients received intravenous infusions of KW-0761 once per week for 8 weeks at a dose of 1.0 mg/kg (Fig. 9.3). Of 28 patients enrolled onto the study, 27 received at least one infusion of KW-0761 (Table 9.3). Objective responses were noted in 13 of 26 evaluable patients, including eight complete responses, with an overall response rate of 50% (95% CI, 30–70%). Median progression-free survival and overall survival were 5.2 and 13.7 months, respectively (Fig. 9.4). The mean half-life period after the eighth infusion was 422 ± 147 h (± standard deviation). The most common adverse events were infusion reactions (89%) and skin rashes (63%), which were manageable and reversible in all cases (Table 9.4). KW-0761 demonstrated clinically meaningful antitumor activity in patients with relapsed ATL, with an acceptable toxicity profile. Further investigation of KW-0761 for treatment of ATL and other T-cell neoplasms is warranted.

Base on these phase I and phase II studies, mogamulizumab was approved and launched on May 2012 in Japan.

Table 9.3 Patient demographics and clinical characteristics in phase II study in relapsed ATL ($n = 27$)[a] (Ref. [16])

Characteristic	No.	%
Age, years		
Median	64	
Range	49-83	
≥65	13	48
Sex		
Male	12	44
Female	15	56
ECOG performance status[b]		
0	15	56
1	7	26
2	5	19
Disease subtype		
Acute	14	52
Lymphoma	6	22
Chronic	7	26
Prior chemotherapy regimens, No.		
1	22	82
2	3	11
3	2	7

ECOG **Eastern Cooperative Oncology Group**
[a]Of 28 patients enrolled, 27 received at least one infusion of KW-0761
[b]ECOG performance status scores range from zero (normal activity) to five (death), with higher scores indicating more severe disability

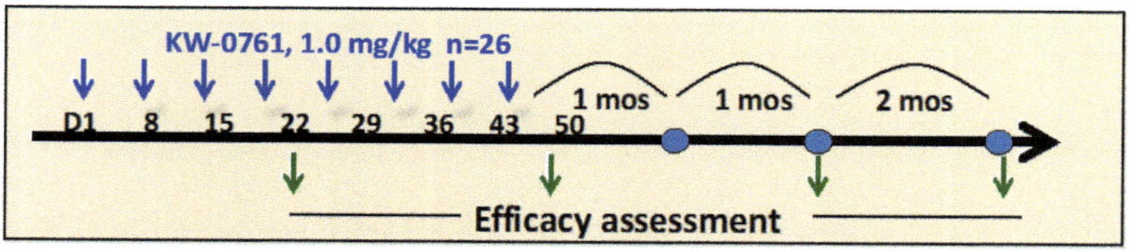

Fig. 9.3 Study design of phase II study. This study was a multicenter, single-arm, phase II trial. Objectives of the study were to evaluate the efficacy, pharmacokinetic profile, and safety of KW-0761 monotherapy. Patients received intravenous infusions of KW-0761 once per week for 8 weeks at a dose of 1.0 mg/kg

9.5 Randomized Phase II Study in Newly Diagnosed ATL

This multicenter, randomized, phase II study was conducted to examine whether the addition of mogamulizumab, a humanized anti-CC chemokine receptor 4 antibody, to mLSG15, a dose-intensified chemotherapy, further increases efficacy without compromising safety of patients with newly diagnosed aggressive adult T-cell leukemia-lymphoma (ATL) (Fig. 9.5). Patients were assigned 1:1 to receive mLSG15 plus mogamulizumab or mLSG15 alone. The primary end point was the complete response rate (%CR); secondary end points included the overall response

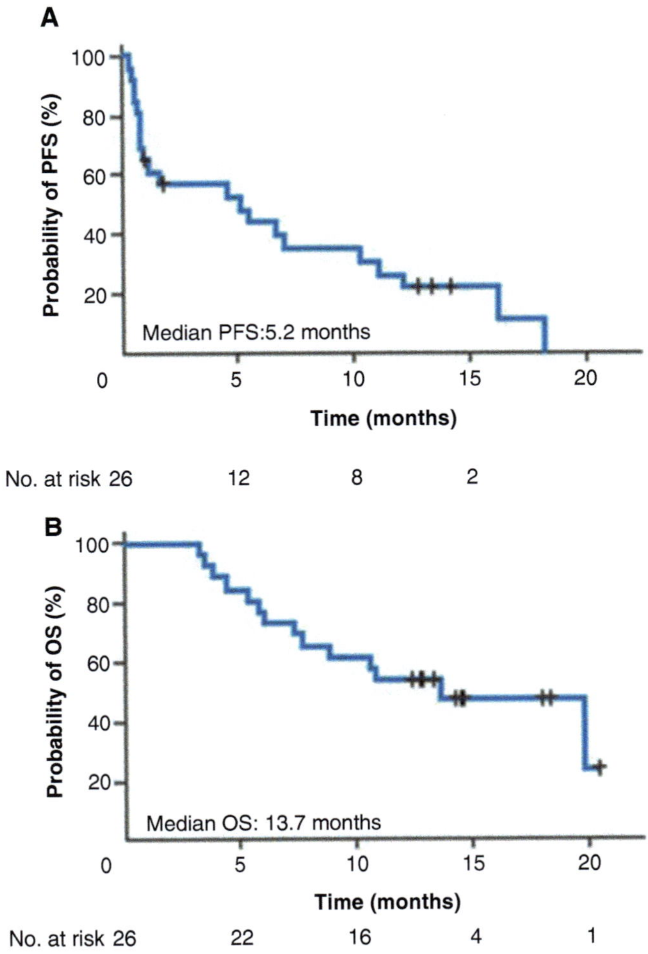

Fig. 9.4 Kaplan-Meier curves of estimated (**a**) progression-free survival (PFS; median, 5.2 months) and (**b**) overall survival (OS; median, 13.7 months) in phase II study in relapsed ATL (Ref. [16])

rate (ORR) and safety. Between August 2010 and September 2011, 54 patients with newly diagnosed aggressive ATL were enrolled at 18 institutions. Of these 54 patients, 29 in the mLSG15-plus-mogamulizumab arm and 24 in the mLSG15 arm received treatment according to our study protocol (Table 9.5). The %CR and ORR in the mLSG15-plus-mogamulizumab arm (n = 29) were 52% [95% confidence interval (CI), 33–71%] and 86%, respectively; the corresponding values in the mLSG15 arm (n = 24) were 33% (95% CI, 16–55%) and 75%, respectively (Table 9.6). The median PFS in the mLSG15-plus-mogamulizumab and mLSG15 arms were 8·5 and 6·3 months, respectively (Fig. 9.6). The median OS was not

Table 9.4 Adverse events ($n = 27$)[a] in phase II study in relapsed ATL (Ref. [16])

Adverse Event	Grade (No. of patients)				All Grades		Infusion Reaction Related (No. of patients)	
	1	2	3	4	No. of Patients	%	All Grades	≥ Grade 2
Nonhematologic								
Infusion reaction	1	22	1	0	24	89		
Fever	20	2	0	0	22	82	18	2
Rash	3	9	5	0	17	63	1	0
Chills	14	2	0	0	16	59	16	2
ALT	5	4	2	0	11	41		
AST	3	5	2	0	10	37		
Tachycardia	9	0	0	0	9	33	9	0
Hypertension	6	2	0	0	8	30	8	1
Albuminemia	7	1	0	0	8	30		
ALP	4	2	0	0	6	22		
Weight gain	5	0	0	0	5	19		
Nausea	4	1	0	0	5	19	5	1
Hyponatremia	5	0	0	0	5	19		
Hypoxemia	0	2	3	0	5	19	4	4
Hypotension	2	2	0	0	4	15	3	1
Pruritus	0	3	1	0	4	15		
γ-GTP	0	1	3	0	4	15		
Hypophosphatemia	0	4	0	0	4	15		
Hyperuricemia	4	0	0	0	4	15		
Hypercalcemia	1	1	0	1	3	11		
Hypokalemia	1	0	2	0	3	11		
Erythema multiforme†	0	0	1	0	1	4		
Hyperglycemia	0	0	1	0	1	4		
Tumor lysis syndrome	0	0	1	0	1	4		
Metabolic/laboratory, other‡	4	7	3	0	14	52		
Hematologic								
Lymphopenia§	0	6	9	11	26	96		
Leukocytopenia	3	7	8	0	18	67		
Thrombocytopenia	7	2	3	2	14	52		
Neutropenia	5	4	5	0	14	52		
Hemoglobin	4	3	1	0	8	30		

ALP **alkaline phosphatase,** *BUN* **blood urea nitrogen,** *CRP* **C-reactive protein,** *GTP* **glutamyl transpeptidase**

[a]Of 28 patients enrolled, 27 received at least one infusion of KW-0761. Listed are adverse events determined as possibly, probably, or definitely KW-0761 related that occurred in at least 15% of patients or were of grade 3–4 severity

[b]One patient diagnosed as having Stevens-Johnson syndrome

[c]Other metabolic and laboratory test abnormalities included hypoproteinemia, BUN elevation, CRP, glycosuria, hypochloremia, and hyperammonemia

[d]Lymphopenia included decrease of abnormal lymphocytes

reached in either arm (Fig. 9.6). Grade ≥3 treatment-emergent adverse events, including anemia, thrombocytopenia, lymphopenia, leukopenia, and decreased appetite, were observed more frequently (≥10% difference) in the mLSG15-plus-mogamulizumab arm. Several adverse events, including skin disorders, cytomegalovirus infection, pyrexia, hyperglycemia, and interstitial lung disease, were

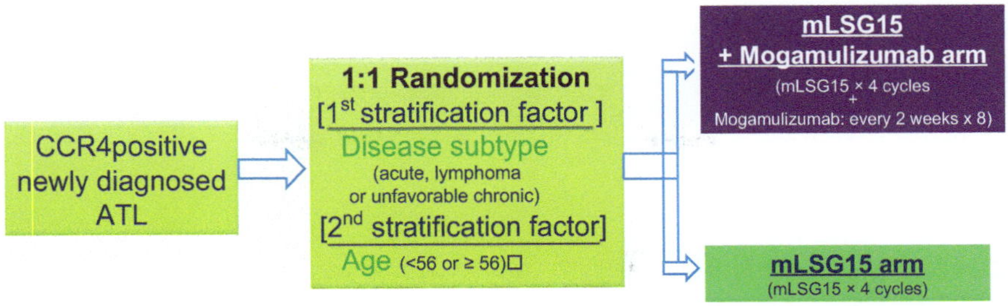

Fig. 9.5 Study design of randomized phase II study in newly diagnosed ATL. The primary end point was the complete response rate (%CR). Eligible patients were randomly assigned in a 1:1 ratio to the two treatment groups based on dynamic allocation and minimization by a central randomization center

Table 9.5 Demographics and clinical characteristics of randomized phase II study (Ref. [17])

	mLSG15 + mogamulizumab (*n* = 29)	mLSG15 (*n* = 24)[a]
ATL subtype		
Acute	20 (69%)	17 (71%)
Lymphoma	6 (21%)	7 (29%)
Chronic[b]	3 (10%)	0 (0%)
Age, years		
Median	61	64
Range	49–81	37–74
<56	11 (38%)	6 (25%)
≥56	18 (62%)	18 (75%)
Sex		
Male	12 (41%)	16 (67%)
Female	17 (59%)	8 (33%)
ECOG PS		
0	16 (55%)	13 (54%)
1	10 (35%)	9 (38%)
2	3 (10%)	2 (8%)

ECOG Eastern Cooperative Oncology Group, *PS* performance status
[a]25 patients were randomized; 24 were treated
[b]Chronic type with poor prognostic factors

observed only in the mLSG15-plus-mogamulizumab arm. Although the combination strategy showed a potentially less favorable safety profile, a higher %CR was achieved, providing the basis for further investigation of this novel treatment for newly diagnosed aggressive ATL. Based on these data of this randomized phase II study, mogamulizumab was approved for the expansion of indication in newly diagnosed CCR4+ ATL on December 2014 in Japan.

Table 9.6 Response to treatment in randomized phase II study in newly diagnosed ATL (Ref. [17])

	mLSG15 + mogamulizumab ($n = 29$)	mLSG15 ($n = 24$)
CR	9	5
CRu	6	3
PR	10	10
CR + CRu	15	8
%CR (95% CI)	52% (33–71)	33% (16–55)
Between-group difference (95% CI)	18·4% (−8·9 to 43·8)	
CR + CRu + PR	25	18
ORR (95% CI)	86% (68–96)	75% (53–90)

CR complete response, *CRu* uncertified complete response, *PR* partial response; *%CR* complete response rate, *CI* confidence interval, *ORR* overall response rate

Recently, the impact of pretransplantation mogamulizumab on clinical outcomes after allogeneic-hematopoietic stem cell transplantation (allo-HSCT) was reported [18]. In this retrospective analysis of 996 allo-HSCT recipients age 70 years or younger with aggressive ATL who were given the diagnosis between 2000 and 2013 and who received intensive chemotherapy by multiple chemotherapeutic drugs as first-line therapy, 82 patients received mogamulizumab with a median interval of 45 days from the last mogamulizumab to allo-HSCT. Pretransplantation mogamulizumab was associated with an increased risk of grade 3–4 acute graft-versus-host disease (GVHD; relative risk, 1.80; $P < 0.01$) and refractoriness to systemic corticosteroid for acute GVHD (relative risk, 2.09; $P < 0.01$). The probability of 1-year overall survival was significantly inferior in patients with pretransplantation mogamulizumab compared with those without (32.3% v 49.4%; $P < 0.01$). Pretransplantation mogamulizumab was significantly associated with an increased risk of GVHD-related mortality, which supports the relevance of CCR4-expressing regulatory T cells after allo-HSCT in humans. Therefore, in clinical practice, mogamulizumab should be cautiously used for patients with ATL who are eligible for allo-HSCT.

Mogamulizumab was also approved in relapsed or refractory peripheral T-cell lymphoma (PTCL) and cutaneous T-cell lymphoma (CTCL) based on the data of a phase II study in relapsed/refractory PTCL/CTCL on April 2014 in Japan [19].

Mogamulizumab is expected to become a core agent with other drugs including molecular targeting drugs such as romidepsin, lenalidomide, forodesine, and darinaparsin or chemotherapeutic drugs including pralatrexate in ATL or PTCL/CTCL.

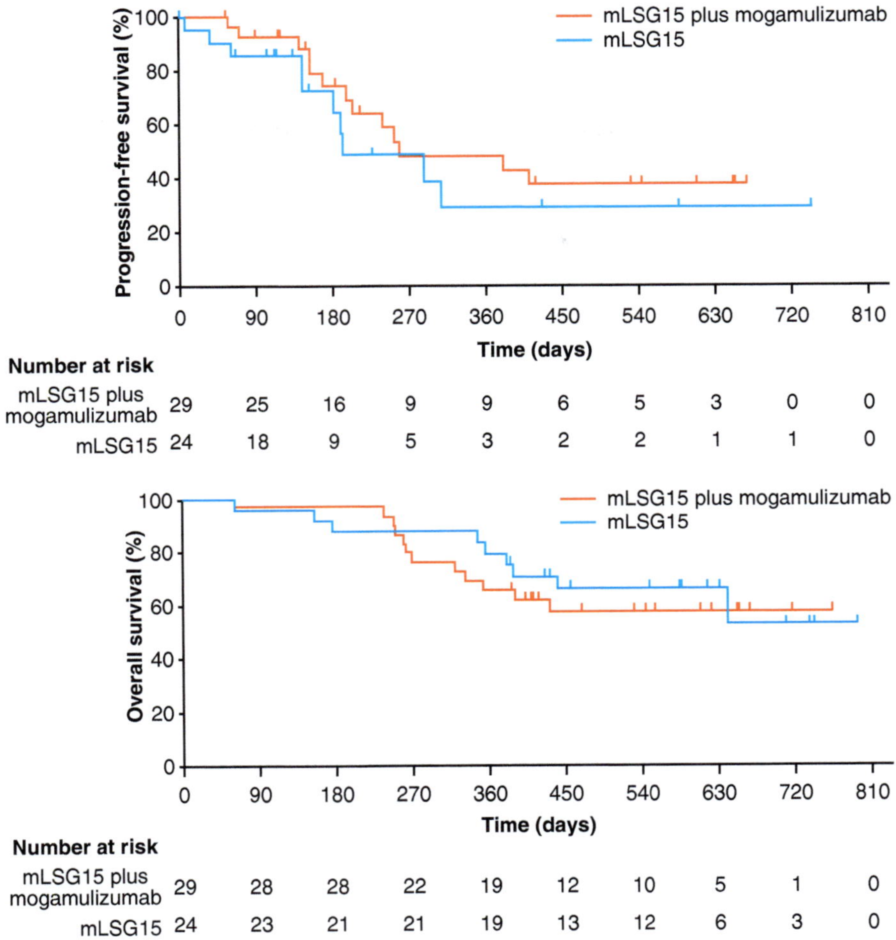

Fig. 9.6 Progression-free survival and overall survival in randomized phase II study. **a** Kaplan-Meier curve of estimated progression-free survival (median, 8•5 and 6•3 months in the mLSG15-plus-mogamulizumab and mLSG15 arms, respectively). **b** Kaplan-Meier curve of estimated overall survival (median, not achieved in either arm). The median follow-up periods in the mLSG15-plus-mogamulizumab and mLSG15 arms were 413 days (range, 63–764 days) and 502 days (range, 62–794 days), respectively. (Ref. [17])

References

1. Shimoyama M. Diagnostic criteria and classification of clinical subtypes of adult T-cell leukaemia-lymphoma: a report from the Lymphoma Study Group (1984–87). Br J Haematol. 1991;79:428–37.
2. Vose J, Armitage J, Weisenburger D. International peripheral T-cell and natural killer/T-cell lymphoma study: pathology findings and clinical outcomes. J Clin Oncol. 2008;26:4124–30.
3. Uchiyama T, Yodoi J, Sagawa K, et al. Adult T-cell leukemia: clinical and hematologic features of 16 cases. Blood. 1977;50:481–92.
4. Tsukasaki K, Hermine O, Bazarbachi A, et al. Definition, prognostic factors, treatment, and response criteria of adult T-cell leukemia-lymphoma: a proposal from an international consensus meeting. J Clin Oncol. 2009;27:453–9.
5. Tsukasaki K, Utsunomiya A, Fukuda H, et al. VCAP-AMP-VECP compared with biweekly CHOP for adult T-cell leukemia-lymphoma: Japan Clinical Oncology Group Study JCOG 9801. J Clin Oncol. 2007;25:5458–64.
6. Utsunomiya A, Miyazaki Y, Takatsuka Y, et al. Improved outcome of adult T cell leukemia/lymphoma with allogeneic hematopoietic stem cell transplantation. Bone Marrow Transplant. 2001;27:15–20.
7. Hishizawa M, Kanda J, Utsunomiya A, et al. Transplantation of allogeneic hematopoietic stem cells for adult T-cell leukemia: a nationwide retrospective study. Blood. 2010;116:1369–76.
8. Ishida T, Utsunomiya A, Iida S, et al. Clinical significance of CCR4 expression in adult T-cell leukemia/lymphoma: its close association with skin involvement and unfavorable outcome. Clin Cancer Res. 2003;9:3625–34.
9. Yoshie O, Fujisawa R, Nakayama T, et al. Frequent expression of CCR4 in adult T-cell leukemia and human T-cell leukemia virus type 1-transformed T cells. Blood. 2002;99:1505–11.
10. Shinkawa T, Nakamura K, Yamane N, et al. The absence of fucose but not the presence of galactose or bisecting N-acetylglucosamine of human IgG1 complex-type oligosaccharides shows the critical role of enhancing antibody-dependent cellular cytotoxicity. J Biol Chem. 2003;278:3466–73.
11. Ishii T, Ishida T, Utsunomiya A, et al. Defucosylated humanized anti-CCR4 monoclonal antibody KW-0761 as a novel immunotherapeutic agent for adult T-cell leukemia/lymphoma. Clin Cancer Res. 2010;16:1520–31.
12. Yano H, Ishida T, Inagaki A, Ishii T, Ding J, Kusumoto S, et al. Defucosylated anti CC chemokine receptor 4 monoclonal anti-body combined with immunomodulatory cytokines: a novel immunotherapy for aggressive/refractory mycosis fungoides and Sezary syndrome. Clin Cancer Res. 2007;13:6494–500.
13. Ishida T, Iida S, Akatsuka Y, et al. The CC chemokine receptor 4 as a novel specific molecular target for immunotherapy in adult T-Cell leukemia/lymphoma. Clin Cancer Res. 2004;10:7529–39.
14. Ishida T, Utsunomiya A, Iida S, et al. Clinical significance of CCR4 expression in adult T-cell leukemia/lymphoma: its close association with skin involvement and unfavorable outcome. Clin Cancer Res. 2003;9:3625–34.
15. Yamamoto K, Utsunomiya A, Tobinai K, et al. Phase I study of KW-0761, a defucosylated humanized anti-CCR4 antibody, in relapsed patients with adult T-cell leukemia-lymphoma and peripheral T-cell lymphoma. J Clin Oncol. 2010;28:1591–8.
16. Ishida T, Joh T, Uike N, et al. Defucosylated anti-CCR4 monoclonal antibody (KW-0761) for relapsed adult T-cell leukemia-lymphoma: a multicenter phase II study. J Clin Oncol. 2012;30:837–42.
17. Ishida T, Jo T, Takemoto S, et al. Dose-intensified chemotherapy alone or in combination with mogamulizumab in newly diagnosed aggressive adult T-cell leukaemia-lymphoma: a randomized phase II study. Br J Haematol. 2015;169:672–82.

18. Fuji S, Inoue Y, Utsunomiya A, et al. Pretransplantation Anti-CCR4 antibody mogamulizumab against adult T-cell leukemia/lymphoma is associated with significantly increased risks of severe and corticosteroid-refractory graft-versus-host disease, nonrelapse mortality, and overall mortality. J Clin Oncol. 2016 Oct 1;34(28):3426–33.
19. Ogura M, Ishida T, Hatake K, et al. Multicenter phase II study of mogamulizumab (KW-0761), a defucosylated anti-cc chemokine receptor 4 antibody, in patients with relapsed peripheral T-cell lymphoma and cutaneous T-cell lymphoma. J Clin Oncol. 2014;32:1157–63.

Part III

Signaling Inhibitors

FLT3 Inhibitors 10

Hitoshi Kiyoi

Abstract

FLT3 is a type III receptor tyrosine kinase and expresses in most acute leukemia cells as well as normal hematopoietic stem/progenitor cells. *FLT3* mutation is the most frequent genetic alteration in acute myeloid leukemia (AML) and is associated with poor prognosis in AML patients. Since high-dose chemotherapy including allogeneic hematopoietic stem cell transplantation cannot overcome a poor prognosis, development of FLT3 inhibitor is highly expected. To date, several FLT3 inhibitors have been developed and evaluated for safety and efficacy in clinical trials; however, no FLT3 inhibitor has been yet approved for the patients with FLT3 mutations. In addition, several problems for clinical use, such as adverse effects, blood concentration, and resistance, have been apparent in clinical trials. FLT3 inhibitors are now developed in two ways: monotherapy and combination therapy with chemotherapy. Although further evaluations are required in each FLT3 inhibitor, I summarize the characteristics of FLT3 inhibitors in clinical development and discuss important issues to be resolved for clinical use.

Keywords

FLT3 • Inhibitors • Leukemia • Tyrosine kinase • Resistance

H. Kiyoi (✉)
Department of Hematology and Oncology, Nagoya University Graduate School of Medicine, 65 Tsurumai-cho, Showa-ku, Nagoya, Aichi 466-8550, Japan
e-mail: kiyoi@med.nagoya-u.ac.jp

T. Ueda (ed.), *Chemotherapy for Leukemia*, DOI 10.1007/978-981-10-3332-2_10

10.1 Introduction

FLT3 (FMS-like receptor tyrosine kinase) is a class III receptor tyrosine kinase (RTK) together with KIT, FMS, and platelet-derived growth factor receptor (PDGFR) [1–3] and consists of five immunoglobulin-like domains in the extracellular region, a juxtamembrane (JM) domain, a tyrosine kinase (TK) domain separated by a kinase insert (KI) domain, and a C-terminal domain in the intracellular region [4]. FLT3 is expressed in hematopoietic stem cells as well as in the brain, placenta, and liver [2, 5]. The ligand to FLT3 (FL) is expressed as a membrane-bound or soluble form by bone marrow stroma cells and stimulates hematopoietic stem/progenitor cells [6–10]. FL-FLT3 interaction, therefore, plays an important role in the survival, proliferation, and differentiation of stem cells. On the other hand, FLT3 is expressed in most acute myeloid leukemia (AML) and B-lineage acute lymphocytic leukemia (ALL) cells [11–16]. Although FL stimulation enhances proliferation and reduces apoptosis in FLT3-expressing leukemia cells, it had not been clear how FLT3-mediating signal is involved in the pathophysiology of leukemia until the discovery of *FLT3* mutations in AML [17]. There are two types of mutations: an internal tandem duplication in the JM domain-coding sequence of the *FLT3* gene (*FLT3*-ITD) [18] and point mutations at the D835 residue and point mutations, deletions, and insertions in the codons surrounding D835 within a TK domain of FLT3 (*FLT3*-KDM) [19–25]. *FLT3*-ITD and *FLT3*-KDM occur in 15–35% and 5–10% adults with AML, respectively, and are associated with a poor prognosis [26–31]. Both FLT3-ITD and FLT3-KDM proteins are ligand independently activated and constitutively activate downstream signaling molecules, such as MAPK, STAT5, and AKT. Therefore, mutated FLT3 serves as a promising molecular target for the treatment of acute leukemia. To date, many potent FLT3 inhibitors have been developed, and some of them have been evaluated clinical efficacy and safety; however, no FLT3 inhibitors have been yet approved for clinical use. In addition, several problems for clinical use, such as adverse effects, blood concentration, and resistance, have been apparent in clinical trials. To overcome these disadvantages, combination therapy with a traditional chemotherapy and next-generation FLT3 inhibitors are clinically developed. Here, I will summarize the characteristics of FLT3 inhibitors, which have been clinically developed, and future problems to be resolved for clinical use.

10.2 Type I and Type II Inhibitors

The binding of FL to the extracellular domain of FLT3 leads to its dimerization, stabilizing a conformation of the catalytic domain with the activation loop (A-loop) in an open conformation. This conformation of the active site accommodates ATP and substrate binding, enabling transphosphorylation of the A-loop, stabilizing the catalytic domain in an active conformation. Dimerization and the subsequent phosphorylation of tyrosine residues are essential for the activation of FLT3, followed by induction of multiple intracellular signaling pathways leading to cell proliferation

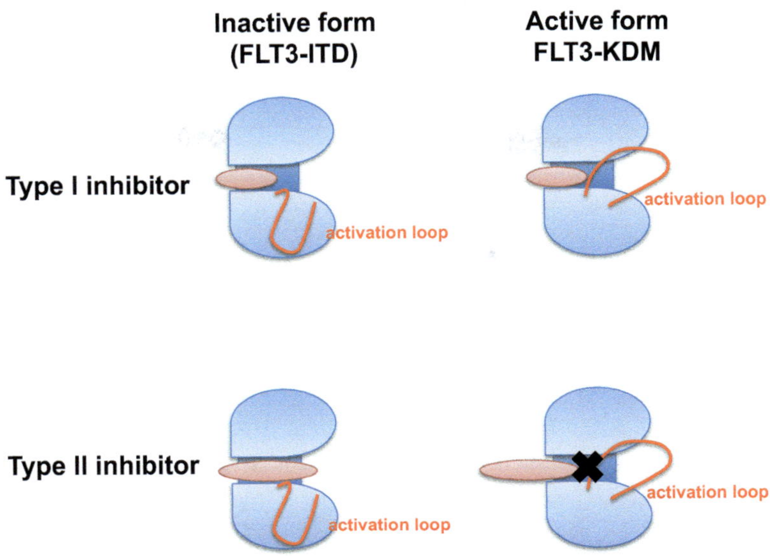

Fig. 10.1 Type I and type II FLT3 inhibitors. The binding of FL to the extracellular domain of wild-type FLT3 leads to its dimerization, stabilizing a conformation in an active conformation. FLT3-ITD takes a form of inactive conformation, while KDMs destabilize the inactive conformation of FLT3 in favor of the active conformation. Type I inhibitor can bond to both active and inactive conformations, while type II inhibitor cannot bind to active conformation

and activation [32]. FLT3 inhibitors compete with ATP for the binding, resulting in the inhibition of kinase activation. FLT3 inhibitors are classified into two types according to the binding potency to inactive and active conformations of FLT3. Type I inhibitors bind both inactive and active conformations of FLT3, while type II inhibitors can only bind the inactive conformation of FLT3 (Fig. 10.1). FLT3-ITD takes a form of inactive conformation, while KDMs destabilize the inactive conformation of FLT3 in favor of the active conformation. Therefore, type I FLT3 inhibitors block activations of both FLT3-ITD and FLT3-KDM, while type II inhibitors cannot block the FLT3-KDM activation.

10.3 First-Generation FLT3 Inhibitors

After the discovery of FLT3 mutations, tyrosine kinase inhibitors (TKIs), which have a potency to inhibit the FLT3 kinase, were firstly subjected to clinical trials (Fig. 10.2) [33].

Tandutinib (Millennium) is a derivative of quinazoline. Although this compound has a high selectivity against FLT3, the IC_{50} value (220 nM) is lower than the other FLT3 inhibitors [34]. Furthermore, it inhibits the FLT3-ITD, but not FLT3-KDM, indicating a type II inhibitor [35]. In a Phase 1 study of 40 patients with relapsed or refractory AML, three patients had 40–50% reduction in the number of bone

Inhibitor	Tandutinib	Lestaurtinib	Midostaurin	Sorafenib
IC_{50} against FLT3 (nM)	220	3	<10	58

Structure

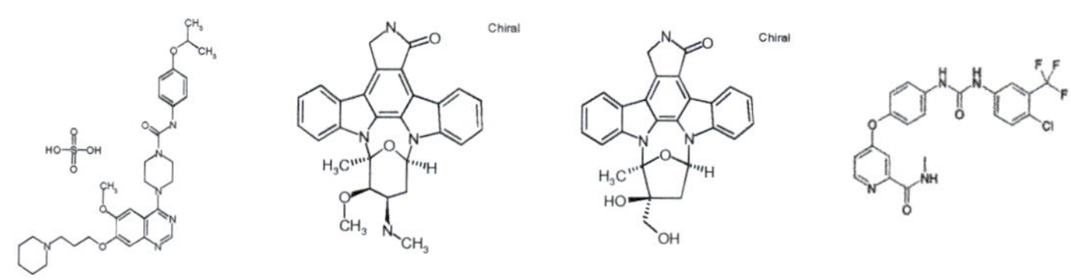

Kinase dendrogram

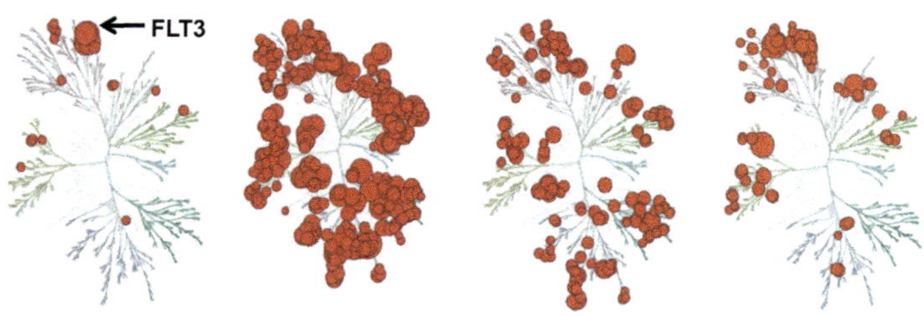

Fig. 10.2 Structure and inhibitory activity of first-generation FLT3 inhibitors. Tandutinib and sorafenib are type II inhibitor. Lestaurtinib and midostaurin are type I inhibitor, but have lower selectivity against FLT3

marrow (BM) blasts. In this study, no adverse effects were observed, while the peak plasma concentration of this compound did not reach to the biologically effective level. In a Phase 2 study of 25 patients with relapsed or refractory AML harboring *FLT3*-ITD, a decrease of peripheral and BM leukemia cells was observed in seven of the 15 patients, while clinical response could not be evaluated in eight patients because of rapid disease progression or the toxicity, such as ptosis and QTc prolongation [36]. Therefore, further clinical development was discontinued.

Sunitinib (Pfizer) is a derivative of indolinone and has been approved for renal cell carcinoma, gastrointestinal stromal tumor (GIST), and neuroendocrine tumor (NET) in Japan. It belongs to a type I inhibitor, has a unique inhibiting property to tyrosine kinases, and inhibits KIT, PDGFR, and KDR kinases more sensitively than FLT3 kinase (Fig. 10.2). In a Phase 1 study of 15 patients with advanced AML, the tentative reduction of peripheral blast cells was observed in seven patients [37]. Since two patients died of cardiotoxicity and the plasma concentration was brought to the biologically effective level, a further clinical development for AML has been discontinued.

Lestaurtinib (Cephalon) was derived from indolocarbazole. This compound is a type I inhibitor with a high potency against FLT3 kinases (IC_{50} is 3 nM), but has potencies against multiple kinases [38, 39]. In a Phase 2a study of 12 AML patients with FLT3 mutations, the reduction of peripheral blast cells under 5% or the loss of BM blasts was observed in four patients, while the complete remission (CR) was not achieved in any patients [40]. Since this compound is also a derivative of indolocarbazole, the plasma concentration is lower than expected. The clinical efficacy of this compound alone seemed to be limited, so a Phase 2 study with a combination of lestaurtinib and conventional chemotherapeutic agents was conducted [41]. In this study, 224 patients with the first relapsed AML harboring FLT3 mutations were randomly assigned to chemotherapy (MEC or high-dose AraC) alone or a combination of chemotherapy and lestaurtinib. The CR/CRp rate in the combination group (16%) was not statistically better than that in the chemotherapy group (21%). Based on these results, further clinical development of lestaurtinib has been discontinued.

Sorafenib (Bayer) is a type II multikinase inhibitor, which has potency against RAF-1, VEGFR, PDGFR, KIT, and FLT3, and has been approved for hepatocellular carcinoma and renal cell cancer (Fig. 10.2) [42]. The IC_{50} value against FLT3 is 58 nM. Although clinical efficacy of sorafenib monotherapy was limited to the transient blast reduction in two Phase 1 studies, a combination with chemotherapy revealed a high CR rate in the relapsed and/or refractory AML patients with *FLT3*-ITD mutations [43]. However, since a combination of chemotherapy and sorafenib did not show better overall and event-free survivals than a chemotherapy alone in elderly AML patients, further studies are required to evaluate the efficacy and safety of the combination therapy [44].

Midostaurin (Novartis) is a benzoylstaurosporine, initially developed as a KDR inhibitor, and belongs to a type I inhibitor (Fig. 10.2) [45]. In a Phase 2 study of 61 patients including 11 *FLT3*-ITD and 4 *FLT3*-KDM patients, half of the enrolled patients showed over a 50% reduction in the number of bone marrow blasts [46]. Although one AML patient with *FLT3*-ITD achieved complete remission, the duration was very short. Pharmacokinetic properties showed that the plasma concentration of this compound could not be maintained at the biologically effective level, because it consists of an indolocarbazole molecule, which is known to be highly associated with acid-α-glycoprotein (AGP) in human plasma. Notably, two patients died of pulmonary edema, which was considered a drug-induced toxicity. Since it was concluded that a monotherapy of midostaurin did not have sufficient clinical activity in AML patients with *FLT3* mutations, a combination with chemotherapeutic regimens is evaluated. A randomized Phase 3 study (CALGB 10603/RATIFY study) was conducted for evaluating the superiority of midostaurin in addition to the conventional induction and consolidation therapies, and the interesting results were reported at the 57th Annual Meeting of ASH in 2015 . Between May 2008 and October 2011, 717 patients (555 FLT3-ITD; 162 FLT3-KDM) were randomized to either the conventional chemotherapy plus midostaurin ($n = 360$) or the conventional chemotherapy plus placebo ($n = 357$). Overall and event-free survivals were significantly superior in the midostaurin group than placebo group ($P = 0.007$ and 0.004, respectively) (Table 10.1). This study firstly demonstrated that the

Table 10.1 Results of CALGB 10603/RATIFY study

	Arm	Median month (95% CI)	*P* value
Overall survival	Midostaurin	74.7 (31.5, not attained)	0.007
	Placebo	26.0 (18.5, 46.5)	
Overall survival (SCT censored)	Midostaurin	Not attained	0.047
	Placebo	Not attained	
Event-free survival	Midostaurin	8.0 (5.3, 10.6)	0.0044
	Placebo	3.0 (1.9, 5.8)	
Event-free survival (SCT censored)	Midostaurin	8.2 (5.5, 10.7)	0.025
	Placebo	3.0 (1.9, 5.8)	

combination of chemotherapy and FLT3 inhibitor improves the long-term prognosis of the AML patients with FLT3 mutations. However, the CR rate of chemotherapy and midostaurin group (59%) was the same as that of chemotherapy and placebo group (54%), indicating that further study is required for fully understanding the significance of midostaurin in the induction therapy.

10.4 Second-Generation FLT3 Inhibitors

Clinical efficacies of first-generation FLT3 inhibitor monotherapy were lower than expected. In addition, several problems, such as maintaining the effective plasma concentration and serious adverse events, have been apparent to be resolved before clinical use. Since the first-generation FLT3 inhibitors were not originally screened for the sensitivity and selectivity against the activated FLT3 kinase, the second-generation FLT3 inhibitors have been developed based on the growth inhibitory effects against leukemia cells with FLT3 mutations (Fig. 10.3).

Quizartinib (Daiichi-Sankyo) has been screened for the affinity against FLT3 using the KinomeScan technique and has a high selectivity and sensitivity to FLT3. Although the IC_{50} value against dephosphorylation of FLT3-ITD is 1.1 nM, this compound does not have a potency against FLT3-KDM (type II inhibitor) [33]. The preclinical study showed the high bioavailability and AUC [47]. In a Phase 1 study, the QTc prolongation was the dose-limiting toxicity, while one CR and four incomplete CR (CRi) were observed in 18 AML patients harboring *FLT3*-ITD. In a Phase 2 study, 40 of the 79 (50.6%) patients with relapsed and/or refractory AML harboring *FLT3*-ITD achieved CRp or CRi. However, no CR was observed due to the BM suppression. The BM suppression is thought to be caused by the KIT inhibition of quizartinib. In addition, the QTc prolongation was also observed even at the recommended dose, which was determined by the Phase 1 study. These results indicated the strong potency of quizartinib against AML cells harboring FLT3-ITD, while it is necessary to determine the optimal dose and/or schedule in the clinical use.

Crenolanib (Arog Pharmaceuticals) is a benzamidine quinolone derivative and developed as a potent inhibitor of PDGFR, while subsequent analysis revealed that

Inhibitor	Quizartinib	Crenolanib	Gilteritinib
IC_{50} against FLT3 (nM)	1.1	1.3	0.29
Structure	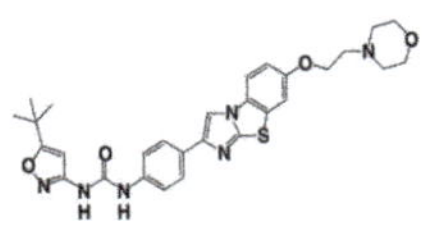	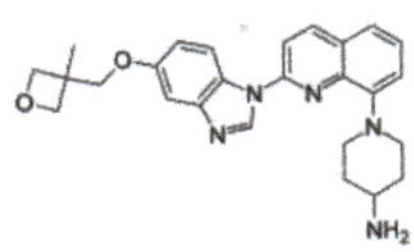	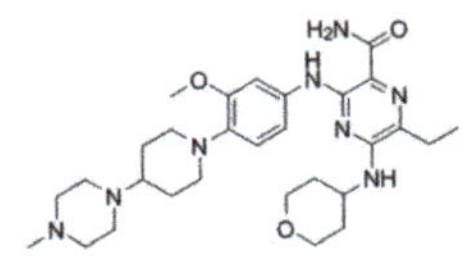
Kinase dendrogram	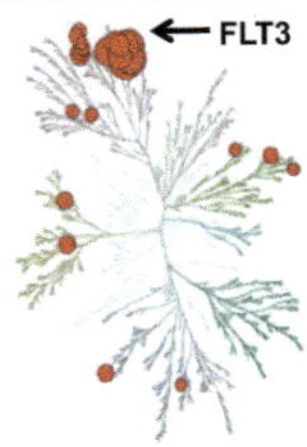	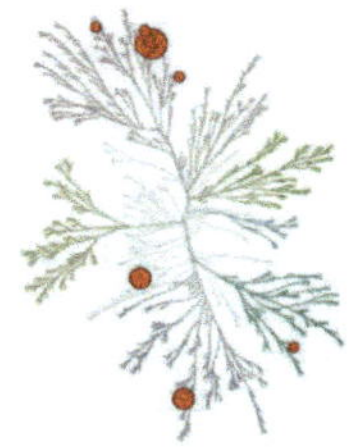	not available

Fig. 10.3 Structure and inhibitory activity of second-generation FLT3 inhibitors. Quizartinib is a highly FLT3 selective type II inhibitor. Crenolanib and gilteritinib are type I inhibitors, and their inhibitory profiles are more FLT3 selective than lestaurtinib and midostaurin

it has a potency against both FLT3-ITD and FLT3-KDM (Fig. 10.3) [48]. Crenolanib is a type I inhibitor and has the same potency against FLT3-ITD (IC_{50} is 1.3 nM) as quizartinib. Although it has a potency against FLT3-KDM, inhibitory activities are different in the types of FLT3-KDM. Of note is that crenolanib inhibits all types of D835-mutated FLT3 kinases, but does not F691L-mutated FLT3 (Table 10.2). Furthermore, recent study demonstrated that the combination with type II inhibitor sorafenib increases antileukemia activity, suggesting that simultaneous type I and type II inhibition may increase efficacy of leukemia cells regardless mutation types of FLT3 [49]. Clinical efficacy and safety of crenolanib is now evaluated by monotherapy and combination therapy with conventional chemotherapy or sorafenib.

Gilteritinib (ASP2215, Astellas) has been developed for a selective inhibitor of AXL and FLT3. It was reported that gilteritinib has a potency against both FLT3-ITD and D835-mutated FLT3 (type I inhibitor). The preliminary data of Phase 1/2 study was reported at the Annual Meeting of ASCO in 2015. Although gilteritinib was well tolerated from 20 to 300 mg, DLT (Grade 3 diarrhea and AST/ALT elevation) was observed in two patients at 450 mg. The MTD was, therefore, determined as 300 mg. It was also reported that composite complete remission (CRc; CR, CRp, and CRi) and overall response (CRc plus partial remission) were observed in 47.2% and 57.5%, respectively, in 106 relapsed or refractory AML patients with FLT3 mutations who were treated with more than 80 mg of gilteritinib. Randomized

Table 10.2 Inhibitory activity of crenolanib against mutant FLT3 kinases

Mutation type	IC50 (nM)
ITD	1.3
D835Y	6.9
D835F	6.5
D835H	19.8
D835N	4.3
D835V	2.3
ITD/D835Y	8.7
ITD/F691L	67.8

Phase III study of gilteritinib versus salvage chemotherapy in patients with relapsed or refractory AML with FLT3 mutation is now conducted.

10.5 Resistance of FLT3 Inhibitors

To date, several FLT3 inhibitors were subjected to the clinical trials. Although each FLT3 inhibitor has a characteristic property about sensitivity and selectivity, resistance has been apparent regardless the character through the early clinical studies. Resistant mechanisms of FLT3 inhibitors are classified into primary and secondary resistances (Table 10.3) [50, 51]. The primary resistance includes a different potency against types of FLT3 mutations, other activating signals, and the lower potency against leukemia stem cells. Although FLT3 inhibitors were classified into type I and type II inhibitor based on the potencies against FLT3-ITD and FLT3-KDM, it remains unclear which type of inhibitor improves the prognosis of the patients with FLT3 mutations. Since the first-generation type I inhibitors, such as lestaurtinib and midostaurin, have potency against many kinases in addition to FLT3, adverse events by off-target effects were thought to be a disadvantage of type I inhibitor. Therefore, clinical efficacy of more FLT3 selective type I inhibitors, such as crenolanib and gilteritinib, is highly expected. However, recent results of Phase 3 study demonstrated that an addition of midostaurin to chemotherapy significantly improved both overall and event-free survivals in AML patients with FLT3 mutations; further study is required to clarify how type I inhibitors should be used for getting the best clinical result.

The secondary resistance includes FL-dependent resistance, an acquisition of resistant mutations, and overexpression of FLT3 (Table 10.3). It was reported that the growth inhibitory effect of FLT3 inhibitors is reduced by the addition of FL in vitro (Table 10.4) [52]. In a Phase 2 study of lestaurtinib, the plasma concentration of FL was increased during the treatment of lestaurtinib, and the high FL concentration was associated with lower clinical efficacy. The most important resistance mechanism is the acquisition of resistant mutations. The resistant mutation was not clearly identified in Phase 1/2 studies of the first-generation FLT3 inhibitors, because their monotherapy did not show sufficient clinical efficacies. However,

Table 10.3 Primary and secondary resistant mechanism of FLT3 inhibitor

Primary resistance	Secondary resistance
Low potency against FLT3-KDM	Acquiring resistant mutations
Other activating signals	FL stimulation
Low potency against leukemia stem cells	Overexpression of FLT3

Table 10.4 Comparison of GI_{50} values of FLT3 inhibitors in the FL present condition

	GI_{50} value against MOLM14 (nM)			
FLT3 inhibitors	FL	0 ng/mL	10 ng/mL	Inhibitory ratio
Lestaurtinib		3.3	6.8	2.1
Midostaurin		7.2	25	3.5
Sorafenib		3.3	12	3.6
Quizartinib		0.38	1.3	3.4

Addition of FL reduces the GI_{50} values of FLT3 inhibitors against *FLT3*-ITD-positive human AML cell line MOLM14

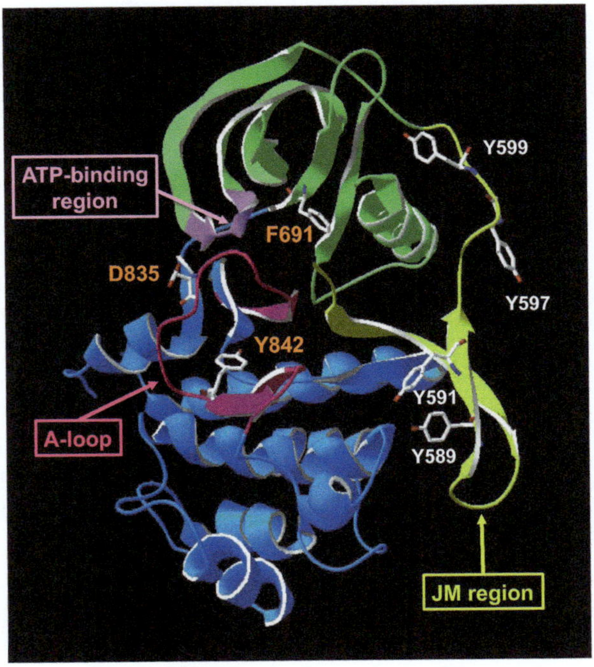

Fig. 10.4 Structure of FLT3 and resistant mutations. In the inactive form of wild-type FLT3, the JM domain blocks activation of the kinase and may inhibit self-dimerization. Mutations of D835 and Y842 residues in the A-loop induce a conformational change blocking the binding of FLT3 inhibitors to the ATP-binding pocket. Since the F691 residue is a gatekeeper of the ATP-binding pocket, its mutation also blocks the binding of FLT3 inhibitors

several resistant mutations were identified in the patients who were treated with quizartinib [53]. It has been reported that D835Y, D835V, D835F, or F691L mutations were additionally acquired at relapse in eight patients with *FLT3*-ITD who achieved CR by the quizartinib monotherapy. Since these mutated residues structurally exist around the ATP-binding pocket and the F691L mutation corresponds to the gatekeeper mutation, T315I, in the *BCR-ABL* gene, the binding of quizartinib to

Table 10.5 GI_{50} values of FLT3 inhibitors against mutation types

	GI_{50} (nM) [relative ratio to ITD]			
Mutation type	Quizartinib	Sorafenib	Ponatinib	Crenolanib
FLT3/ITD	0.13 [1]	1.3 [1]	3.0 [1]	1.3 [1]
FLT3/ITD+F691L	102 [785]	1189 [915]	52 [17]	67.8 [52.2]
FLT3/ITD+F691I	122 [938]	648 [498]	4.2 [1.4]	–
FLT3/ITD+D835V	120 [923]	2209 [1699]	349 [116]	–
FLT3/ITD+D835Y	28 [215]	675 [519]	284 [95]	8.7 [6.7]
FLT3/ITD+D835F	166 [1277]	2374 [1826]	414 [138]	–
FLT3/ITD+D835H	5.5 [42]	164 [126]	211 [70]	–
FLT3/ITD+D839G	1.9 [15]	112 [86]	54 [18]	–
FLT3/ITD+Y842C	33 [254]	469 [361]	229 [76]	–
FLT3/ITD+Y842H	18 [138]	260 [200]	80 [27]	–

mutant FLT3 is blocked (Fig. 10.4). Consistently, most resistant mutations acquired after the treatment of quizartinib are resistant to another type II inhibitor sorafenib, while novel type I inhibitor, such as ponatinib and crenolanib, shows inhibitory activities against those resistant mutations (Table 10.5). Since the clinical efficacies and selectivity of first-generation FLT3 inhibitors were lower, more selective and sensitive FLT3 inhibitors are thought to be better for clinical use. However, resistant mutation was easily induced by quizartinib, which showed the best clinical efficacy in clinically developed FLT3 inhibitors. Therefore, it remains unclear whether FLT3-selective inhibitor is clinically better than multikinase inhibitor.

10.6 Conclusion

Since *FLT3* mutation is the most frequent genetic alteration and a poor prognostic factor for the long-term survival in AML patients, FLT3 is a promising therapeutic target. Although clinical efficacies of the first-generation FLT3 inhibitors were unimpressive, it has been proved by the quizartinib study that selective and continuous FLT3 inhibition could provide patients with CR. Several novel type I FLT3 inhibitors are now clinically investigated. It is highly expected that next-generation FLT3 inhibitors will make for a more efficacious therapeutic strategy for leukemia therapy.

References

1. Rosnet O, Marchetto S, de Lapeyriere O, Birnbaum D. Murine Flt3, a gene encoding a novel tyrosine kinase receptor of the PDGFR/CSF1R family. Oncogene. 1991;6(9):1641–50.
2. Rosnet O, Schiff C, Pebusque MJ, Marchetto S, Tonnelle C, Toiron Y, et al. Human FLT3/FLK2 gene: cDNA cloning and expression in hematopoietic cells. Blood. 1993;82(4):1110–9.

3. Lyman SD, James L, Zappone J, Sleath PR, Beckmann MP, Bird T. Characterization of the protein encoded by the flt3 (flk2) receptor-like tyrosine kinase gene. Oncogene. 1993;8(4):815–22.
4. Matthews W, Jordan CT, Wiegand GW, Pardoll D, Lemischka IR. A receptor tyrosine kinase specific to hematopoietic stem and progenitor cell-enriched populations. Cell. 1991;65(7):1143–52.
5. Rosnet O, Buhring HJ, de Lapeyriere O, Beslu N, Lavagna C, Marchetto S, et al. Expression and signal transduction of the FLT3 tyrosine kinase receptor. Acta Haematol. 1996a;95(3–4):218–23.
6. Hannum C, Culpepper J, Campbell D, McClanahan T, Zurawski S, Bazan JF, et al. Ligand for FLT3/FLK2 receptor tyrosine kinase regulates growth of haematopoietic stem cells and is encoded by variant RNAs. Nature. 1994;368(6472):643–8.
7. McKenna HJ, Smith FO, Brasel K, Hirschstein D, Bernstein ID, Williams DE, et al. Effects of flt3 ligand on acute myeloid and lymphocytic leukemic blast cells from children. Exp Hematol. 1996;24(2):378–85.
8. Rusten LS, Lyman SD, Veiby OP, Jacobsen SE. The FLT3 ligand is a direct and potent stimulator of the growth of primitive and committed human CD34+ bone marrow progenitor cells in vitro. Blood. 1996;87(4):1317–25.
9. Lyman SD. Biology of flt3 ligand and receptor. Int J Hematol. 1995;62(2):63–73.
10. Lyman SD, Jacobsen SE. c-kit ligand and Flt3 ligand: stem/progenitor cell factors with overlapping yet distinct activities. Blood. 1998;91(4):1101–34.
11. Dehmel U, Zaborski M, Meierhoff G, Rosnet O, Birnbaum D, Ludwig WD, et al. Effects of FLT3 ligand on human leukemia cells. I. Proliferative response of myeloid leukemia cells. Leukemia. 1996a;10(2):261–70.
12. Dehmel U, Quentmeier H, Drexler HG. Effects of FLT3 ligand on human leukemia cells. II. Agonistic and antagonistic effects of other cytokines. Leukemia. 1996b;10(2):271–8.
13. DaSilva N, Hu ZB, Ma W, Rosnet O, Birnbaum D, Drexler HG. Expression of the FLT3 gene in human leukemia-lymphoma cell lines. Leukemia. 1994;8(5):885–8.
14. Drexler HG. Expression of FLT3 receptor and response to FLT3 ligand by leukemic cells. Leukemia. 1996;10(4):588–99.
15. Drexler HG, Meyer C, Quentmeier H. Effects of FLT3 ligand on proliferation and survival of myeloid leukemia cells. Leuk Lymphoma. 1999;33(1–2):83–91.
16. Rosnet O, Buhring HJ, Marchetto S, Rappold I, Lavagna C, Sainty D, et al. Human FLT3/FLK2 receptor tyrosine kinase is expressed at the surface of normal and malignant hematopoietic cells. Leukemia. 1996;10(2):238–48.
17. Zheng R, Levis M, Piloto O, Brown P, Baldwin BR, Gorin NC, et al. FLT3 ligand causes autocrine signaling in acute myeloid leukemia cells. Blood. 2004;103(1):267–74.
18. Nakao M, Yokota S, Iwai T, Kaneko H, Horiike S, Kashima K, et al. Internal tandem duplication of the flt3 gene found in acute myeloid leukemia. Leukemia. 1996;10(12):1911–8.
19. Yamamoto Y, Kiyoi H, Nakano Y, Suzuki R, Kodera Y, Miyawaki S, et al. Activating mutation of D835 within the activation loop of FLT3 in human hematologic malignancies. Blood. 2001;97(8):2434–9.
20. Abu-Duhier FM, Goodeve AC, Wilson GA, Care RS, Peake IR, Reilly JT. Identification of novel FLT-3 Asp835 mutations in adult acute myeloid leukaemia. Br J Haematol. 2001;113(4):983–8.
21. Stirewalt DL, Kopecky KJ, Meshinchi S, Appelbaum FR, Slovak ML, Willman CL, et al. FLT3, RAS, and TP53 mutations in elderly patients with acute myeloid leukemia. Blood. 2001;97(11):3589–95.
22. Thiede C, Steudel C, Mohr B, Schaich M, Schakel U, Platzbecker U, et al. Analysis of FLT3-activating mutations in 979 patients with acute myelogenous leukemia: association with FAB subtypes and identification of subgroups with poor prognosis. Blood. 2002;99(12):4326–35.

23. Spiekermann K, Bagrintseva K, Schoch C, Haferlach T, Hiddemann W, Schnittger S. A new and recurrent activating length mutation in exon 20 of the FLT3 gene in acute myeloid leukemia. Blood. 2002;100(9):3423–5.
24. Kindler T, Breitenbuecher F, Kasper S, Estey E, Giles F, Feldman E, et al. Identification of a novel activating mutation (Y842C) within the activation loop of FLT3 in patients with acute myeloid leukemia (AML). Blood. 2005;105(1):335–40.
25. Taketani T, Taki T, Sugita K, Furuichi Y, Ishii E, Hanada R, et al. FLT3 mutations in the activation loop of tyrosine kinase domain are frequently found in infant ALL with MLL rearrangements and pediatric ALL with hyperdiploidy. Blood. 2004;103(3):1085–8.
26. Kiyoi H, Naoe T. FLT3 in human hematologic malignancies. Leuk Lymphoma. 2002;43(8):1541–7.
27. Stirewalt DL, Radich JP. The role of FLT3 in haematopoietic malignancies. Nat Rev Cancer. 2003;3(9):650–65.
28. Levis M, Small D. FLT3: ITDoes matter in leukemia. Leukemia. 2003;17(9):1738–52.
29. Kottaridis PD, Gale RE, Linch DC. Flt3 mutations and leukaemia. Br J Haematol. 2003;122(4):523–38.
30. Naoe T, Kiyoi H. Normal and oncogenic FLT3. Cell Mol Life Sci. 2004;61(23):2932–8.
31. Kiyoi H, Yanada M, Ozekia K. Clinical significance of FLT3 in leukemia. Int J Hematol. 2005;82(2):85–92.
32. Weiss A, Schlessinger J. Switching signals on or off by receptor dimerization. Cell. 1998;94(3):277–80.
33. Karaman MW, Herrgard S, Treiber DK, Gallant P, Atteridge CE, Campbell BT, et al. A quantitative analysis of kinase inhibitor selectivity. Nat Biotechnol. 2008;26(1):127–32. doi:10.1038/nbt1358.
34. Kelly LM, Yu JC, Boulton CL, Apatira M, Li J, Sullivan CM, et al. CT53518, a novel selective FLT3 antagonist for the treatment of acute myelogenous leukemia (AML). Cancer Cell. 2002;1(5):421–32.
35. Pandey A, Volkots DL, Seroogy JM, Rose JW, Yu JC, Lambing JL, et al. Identification of orally active, potent, and selective 4-piperazinylquinazolines as antagonists of the platelet-derived growth factor receptor tyrosine kinase family. J Med Chem. 2002;45(17):3772–93.
36. DeAngelo DJ, Stone RM, Heaney ML, Nimer SD, Paquette R, Bruner-Klisovic R, et al. Phase II evaluation of the tyrosine kinase inhibitor MLN518 in patients with acute myeloid leukemia (AML) bearing a FLT3 internal tandem duplication (ITD) mutation. Blood. 2004;104:abstract 1792.
37. Fiedler W, Serve H, Dohner H, Schwittay M, Ottmann OG, O'Farrell AM, et al. A phase 1 study of SU11248 in the treatment of patients with refractory or resistant acute myeloid leukemia (AML) or not amenable to conventional therapy for the disease. Blood. 2005;105(3):986–93.
38. George DJ, Dionne CA, Jani J, Angeles T, Murakata C, Lamb J, et al. Sustained in vivo regression of Dunning H rat prostate cancers treated with combinations of androgen ablation and Trk tyrosine kinase inhibitors, CEP-751 (KT-6587) or CEP-701 (KT-5555). Cancer Res. 1999;59(10):2395–401.
39. Levis M, Allebach J, Tse KF, Zheng R, Baldwin BR, Smith BD, et al. A FLT3-targeted tyrosine kinase inhibitor is cytotoxic to leukemia cells in vitro and in vivo. Blood. 2002;99(11):3885–91.
40. Smith BD, Levis M, Beran M, Giles F, Kantarjian H, Berg K, et al. Single-agent CEP-701, a novel FLT3 inhibitor, shows biologic and clinical activity in patients with relapsed or refractory acute myeloid leukemia. Blood. 2004;103(10):3669–76.
41. Levis M, Ravandi F, Wang ES, Baer MR, Perl A, Coutre S, et al. Results from a randomized trial of salvage chemotherapy followed by lestaurtinib for patients with FLT3 mutant AML in first relapse. Blood. 2011;117(12):3294–301. doi:10.1182/blood-2010-08-301796.
42. Wilhelm SM, Carter C, Tang L, Wilkie D, McNabola A, Rong H, et al. BAY 43-9006 exhibits broad spectrum oral antitumor activity and targets the RAF/MEK/ERK pathway and receptor

tyrosine kinases involved in tumor progression and angiogenesis. Cancer Res. 2004;64(19):7099–109. doi:10.1158/0008-5472.CAN-04-1443.
43. Ravandi F, Cortes JE, Jones D, Faderl S, Garcia-Manero G, Konopleva MY, et al. Phase I/II study of combination therapy with sorafenib, idarubicin, and cytarabine in younger patients with acute myeloid leukemia. J Clin Oncol. 2010;28(11):1856–62. doi:10.1200/JCO.2009.25.4888.
44. Serve H, Krug U, Wagner R, Sauerland MC, Heinecke A, Brunnberg U, et al. Sorafenib in combination with intensive chemotherapy in elderly patients with acute myeloid leukemia: results from a randomized, placebo-controlled trial. J Clin Oncol. 2013;31(25):3110–8. doi:10.1200/JCO.2012.46.4990.
45. Meyer T, Regenass U, Fabbro D, Alteri E, Rosel J, Muller M, et al. A derivative of staurosporine (CGP 41 251) shows selectivity for protein kinase C inhibition and in vitro antiproliferative as well as in vivo anti-tumor activity. Int J Cancer. 1989;43(5):851–6.
46. Stone RM, DeAngelo DJ, Klimek V, Galinsky I, Estey E, Nimer SD, et al. Patients with acute myeloid leukemia and an activating mutation in FLT3 respond to a small-molecule FLT3 tyrosine kinase inhibitor, PKC412. Blood. 2005;105(1):54–60.
47. Zarrinkar PP, Gunawardane RN, Cramer MD, Gardner MF, Brigham D, Belli B, et al. AC220 is a uniquely potent and selective inhibitor of FLT3 for the treatment of acute myeloid leukemia (AML). Blood. 2009;114(14):2984–92. doi:10.1182/blood-2009-05-222034.
48. Galanis A, Ma H, Rajkhowa T, Ramachandran A, Small D, Cortes J, et al. Crenolanib is a potent inhibitor of FLT3 with activity against resistance-conferring point mutants. Blood. 2014;123(1):94–100. doi:10.1182/blood-2013-10-529313.
49. Zimmerman EI, Turner DC, Buaboonnam J, Hu S, Orwick S, Roberts MS, et al. Crenolanib is active against models of drug-resistant FLT3-ITD-positive acute myeloid leukemia. Blood. 2013;122(22):3607–15. doi:10.1182/blood-2013-07-513044.
50. Kindler T, Lipka DB, Fischer T. FLT3 as a therapeutic target in AML: still challenging after all these years. Blood. 2010;116(24):5089–102. doi:10.1182/blood-2010-04-261867.
51. Weisberg E, Sattler M, Ray A, Griffin JD. Drug resistance in mutant FLT3-positive AML. Oncogene. 2010;29(37):5120–34. doi:10.1038/onc.2010.273.
52. Sato T, Yang X, Knapper S, White P, Smith BD, Galkin S, et al. FLT3 ligand impedes the efficacy of FLT3 inhibitors in vitro and in vivo. Blood. 2011;117(12):3286–93. doi:10.1182/blood-2010-01-266742.
53. Smith CC, Wang Q, Chin CS, Salerno S, Damon LE, Levis MJ, et al. Validation of ITD mutations in FLT3 as a therapeutic target in human acute myeloid leukaemia. Nature. 2012;485(7397):260–3. doi:10.1038/nature11016.

Part IV

Differentiating Agents

Retinoic Acid, All-*trans* Retinoic Acid (ATRA), and Tamibarotene

11

Norio Asou

Abstract

Retinoids, all-*trans* retinoic acid (ATRA), and tamibarotene can induce differentiation of leukemic cells that carry t(15;17) and potentially lead to complete remission (CR) in patients with acute promyelocytic leukemia (APL). Although introduction of ATRA as a differentiating agent has been a major breakthrough in the treatment of APL, ATRA is currently recognized as a molecular-targeted therapy directed at the PML-RARα chimeric protein, which is generated by the specific chromosomal translocation t(15;17). In several multicenter trials, more than 90% of newly diagnosed APL patients treated with ATRA and chemotherapy achieved CR, of whom 20–30% subsequently relapsed, and then approximately 80% of patients had overall survival. However, several problems still account for treatment failure including early death, death during consolidation, and disease relapse. Tamibarotene demonstrated efficacy in both untreated APL patients and relapsed patients who have been treated with ATRA and chemotherapy. Retinoids are a model of the development of new molecular-targeted agents for other malignant tumors.

Keywords

Acute promyelocytic leukemia (APL) • All-*trans* retinoic acid (ATRA) • Tamibarotene (Am80) • Differentiating agent • Molecular-targeted therapy

N. Asou (✉)
Department of Hematology, International Medical Center, Saitama Medical University, 1397-1 Yamane, Hidaka, Saitama 350-1298, Japan
e-mail: ktcnasou@saitama-med.ac.jp

T. Ueda (ed.), *Chemotherapy for Leukemia*, DOI 10.1007/978-981-10-3332-2_11

11.1 Introduction

Acute promyelocytic leukemia (APL) is a distinct subtype of acute myeloid leukemia (AML), which is characterized by unique morphology and coagulopathy [1–4]. Patients with APL represent a marked hemorrhagic diathesis caused by disseminated intravascular coagulation (DIC) and excessive primary fibrinolysis. APL cells in the vast majority of patients have a characteristic chromosomal translocation t(15;17)(q22;q21) that produces the fusion gene consisted of *promyelocytic leukemia (PML)* and *retinoic acid receptor α (RARα)* [5–9]. The advent of all-*trans* retinoic acid (ATRA) has been the major breakthrough in the treatment of APL [10]. ATRA can induce differentiation of APL cells, resulting in apoptosis of leukemic cells and achievement of complete remission (CR) in APL patients [11–15]. ATRA is currently recognized as the molecular-targeted therapy directed at the chimeric protein PML-RARα, which is generated by the specific chromosomal translocation, although the drug target was demonstrated after ATRA had been clinically used as a differentiating agent [16–18]. In the history of cancer treatment, ATRA is the first successful molecular-targeted drug and provides a development model for new agents targeted at many other malignancies. Tamibarotene (also called Am80) is a synthetic retinoid that induces differentiation of HL-60 and NB-4 cells with approximately ten times stronger in vitro activity than that of ATRA [19, 20]. Phase II studies of tamibarotene demonstrated its efficacy and safety in patients with APL who had relapsed after ATRA-containing therapy [19]. Phase III studies have also compared tamibarotene with ATRA in the maintenance phase and reinduction phase for APL patients [21, 22].

In this chapter, differentiating agents ATRA and tamibarotene in the treatment of APL are reviewed.

11.2 Acute Promyelocytic Leukemia

APL is a distinct subtype of AML that is characterized by the morphology of its leukemic cells, a life-threatening coagulopathy caused by DIC and fibrinolysis, and a specific chromosomal translocation t(15;17) [1–6]. APL represents approximately 10% of adult AML. APL cells have unique morphological characteristics such as a large amount of azurophilic granules and Auer rods (faggot cells) [1, 2]. Azurophilic granules in APL cells contain tissue factor, which can cause DIC [3, 4]. APL cells also express high levels of annexin II, which can increase fibrinolytic activity. In patients with APL, cytotoxic chemotherapy often exacerbates extreme bleeding diathesis, such as intracranial hemorrhage, resulting in a high rate of early mortality [14, 15, 23]. Patients with APL frequently present with pancytopenia. Median WBC count at diagnosis is approximately 2.0×10^9/L, and only 20% of patients showed initial WBC count $>10\times10^9$/L [11, 14, 24]. Usually, APL cells express CD13 and CD33, but are negative for HLA-DR or CD34 [14, 25, 26]. Approximately 10% of patients with APL have the microgranular variant, designated as M3v in FAB classification, characterized by leukemic cells that are devoid of or have sparse fine granules [2]. M3v is generally associated with higher WBC count at presentation and expression of CD2 as well as CD34 and HLA-DR [25–27]. In addition, internal tandem duplications of the *FLT3* gene (*FLT3*-ITD) are frequently detected in patients with M3v [28, 29]. Accurate diagnosis of M3v may be difficult by means of morphology. However, it is of note that leukemic cells with M3v also harbor t(15;17) and respond to ATRA.

Most patients with APL harbored t(15;17) leading to *PML-RARA* fusion gene. PML-RARα chimeric protein retains critical domains of PML and RARα and plays a key role in the pathogenesis of APL (Fig. 11.1) [9, 30, 31]. In addition, PML-RARα is a specific targeted molecule for the differentiating effect of ATRA and the pro-apoptotic effect of arsenic derivatives such as arsenic trioxide (ATO) [30–34]. However, a small number of APL patients have different chromosomal aberrations that interestingly contain 17q (*RARA*) translocations (Table 11.1) [35–38]. Among these variant translocations, it is well documented that PLZF-RARα and STAT5B-RARα are resistant to ATRA [37, 38]. Therefore, identification of the *PML-RARA* fusion gene by FISH and RT-PCR analyses at diagnosis is critical to assure clinical response to ATRA and ATO.

In addition to the presence of chromosomal translocation t(15;17) that produces PML-RARα, other genetic alterations have also been implicated in the development of APL [28, 29, 39, 40]. Expression of *PML-RARA* in mice is associated with long latency of onset of the disease and variable penetrance [41–44]. This indicates that secondary genetic abnormalities contribute to the pathogenesis of APL. A comprehensive mutational analysis of APL revealed that primary APL cells harbored *FLT3*-ITD (27%), *FLT3* (16%), *WT1* (14%), *NRAS* (10%), *KRAS* (4%), *ARID1A*

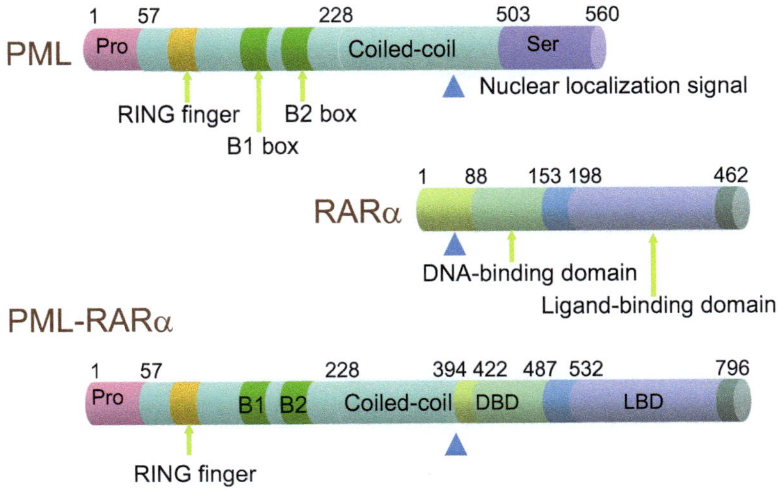

Fig. 11.1 PML-RARα chimeric protein generated by t(15;17)(q22;q21) in APL. The chimeric PML-RARα protein retains critical domains of PML and RARα and promotes development of APL. PML-RARα fusion protein affects both nuclear receptor signaling and assembly of PML nuclear bodies

Table 11.1 Chromosomal translocations in APL and response to all-*trans* retinoic acid (ATRA)

Chromosome	Fusion gene	Incidence	Response to ATRA
t(15;17)(q22;q21)	*PML-RARA*	>98%	+
t(11;17)(q23;q21)	*PLZF(ZBTB16)-RARA*	0.8%	-
t(5;17)(q35;q21)	*NPM1-RARA*	<0.5%	+
t(11;17)(q13;q21)	*NuMA-RARA*	Rare	+
t(17;17)(q11;q21)	*STAT5B-RARA*	Rare	-
t(4;17)(q12;q21)	*FIP1L1-RARA*	Rare	+
Cryptic	*PRKAR1A-RARA*	Rare	+
t(X;17)(p11;q12)	*BCOR-RARA*	Rare	+
t(2;17)(q32;q21)	*OBFC2A-RARA*	Rare	+
t(3;17)(q26;q21)	*TBLR1-RARA*	Rare	+

(4.8%), and *ARID1B* (3%) mutations in 165 initial diagnosis samples [40]. These mutations, which cooperate with PML-RARα, appear to play a role in the pathogenesis of APL. On the other hand, the absence of mutations in other common AML-associated genes including *DNMT3A*, *NPM1*, *TET2*, *ASXL1*, and *IDH1/2* was observed.

11.3 Molecular Mechanism of Action for ATRA

RARα is a member of the nuclear hormone receptor superfamily that acts as ligand-inducible transcriptional regulators [30, 31, 45]. RARα requires heterodimerization with retinoid X receptor α (RXRα) to bind the retinoic acid response element (RARE) located in the promoter regions of the target genes [31, 45]. Unliganded RARα can bind RARE and represses transcriptions through chromatin remodeling by recruiting transcription corepressors including mSin3A, NcoR, and SMRT [16, 46, 47]. These corepressors recruit histone deacetylase (HDAC) complex, resulting in histone deacetylation that leads to transcriptional silencing [16–18]. Retinoic acid (RA) binding to RARα induces dissociation of the HDAC complex and recruits coactivators such as p300/CBP, leading to histone acetylation and activation of transcription [18, 31]. One of the potential RA/RARα target genes is a transcription factor *C/EBPε*, which affects myeloid differentiation [48].

PML is the organizer of nuclear domains called PML nuclear bodies (NBs), which show a speckled pattern in the nucleus by PML antibody staining (Fig. 11.2) [30, 49–52]. Formation of PML NBs is associated with several stress responses, including telomere shortening, DNA damage, aggregation of misfolded proteins, deregulation of ribosome biogenesis, senescence, and proteasome inhibition [53]. NBs appear as domains assembled by oxidative stress and SUMO (small ubiquitin-like modifier)-ylation, whose assembly controls stress-induced posttranslational modification of various proteins. PML overexpression induces cell senescence,

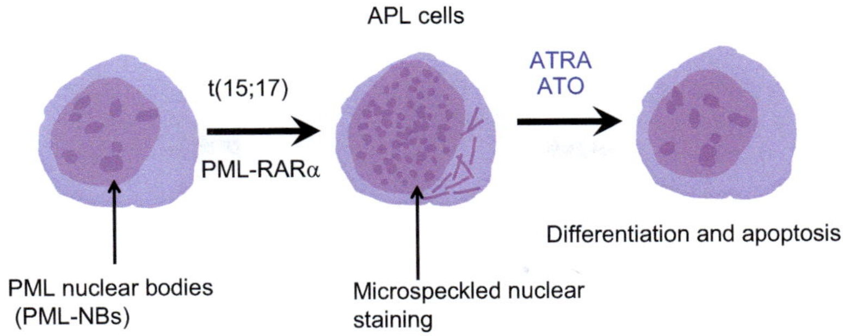

Fig. 11.2 Schematic representation of the nuclear bodies and the effects of ATRA and arsenic trioxide (ATO). In normal myeloid cells, PML nuclear bodies (NBs) show a speckled pattern when stained by PML antibodies. In APL cells, PML-RARα disrupts PML NBs, leading to a microgranular pattern of NBs. Both ATRA and ATO elicit PML-RARα degradation, resulting in reformation of normal NBs and cell differentiation

growth arrest, or apoptosis. In addition, PML NB formation is associated with self-renewal of normal or cancer stem cells [54].

APL is driven by a PML-RARα fusion protein that affects both nuclear receptor signaling and PML NB assembly [30–32, 51]. In APL cells, PML-RARα binds RARE through the DNA-binding domain of RARα in a dominant manner [30, 55]. PML-RARα mediates transcriptional repression of RARα target genes by recruiting corepressors, HDAC and DNA methyltransferase. Physiological dose of RA cannot dissociate the HDAC complex, leading to a maturational block in myeloid differentiation, which is thought to be an initial step of leukemogenesis [16–18]. In contrast, pharmacological doses of ATRA trigger dissociation of the HDAC complex and recruitment of coactivators [16–18, 56]. Thus, PML-RARα is a potent repressor of nuclear hormone receptor signaling, but it also disrupts PML NBs, resulting in a microgranulation pattern (Fig. 11.2) [30, 49–51]. PML-RARα can be SUMOylated at K160 residue of the PML protein to recruit death domain-associated protein (DAXX), which transcriptionally represses target genes [57].

ATRA and ATO target RARα and PML, respectively, the two distinct moieties of the disease-specific oncoprotein PML-RARα [30, 32]. Both ATRA and ATO elicit PML-RARα degradation, leading to reformation of normal NBs mediated by non-rearranged PML and cell differentiation (Fig. 11.2) [49–51, 56]. Arsenic-elicited PML degradation is initiated by SUMOylation of K160 [58]. ATO directly binds with PML at the C-C motif in the B2 domain, and PML SUMOylation can be induced by enhancing ubiquitin-conjugating enzyme 9 (UBC9) binding at the PML RING domain (Fig. 11.1) [59]. ATO induces SUMOylation of PML that recruits a SUMO-dependent ubiquitin ligase, RING finger protein 4 (RNF4), which enforces PML polyubiquitination [33, 34, 59]. PML is also required for some activities of p53. PML-RARα expression impedes p53 signaling and blocks the effects of p53 activation on cell death or clonogenic growth. Thus, NB disruption by PML-RARα impairs p53 key functions in controlling stemness or self-renewal, mediated by enforcing G0 arrest of stem cells, resulting in proliferation and aberrant stem cell self-renewal [58]. NB reformation in response to ATRA or ATO treatments precipitates apoptosis or senescence [60]. Moreover, ATRA induces degradation of PML-RARα and activates normal RARα and PML, resulting in differentiation of APL cells.

11.4 ATRA in the Treatment of Newly Diagnosed APL Patients

11.4.1 ATRA as a Differentiating Agent for APL

In the late 1980s, investigators in Shanghai demonstrated that the active form of retinoids, ATRA, could induce differentiation in APL cells, resolve life-threatening coagulopathy, and achieve a high CR rate [10]. Early studies of ATRA documented marked clinical efficacy in patients with both relapsed and newly diagnosed APL, indicating that ATRA has no cross-resistance against chemotherapeutic agents [61–63]. However, rapid increase of leukocytes is common, which is often accompanied by APL differentiation syndrome (DS; formerly RA or ATRA syndrome) [64]. Furthermore, most patients treated with ATRA alone after achieving CR suffer relapse [62]. Therefore, the combination of ATRA and cytotoxic chemotherapy has been incorporated in the frontline therapy for newly diagnosed APL.

11.4.2 ATRA in Induction Therapy

11.4.2.1 ATRA for Newly Diagnosed APL Patients in Multicenter Trials

In the US intergroup study, previously untreated APL patients were randomly assigned to receive ATRA or chemotherapy which consisted of daunorubicin (DNR) plus cytarabine (Ara-C) during induction [65]. Although CR rates between the two groups were not different, 3-year disease-free survival (DFS) rates were 32% in the chemotherapy group ($n = 174$) and 67% in the ATRA group ($n = 172$) ($P < 0.001$). The 3-year overall survival (OS) rates were 50% for patients assigned to chemotherapy and 71% for patients who received induction with ATRA ($P < 0.001$). In European APL91 study, a multicenter randomized trial compared chemotherapy with DNR plus Ara-C and ATRA combined with the same chemotherapy during induction in newly diagnosed APL patients aged 65 years or younger [66]. The trial was terminated early after the first interim analysis, as 1-year event-free survival (EFS) was significantly higher in the ATRA group (79% vs. 50%, $P = 0.001$). These initial randomized studies indicate that ATRA should be incorporated in frontline therapy for newly diagnosed APL.

Thereafter, several multicenter studies conducted during the past decade have contributed to optimizing the antileukemic efficacy of ATRA when used in combination with chemotherapy for induction therapy (Table 11.2) [21, 65, 67–78]. In the GIMEMA and PETHEMA studies, simultaneous use of ATRA and idarubicin

Table 11.2 ATRA and chemotherapy for newly diagnosed APL in multicenter trials

Study group	Induction therapy	No. of patients	CR (%)	DFS (%)	EFS (%)	OS (%)
Euro APL93	ATRA+DNR/Ara-C	576	93	-		77 (10)
Euro APL2000	ATRA+DNR/Ara-C	340	96	-	84.5 (2)	91.9 (2)
GIMEMA AIDA0493	ATRA+IDR	642	94	70 (6)	-	78 (6)
GIMEMA AIDA2000	ATRA+IDR	453	94	86 (6)	-	87 (6)
PETHEMA LPA96	ATRA +IDR	175	90	81 (3)	-	78 (3)
PETHEMA LPA99	ATRA +IDR	511	91	84 (4)	-	83 (4)
US Intergroup	ATRA +HU	172	72	69 (5)	-	69 (5)
US Intergroup	ATRA +DNR/Ara-C	244	90	90 (3)	80 (3)	86 (3)
JALSG APL97	ATRA +IDR/Ara-C	283	94	69 (6)	-	84 (6)
JALSG APL204	ATRA +IDR/Ara-C	344	93	-	-	89 (4)

CR complete remission, *DFS* disease-free survival, *EFS* event-free survival, *OS* overall survival, *DNR* daunorubicin, *Ara-C* cytarabine, *IDR* idarubicin, *HU* hydroxyurea, parentheses represent observation times (years)

(IDR) (AIDA) during induction was highly effective and led to CR in 90–95% of patients; resistance to AIDA therapy was reported only infrequently [71–74]. In the Japan Adult Leukemia Study Group (JALSG) studies, ATRA was administered to all patients at a 45 mg/m²/day until CR or for 60 days [21, 24, 63, 77]. Addition of chemotherapy during induction depends on the initial WBC count and leukemic cell count in the peripheral blood (Fig. 11.3) [21]. Subsequent consolidation therapy consisted of three courses of intensive chemotherapy with anthracyclines and Ara-C. In the JALSG AML87 and AML89 studies, 6-year DFS rates in CR patients who were treated with chemotherapy alone were 40% and 45%, respectively [63]. In the JALSG APL92 and APL97 studies, which included ATRA plus chemotherapy during induction followed by consolidation chemotherapy, the 6-year DFS were 59% and 68.5%, respectively (Fig. 11.4) [24, 77, 78].

In current multicenter trials, more than 90% of newly diagnosed APL patients treated with ATRA plus chemotherapy achieve CR, of whom 20–30% subsequently relapse and then approximately 60–80% of patients have DFS (Table 11.2) [67–78]. Non-cross-resistance between ATRA and chemotherapeutic drugs appears to contribute to the significant improvement in EFS. However, several major clinical problems still account for treatment failure, including early death, death during consolidation, and disease relapse. Induction failure is mainly caused by hemorrhage, DS, or infection [3, 4, 23, 64]. Another sizable subset of patients dies in CR from complications of consolidation, mainly from infection due to chemotherapy-associated myelosuppression [67–78]. Optimal chemotherapy during induction and post-remission in these high-risk groups remains to be determined. Because of the excellent response with ATRA plus chemotherapy, hematopoietic stem cell transplantation (HSCT) is generally not indicated in first CR but might be considered for second CR patients [79, 80].

These multicenter studies led to a proposal to assess relapse risk in APL patients treated with ATRA and chemotherapy. The JALSG APL92 study revealed that

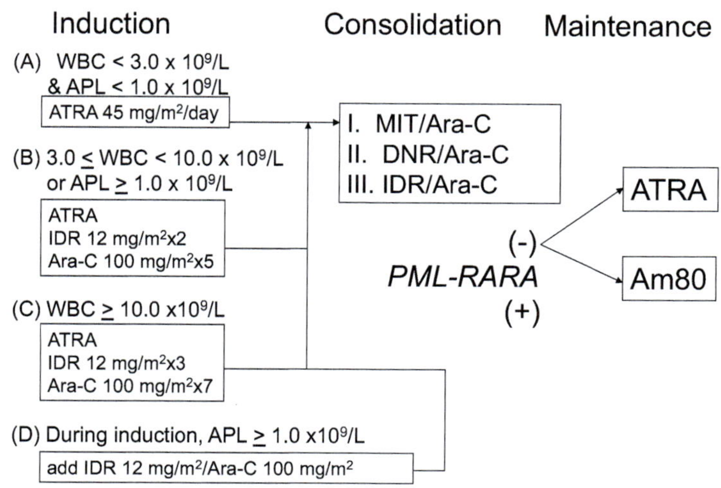

Fig. 11.3 Therapeutic protocol in the JALSG APL204 study. ATRA was administered to all patients at a daily dose of 45 mg/m^2 until the patients achieved complete remission or for 60 days, whichever occurred first. Chemotherapy regimen depended on initial WBC count and APL cell count in the peripheral blood. For example, patients whose pretreatment WBC counts were 3.0–10.0×10^9/L and/or the APL cell count exceeded 1.0×10^9/L (group B) received idarubicin and cytarabine. Consolidation therapy consisted of three courses of intensive chemotherapy. After completion of the third consolidation course, patients in molecular remission of *PML-RARA* were then randomly assigned to either oral administration of ATRA (45 mg/m^2/day) or to oral tamibarotene (Am80; 6 mg/m^2/day), both for 14 days every 3 months. Maintenance therapy was continued for up to 2 years for a total of up to eight courses in both groups

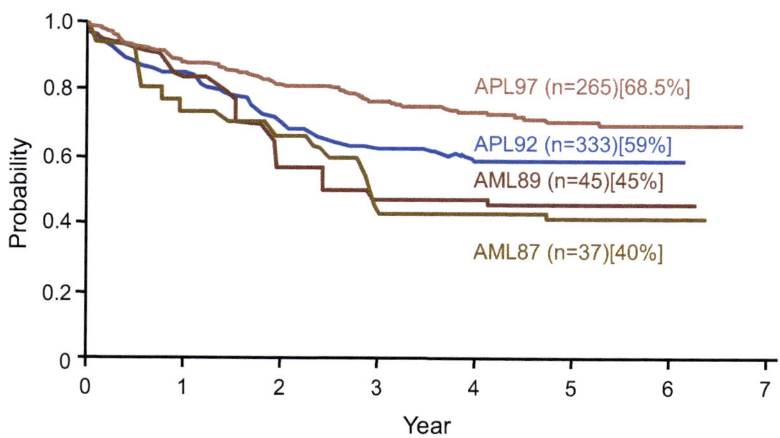

Fig. 11.4 Disease-free survival in APL patients who achieved complete remission in the Japan Adult Leukemia Study Group (JALSG) APL studies. In the JALSG AML87 and AML89 studies, APL patients were treated with chemotherapy alone, whereas APL patients registered in the JALSG APL92 and APL97 studies were treated with ATRA and chemotherapy. In the APL97 study, chemotherapy regimens during induction and consolidation consisted of anthracyclines and cytarabine instead of anthracyclines and biphenyl cytarabine in the APL92 study

initial WBC count at diagnosis can independently predict DFS [24]. The predicted 4-year DFS rate was 68% in patients whose initial WBC count was less than 10×10^9/L and 42% in those whose initial WBC count was $>10 \times 10^9$/L ($P = 0.0007$). Relapse-risk groups proposed by the PETHEMA group were as follows: low risk, WBC count $<10 \times 10^9$/L and platelet count $\geq 40 \times 10^9$/L; intermediate risk, WBC count $<10 \times 10^9$/L and platelet count $<40 \times 10^9$/L; and high risk, WBC count $\geq 10 \times 10^9$/L [81]. This so-called Sanz risk score, essentially based on WBC and platelet counts at diagnosis, allowed further refinement of frontline APL therapy through up-front risk assessment and use of risk-adapted ATRA and chemotherapy.

To decrease mortality in CR, the PETHEMA group reduced the intensity of consolidation by avoiding Ara-C in the LPA99 study (Table 11.2) [74]. They observed a lower rate of death in CR (2%) and a low cumulative incidence of relapse (CIR) (10%). On the other hand, the APL2000 trial conducted by the French-Belgian-Swiss APL group in patients with WBC count less than 10×10^9/L, which examined the role of Ara-C in addition to ATRA and anthracyclines, found a significantly higher 2-year CIR (15.9% in the no Ara-C group vs. 4.7% in the Ara-C group, $P = 0.011$) and lower 2-year OS (89.6% vs. 97.9%, $P = 0.0066$) in patients treated without Ara-C [69]. To assess these discrepancies between the LPA99 and APL2000 studies, particularly regarding the effect of Ara-C, these two studies were jointly analyzed [82]. In the low- and intermediate-risk groups, 3-year CIR was 14.3% and 4.2% ($P = 0.03$) in the APL2000 and LPA99 trials, respectively. OS were 95.6% and 93.8% ($P = 0.53$) in the APL2000 ($n = 96$) and LPA99 ($n = 402$) trials, respectively. In the high-risk group, 3-year CIR was 9.9% and 18.5% ($P = 0.12$), and 3-year OS was 91.5% and 80.8% ($P = 0.026$) in the APL2000 ($n = 82$) and LPA99 ($n = 104$) trials, respectively. These results suggest that ATRA combined with a high cumulative dose of IDR without Ara-C but with a maintenance treatment like the PETHEMA approach may give excellent results with limited toxicity in low- and intermediate-risk APL, whereas the addition of Ara-C to ATRA and anthracyclines in high-risk patients may result in a trend toward lower CIR and a better OS.

11.4.2.2 Hemorrhage

Recent registry studies show that hemorrhage is still a major problem, as many patients fail to be promptly diagnosed and/or receive appropriate treatment in time [83]. Remission induction failures are a major stumbling block even in current APL therapy. Although infection is the predominant cause of death in AML, hemorrhage is the most common cause of death during induction in APL patients, followed by DS and infection [23]. The majority of lethal hemorrhages occurred early during induction. Repletion of coagulation factors and platelet with blood products is the mainstay of supportive treatment in APL patients. In most multicenter studies, platelet transfusions are given to maintain a platelet count of at least 30×10^9/L until resolution of the coagulopathy [14]. Patients with active coagulopathy also receive fresh-frozen plasma, cryoprecipitate, or fibrinogen to maintain a fibrinogen level above 1.5 g/L. Nevertheless, fatal hemorrhagic events have been seen in 2–5% of patients treated with ATRA and chemotherapy [23]. APL cells mediate hemorrhagic diathesis through multiple mechanisms that lead to a combination of consumptive coagulopathy and primary hyperfibrinolysis. Exposure of tissue factor, annexin II, and microparticles from the leukemic cells has been implicated in the coagulopathy [3, 4]. Therefore, not only aggressive supportive care but also prompt treatment with ATRA (with or without ATO) is the most important step in preventing bleeding complications [14]. In a randomized comparison of ATRA plus chemotherapy vs. ATRA plus ATO, the ATRA and ATO combination resulted in decreased early death, which suggests that ATO exerts a better counteractive effect on coagulopathy compared with chemotherapy [84, 85].

In the JALSG APL97 study, 18 patients (6.5%) suffered severe hemorrhage and nine of them succumbed to early deaths [86]. Although most of them were receiving frequent transfusions, the targeted levels of platelet counts (30×10^9/L) and plasma fibrinogen (1.5 g/L) were reached at the day of bleeding in only 71% and 40%, respectively. Risk factor analysis identified three pretreatment variables associated with severe hemorrhage, initial fibrinogen level, WBC count, and performance status. In addition, patients with severe hemorrhage were more likely to develop DS or pneumonia than patients without hemorrhage. In the PETHEMA study, a multivariate analysis of pretreatment characteristics showed that abnormal creatinine level, high peripheral leukemic cells, and the presence of coagulopathy were associated with an increased risk of fatal hemorrhage [23].

11.4.2.3 Differentiation Syndrome (DS)

DS, formerly known as ATRA syndrome, is a life-threatening complication in patients with APL who undergo induction therapy with ATRA or arsenics [64, 87, 88]. The syndrome is clinically characterized by unexplained fever, weight gain, peripheral edema, dyspnea with interstitial pulmonary infiltrates, pleural or pericardial effusion, hypotension, and renal failure. The reported incidence of this syndrome ranges from 2% to 27% [67–78]. This wide range is probably because of the different criteria used to diagnose DS and differences in induction therapy and prophylaxis. Early addition of chemotherapy to ATRA and administration of high-dose dexamethasone at the onset of the first symptoms appeared to reduce the DS-related mortality to 1% or less in the recent trials. Although predictive factors of DS have not been determined, DS is associated with increased differentiated neutrophils that secrete inflammatory cytokines such as IL-6, IL-8, and TNFα. Prevention of hemorrhage and DS during induction is critical to achieve CR, because primary resistance to ATRA is an exception in newly diagnosed APL with t(15;17).

The Spanish PETHEMA group analyzed the incidence, characteristics, prognostic factors, and outcome in 739 patients treated with AIDA in the LPA96 and LPA99 studies (Table 11.2) [89]. Diagnosis of DS was made according to the presence of the following signs and symptoms described by Frankel et al. [64]: dyspnea, unexplained fever, weight gain greater than 5 kg, unexplained hypotension, acute renal failure, and particularly a chest radiograph demonstrating pulmonary infiltrates or pleuropericardial effusion. In this study, patients with four or more of the above signs or symptoms were classified as having severe DS, while those with two or three signs or symptoms were considered to have moderate DS. Of the 739 patients,

Table 11.3 Management and outcomes of APL differentiation syndrome (DS) in the PETHEMA LPA96 and LPA99 studies

	No DS	Moderate	Severe	Total of DS
No. of signs and symptoms	0-1	2-3	≥4	≥2
No. of patients	556	90 (12%)	93 (13%)	183 (25%)
Median age (range)	39 (2-83)	-	-	43 (3-78)
Leukocyte count (x10^9/L)	2.0 (0.2-460)	-	-	3.3 (0.4-133)
ATRA withdraw	87 (16%)	54 (60%)	60 (64%)	114 (62%)*
DEXA i.v.	90 (16%)	74 (82%)	84 (90%)	158 (86%)*
Dialysis	NA	1 (1%)	11 (12%)	12 (6.6%)*
Ventilation	NA	7 (8%)	24 (26%)	31 (17%)*
Induction death	37 (7%)	5 (6%)	24 (26%)	29 (16%)*
Death due to DS	0	0	10 (11%)	10 (5%)*
Death (Bleeding)	22 (4%)	5 (6%)	10 (11%)	15 (8%)*
Death (Infection)	14 (2%)	0	3 (3%)	3 (2%)
Thrombosis	18 (3%)	3 (3%)	9 (10%)	12 (7%)*

*$P < 0.05$

183 (24.8%) experienced DS including 93 (12.6%) with severe DS and 90 (12.2%) with moderate DS (Table 11.3). The most common manifestations of severe DS were dyspnea (95%), pulmonary infiltrates (81%), unexplained fever (74%), weight gain of more than 5 kg (68%), pleural effusion (58%), and renal failure (46%). DS occurred at a median of 12 days after starting ATRA treatment (range, 0–46 days). Severe DS occurred comparatively early, at a median of 6 days, while moderate DS appeared after a median of 15 days. The first peak occurred during the first week of ATRA treatment in 47% of patients with DS, and subsequently later cases of DS developed in the third week (25%), in the fourth week (19%), and after day 29 (3%). Development of moderate DS had no impact on the mortality during induction (6% with moderate DS vs. 7% without DS, $P = 0.82$), but severe DS was associated with an increased mortality (26%, $P < 0.001$) (Table 11.3). Notably, hemorrhagic mortality was also higher in patients who developed severe DS than in those with moderate DS or no DS ($P = 0.02$). In addition, severe DS was also significantly associated with a higher frequency of thrombosis. WBC counts greater than 5×10^9/L and serum creatinine levels greater than 1.4 mg/dL at diagnosis were identified as independent predictors of severe DS. Renal failure due to capillary leak syndrome caused by cytokine release in DS may explain the association between high serum creatinine and severe DS. Although the preemptive use of corticosteroids at the earliest clinical manifestations of DS has been adopted as the standard management, their prophylactic use is controversial [14]. A statistically significant reduction in the incidence of severe DS, but not in DS-related mortality, was probably associated with prophylactic use of prednisolone during an early 15-day interval in the LPA99 study [74]. As severe DS is associated with higher morbidity and mortality during induction, risk-adapted strategies that focus on patients with adverse risk factors deserve further investigation.

Table 11.4 ATRA in consolidation therapy

Study	Induction	Consolidation	Risk group	No. of Pts	CR (%)	CIR (%)	DFS (%)	OS (%)
LPA96	ATRA+IDR	CTx3	All	172	91	18 (5)	77 (5)	76 (5)
			Int./High	138	-	21 (5)	75 (5)	75 (5)
LPA99	ATRA+IDR	CT+ATRAx3**	All	560	91	11 (5)*	84 (5)*	82 (5)
			Int./High	453	-	13 (5)*	83 (5)*	81 (5)
AIDA-0493	ATRA+IDR	CTx3	All	642	94.3	27.7 (6)	69.5 (6)	78.1 (6)
			Low/Int.	461	-	19.9 (6)	76.6 (6)	84.7 (6)
			High	176	-	49.7 (6)	49.6 (6)	61.3 (6)
AIDA-2000	ATRA+IDR	CT+ATRAx3	All	453	94.4	10.7 (6)*	85.6 (6)*	87.4 (6)*
			Low/Int.	324	-	11.2 (6)*	85.9 (6)*	89.1 (6)
			High	129	-	9.3 (6)*	84.5 (6)*	83.4 (6)*

CR complete remission, *CIR* cumulative incidence of relapse, *DFS* disease-free survival, *OS* overall survival, *IDR* idarubicin, *CT* chemotherapy, parentheses represent observation years
*$P < 0.05$
**In the LPA99 trial, only intermediate- and high-risk patients received ATRA combined with the reinforced single-agent chemotherapy courses

11.4.3 ATRA in Consolidation Therapy

In the LPA99 trial, the Spanish PETHEMA group reported that a risk-adapted strategy combined with ATRA and anthracycline monochemotherapy for both induction and consolidation, followed by maintenance with ATRA and low-dose methotrexate (MTX) and mercaptopurine (6MP), resulted in a higher antileukemic efficacy than in the previous LPA96 trial (Table 11.4) [74]. Intermediate- and high-risk patients received ATRA (45 mg/m^2/day for 15 days) combined with anthracycline for three courses during the consolidation phase in the LPA99 study. This risk-adapted strategy combining ATRA and anthracycline monotherapy for consolidation led to significantly improved 5-year CIR and DFS rates in the intermediate-/high-risk patients (Table 11.4).

In the Italian GIMEMA Cooperative Group, the risk-adapted AIDA-2000 trial was designed to investigate the effects on patients' outcomes of two main modifications from the original AIDA-0493 study: the omission of Ara-C in the low-/intermediate-risk group and the addition of ATRA (45 mg/m^2/day for 15 days) during three courses of consolidation for all risk categories [72]. A total of 642 and 453 adult patients, aged 18–60 years, were enrolled in the AIDA-0493 and AIDA-2000 trials, respectively. The 6-year DFS rates were 69.5% in the AIDA-0493 and 85.6% in the AIDA-2000 ($P < 0.0001$) (Table 11.4). The 6-year CIR rates were 27.7% and 10.7% for all risk groups in the AIDA-0493 and AIDA-2000 studies, respectively ($P < 0.0001$). Percentages of CNS relapses were 2.5% and 2.1% in the two studies. This study shows that a risk-adapted post-remission strategy using variable chemotherapy intensity and addition of ATRA for consolidation resulted in significantly improved outcomes in patients with newly diagnosed APL. The benefit appears to

Table 11.5 ATRA in maintenance therapy

Study group		None	ATRA	MTX+6MP	ATRA+MTX+6MP	Am80
US Intergroup	No. of patients	54	46	-	-	-
	No. of relapses	21	10	-	-	-
	5-yearRFS (%)	55	74*	-	-	-
Euro-APL93	No. of patients	79	76	117	129	-
	No. of relapses	35	26	29	18	-
	10-year CIR (%)	43	33*	23*	13*	-
GIMEMA AIDA0493	No. of patients	76	83	78	81	-
	No. of events	22	25	22	23	-
JALSG APL204	No. of standard-risk patients	-	109	-	-	108
	4-year RFS (%)	-	90	-	-	92
	No. of high-risk patients	-	26	-	-	26
	4-year RFS (%)	-	58	-	-	87*

ATRA all-trans retinoic acid, *MTX* methotrexate, *6MP* 6-mercaptopurine, *Am80* tamibarotene, *RFS* relapse-free survival, *CIR* cumulative incidence of relapse
$^{*}P < 0.05$

result both from reduced toxicity and from increased antileukemic efficacy in the AIDA-2000 study. In the high-risk group, especially, addition of ATRA during each consolidation cycle significantly improved DFS and CIR rates in the AIDA-2000 compared with the AIDA-0493 study (Table 11.4). These Italian and Spanish studies document that the combination of ATRA plus chemotherapy in both induction and consolidation phases may contribute to improvement of CIR and DFS in high-risk group patients.

11.4.4 ATRA in Maintenance Therapy

The US intergroup study showed that maintenance treatment with continuous ATRA during 1 year significantly reduced relapses and improved survival (Table 11.5) [65]. On the other hand, the JALSG APL97 study showed that intensified maintenance with six courses of chemotherapy including biphenyl Ara-C and anthracyclines did not improve DFS in patients who achieved molecular remission after three courses of consolidation [77].

Of the 401 patients randomized for maintenance treatment on the European APL93 study, the 10-year CIR rates were 43.2%, 33%, 23.4%, and 13.4% in patients with no maintenance, maintenance with ATRA alone, maintenance with chemotherapy (6MP and MTX) alone, and both, respectively ($P < 0.001$) (Table 11.5) [67, 68]. Maintenance with 6MP and MTX significantly improved 10-year OS (85.2% vs. 79.2%; $P = 0.02$), but OS was not significantly modified by maintenance with ATRA (82.7% vs. 79.4%; $P = 0.44$). Among patients with WBC counts $\geq 5 \times 10^9$/L, the 10-year CIR rates were 68.4%, 53.1%, 32.8%, and 20.6% with no maintenance, ATRA alone, chemotherapy alone, and both, respectively ($P < 0.001$). In patients with WBC counts $<5 \times 10^9$/L, the 10-year CIR rates were 29.2%, 22.9%, 21.0%, and 11.5% with no maintenance, ATRA alone, chemotherapy alone, and both, respectively ($P = 0.069$). The beneficial effect of maintenance with intermittent ATRA and continuous 6MP + MTX, with an additive effect of the two modalities, was particularly clear in patients with WBC counts higher than 5×10^9/L; the relapse rate dropped from 68.4% with no maintenance to 20.6% with combined maintenance.

An updated Italian GIMEMA group study, using the same randomization design as in the APL93 trial for maintenance (i.e., no maintenance vs. ATRA vs. 6MP + MTX vs. both), showed no difference in relapse among maintenance arms (Table 11.5) [71]. The benefit of maintenance may in fact depend on prior induction and consolidation therapy. For example, both GIMEMA0493 and JALSG APL97 studies used IDR as anthracycline for induction and consolidation chemotherapy, whereas the US and European studies, which showed a large benefit for maintenance, used DNR, which may be less effective than IDR for APL [65, 67, 71, 77]. In addition, it should be noted that in the GIMEMA and JALSG studies, only patients with molecular remission after three courses of consolidation were enrolled to the randomized study for maintenance, whereas patients with hematological remission after two courses of consolidation were randomized to maintenance in both the US and European studies. These conflicting evidences indicate that the relative benefit of maintenance depends on the prior induction and consolidation therapies. Therefore, it is appropriate to use maintenance in conjunction with treatment protocols in which it has been shown to confer benefit [14].

11.4.5 Long-Term Follow-Up for Newly Diagnosed APL

The European APL group reported very long-term outcomes of APL after treatment with ATRA and chemotherapy [68]. In the APL93 trial, 576 newly diagnosed APL patients were enrolled from 97 European centers. A total of 533 (92.5%) patients achieved CR, 42 (7.3%) had early deaths, and one (0.2%) had resistant leukemia. With a median follow-up of 121 months, 142 (26.6%) of the 533 patients who achieved CR had relapsed, 59 (11%) had died in CR, and 329 (61.7%) remained in first CR (Table 11.6). The 10-year CIRs were 16.5% in the 306 patients <65 years with WBC count $<5 \times 10^9$/L, 37.9% in the high WBC count group, and 9.3% in the elderly group ($P < 0.001$). The estimated 10-year OS in the APL93 study was 77%. Most relapses occurred before the arsenic era, and 79% were treated with chemotherapy combined with ATRA. A total of 88% of the patients achieved second CR, and 63% of them subsequently underwent autologous or allogeneic HSCT. Of the 533 patients who achieved CR, 59 (11%) died in first CR, including 23 who died during consolidation, 10 during maintenance, and 26 after the end of maintenance treatment. Sepsis was the leading cause of death in CR ($n = 23$), followed by secondary tumors ($n = 10$). Among the 23 fatal infections, 17 occurred during consolidation, but six occurred during maintenance.

The updated results of the JALSG APL97 study with a median follow-up of 7.7 years also confirmed favorable long-term antileukemic effects of ATRA combined with chemotherapy in newly diagnosed APL (Table 11.6) [78]. Interestingly, long-term observation in the European APL93 and JALSG APL97 studies showed similar results for CR rates, death in CR rates, 10-year CIR, and 10-year OS rates (Table 11.6). The major cause of death was sepsis secondary to myelosuppression, especially after consolidation courses and in elderly patients. Long-term outcome in the European APL93 and JALSG APL97 studies confirms that the combination of ATRA with chemotherapy can cure at least three-quarter of APL patients (Fig. 11.5).

Table 11.6 Long-term follow-up for APL patients treated with ATRA and chemotherapy

	Euro APL93	JALSG APL97
No. of patients	576	283
Median age (range)	46 (28-72)	48 (15-70)
Median initial leukocyte count (x10^9/L)	-	1.7 (0.03-257.0)
Median platelet count (x10^9/L)	-	30 (2-238)
M3v	81 (15%)	18 (6%)
Complete remission	533 (92.5%)	267 (94%)
10-year cumulative incidence of relapse (CIR)	26.6%	26.5%
10-year cumulative incidence of non-relapse mortality	11%	8.6%
10-year event-free survival (EFS)	61.7%	-
10-year disease-free survival (DFS)	-	67%
10-year overall survival (OS)	77%	78.8%

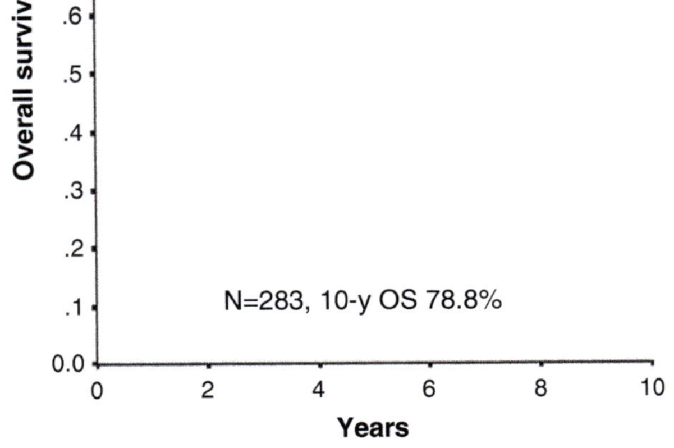

Fig. 11.5 10-year overall survival in patients with APL treated with ATRA and chemotherapy in the JALSG APL97 study. Of 283 patients, 267 (94%) achieved complete remission in the JALSG APL97 study. The 10-year cumulative incidences of non-relapse mortality and relapse were 8.6% and 26.5%, respectively. Estimated 10-year disease-free survival and overall survival rates were 67% and 78.8%

However, reduction of the incidence of non-relapse mortality (NRM) during consolidation in this highly curable disease is mandatory and requires reduction in the use of myelosuppressive drugs. In addition, the 10-year CIR was observed approximately one-quarter of APL patients treated with ATRA and chemotherapy (Table 11.6). Arsenic derivatives appear to have a growing role to play in these situations. Arsenic compounds are generally not myelosuppressive, and their use in first-line treatment of APL may reduce the total amount of chemotherapy and fatal infections [84, 85, 90, 91].

11.4.6 Unsolved Issues in APL Treated with ATRA and Chemotherapy

11.4.6.1 Relapse

In the European APL93 and JALSG APL97 studies, 10-year CIR rates were 26.6% and 26.5%, respectively (Table 11.6) [68, 78]. Relapse is still the main issue in APL patients treated with ATRA and chemotherapy, and drug resistance to ATRA is a critical problem. Relapse at extramedullary sites occurs up to 3–5% of APL patients treated with ATRA and chemotherapy [92, 93]. Extramedullary relapse such as the central nervous system (CNS) involvement can occur either in isolation or associated with marrow relapse. Management of relapse in the CNS and other extramedullary sites is a challenging issue. European LeukemiaNet recommends that CNS prophylaxis can be considered only for patients with hyperleukocytosis during induction [14]. Notably, first late relapse (>4 years) was also seen in about 3% of APL patients treated with ATRA and intensive chemotherapy [77, 94].

Inferior prognostic factor for relapse is high presenting WBC count (>10×10^9/L) in APL patients who received ATRA and chemotherapy [24, 81]. This high-risk group is also related to *FLT3*-ITD, *PML* break point (bcr3 isoform), and M3v [28, 29]. Expression of CD56 in APL cells has been associated with short DFS and extramedullary relapses [95–98]. A total of 72 (11%) of 651 patients were CD56+ (expression of CD56 in >20% APL cells) in the PETHEMA studies [97]. CD56 + APL was significantly associated with high WBC counts, bcr3 isoform, and extramedullary relapse. Moreover, 5-year CIR rates were 22% and 10% for CD56+ and CD56- APL patients (P = 0.006). In the JALSG APL97 study, expression of CD56 was found in 23 (9.6%) of 239 patients [98]. The CIR and EFS showed an inferior trend in CD56+ APL.

Detection of minimal residual disease (MRD) by RT-PCR or real-time quantitative PCR of *PML-RARA* in the marrow cells has suggested a benefit for preemptive therapy in patients who develop molecular relapse compared with treatment initiated at the time of hematological relapse [6, 99–102]. The risks of hemorrhagic early death and development of DS when patients present with overt disease argue strongly in favor of starting therapy as early as possible in cases of emergent relapse. This has provided the rationale for sequential MRD assessment by every 3 months during first 3 years after completion of consolidation therapy [14].

Several mechanisms of resistance to ATRA have been proposed, including the development of mutations in the ligand-binding domain (LBD) of the RARα, accelerated ATRA catabolism, and increased levels of cellular retinoic acid binding protein (CRABP), which induces retinoic acid metabolism [103, 104]. Genetic mutations that result in amino acid substitution in the RARα LBD are reported as underlying mechanisms in resistance to ATRA [105, 106]. In the *RARA* mutation, ATRA binding with LBD is generally impaired, and then ligand-dependent corepressor dissociation and degradation of PML-RARα by the proteasome pathway are inhibited. As a result, a maturational block in cell differentiation is observed in APL patients resistant to ATRA. Gallagher et al. [106] reported that LBD mutations were observed in 18 of 45 (40%) relapse patients treated with ATRA and chemotherapy.

About 25% of patients eventually relapse and are possibly refractory to further ATRA and chemotherapy. In addition, second CR achieved with ATRA lacks durability. The new retinoid, tamibarotene, developed in Japan has more potent in vitro differentiation activity than ATRA [19]. Tamibarotene induced second CR in approximately 60% of patients with relapsed APL after ATRA treatment.

Currently, ATO is considered a first-line therapy for relapsed APL patients who were previously treated with ATRA and chemotherapy [90]. ATO induces CR in more than 80% of patients after treatment with ATRA and chemotherapy. Since ATO does not appear to completely eradicate leukemic cells in all patients, the best post-remission therapy remains to be examined. Outcomes of autologous HSCT in patients with second molecular remission after arsenic therapy were excellent [79, 80, 107, 108]. Although tamibarotene, ATO, and gemtuzumab ozogamicin (GO: CD33 antibody conjugated with calicheamicin) are effective for relapsed patients, their optimal scheduling and benefits when combined with other therapies for newly diagnosed APL remain to be determined [101, 109].

11.4.6.2 Elderly APL Patients

APL shows a more even age distribution and is less frequently diagnosed in the elderly compared with other AML subtypes. Only 15–20% of APL patients are older than 60 years, and only 1–6% are older than 70 years [110, 111]. The introduction of ATRA combined with chemotherapy has led to considerable improvement in disease outcome by allowing significantly higher CR and DFS rates with respect to the pre-ATRA era. However, compared with younger patients, elderly patients had less favorable outcomes because of poor tolerance to intensive chemotherapy during induction and consolidation phases. CR rates among elderly patients are lower than in younger patients, because of higher rates of early death (Table 11.7) [78, 110–112]. In the GIMEMA study, 43 of 67 elderly patients (64%) completed three courses of consolidation chemotherapy, while seven (11%) and 17 (25%) patients withdrew after their first and second courses, respectively; nine (13%) died in CR and 12 (18%) relapsed [110]. After amending the protocol to include only the first cycle, all patients received their assigned treatment; two (5%) died in CR and six (15%) relapsed. This highlighted the frequency and severity of complications associated with intensive chemotherapy and indicated that less intensive post-remission therapy allows significant reduction of therapy-related toxicity in APL of

Table 11.7 Elderly patients with APL treated with ATRA and chemotherapy in multicenter trials

Study	GIMEMA AIDA0493	PETHEMA LPA96&99	European APL93	JALSG APL97
No. of patients	134	104	129	46
Median age (range)	66 (60-75)	68 (60-83)	66 (62-70)	63 (60-70)
High-risk	21 (16%)	21 (20%)	0	9 (20%)
Complete remission	116 (87%)	87 (84%)	111 (86%)	41 (89%)
Death during induction	16 (12%)	16 (15%)	18 (14%)	5 (11%)
Hemorrhage	4 (3%)	6 (6%)	-	1 (2%)
Differentiation synd.	4 (3%)	1 (1%)	-	2 (4%)
Infection	2 (1.5%)	9 (9%)	-	1 (2%)
Death during consolidation	11 (10%)	3 (3%)	10 (9%)	5 (13%)
Disease-free survival (DFS)	59% (6)	79% (6)	53% (4)*	65% (10)
CIR	20%	8.5% (6)	15.6% (4)	15% (10)
Cumulative incidence of NRM	-	-	18.6%	20% (10)
Overall survival (OS)	56% (6)	-	57.8% (4)	63% (10)

CIR cumulative incidence of relapse, *NRM* non-relapse mortality
*Event-free survival

the elderly. In the PETHEMA LPA66 and LPA99 studies using anthracycline monotherapy for consolidation, excellent tolerance and a high degree of compliance were observed (Table 11.7) [111]. In both European APL93 and JALSG APL97 studies, a significantly higher cumulative incidence of NRM, particularly during consolidation, was observed in the elderly patients than in younger patients (Table 11.7) [78, 112]. In addition, the PETHEMA studies show that a significantly higher incidence of low-risk patients among the elderly cohort may partially account for their low CIR compared with younger patients [111]. However, CIR rates in other studies did not significantly differ between the elderly and younger patients. These observations suggest that high incidence of NRM during induction and consolidation therapy is the main cause of poor long-term outcome in elderly patients [78, 110–112]. ATO, which is only mildly myelosuppressive, may be a better choice to reduce NRM risk in elderly patients.

11.4.6.3 Therapy-Related Myelodysplastic Syndromes and Leukemia After Treatment for APL with ATRA and Chemotherapy

The use of ATRA in combination with chemotherapy has markedly improved outcomes for APL patients. However, a significant number of patients developed therapy-related myelodysplastic syndromes (MDS) or AML [113]. The Rome group firstly reported 5 of 77 APL patients (6.5%) who acquired therapy-related MDS or AML [113]. Of 677 patients treated in the European APL91 and APL93 studies, 6 (0.97%) developed MDS during a median follow-up of 51 months [114]. In the PETHEMA studies, 17 of 918 patients (1.9%) who achieved CR developed therapy-related MDS and AML after a median of 43 months from CR [115]. Partial and complete deletions of chromosomes 5 and 7 and 11q23 (*MLL*) rearrangements were the most common cytogenetic abnormalities in these therapy-related MDS and AML cases. In addition, clinical outcomes for patients with therapy-related MDS and AML were extremely poor. Median OS after development of therapy-related MDS or AML was approximately 10 months. Allogeneic HSCT can barely rescue these patients. Thus, the occurrence of therapy-related MDS and AML after successful treatment of APL is an emerging problem. The prognostic scoring system at initial diagnosis and monitoring of MRD by RT-PCR might allow better tailoring of treatment intensity in APL patients to spare unnecessary toxicity and to minimize the risk of therapy-related MDS and AML. The choice of ATO instead of chemotherapy during induction and consolidation could avoid development of these late complications in this curable disease.

11.5 Tamibarotene

11.5.1 Properties of Tamibarotene

Tamibarotene (formerly Am80) is a synthetic retinoid that induces differentiation of myeloid cell lines such as HL-60 and NB-4 cells with in vitro activity approximately ten times more potent than that of ATRA [19, 20]. Tamibarotene has a low affinity for the CRABP, the overexpression of which is associated with ATRA resistance [103, 104]. As tamibarotene also has a lower affinity for the dermal retinoic acid receptor-γ (RARγ), it may have lower rates of dermatological adverse events than ATRA. In addition, unlike ATRA, plasma levels of tamibarotene do not decline after daily administration, so it has a more favorable pharmacokinetic profile. These properties imply that tamibarotene is superior to ATRA in APL treatment. Tamibarotene has been shown to be effective for both untreated APL patients and those who have relapsed after ATRA and chemotherapy [19, 21, 22].

11.5.2 Tamibarotene in Reinduction Therapy for Relapsed APL Patients

Tobita et al. [19] reported that 24 patients with APL who relapsed after combination therapy with ATRA and chemotherapy were treated with tamibarotene alone (6 mg/m^2/day). Most patients had not received ATRA as consolidation or maintenance therapy in their previous treatment, and none had received ATO. In this trial, 14 (58%) patients achieved second CR after induction therapy with tamibarotene. After a maximum follow-up of 14 months, five patients who achieved CR received an allogeneic HSCT and none relapsed. Eight received additional consolidation with conventional chemotherapy and one had relapsed. One who had continued with tamibarotene therapy alone relapsed after 2 months. Adverse effects of tamibarotene included DS ($n = 1$), hyperleukocytosis ($n = 1$), xerosis ($n = 9$), cheilitis ($n = 8$), hyperglyceridemia ($n = 16$), and hypercholesterolemia ($n = 15$). Thus, tamibarotene is active for APL after relapse from ATRA-induced CR.

Sanford et al. [22] reported on the use of tamibarotene in patients who had relapsed after use of both ATRA and ATO. In this phase II study, 14 adults with relapsed or refractory APL after treatment with ATRA and ATO were treated with tamibarotene (6 mg/m^2/day) during induction and for up to six cycles of consolidation. The overall response rate was 64%, but seven of the nine responders relapsed again after a median of 4.6 months (range, 1.6–26.8 months). This study demonstrates that single-agent tamibarotene was well tolerated and resulted in a relatively better response rate in patients with relapsed and refractory APL. Optimal management for patients who relapsed after ATRA and ATO treatment is currently unknown. Clinical trials of tamibarotene for relapsed patients should consider incorporating other agents such as anthracyclines, ATO, and GO.

11.5.3 Tamibarotene in Maintenance Therapy

A recently published randomized trial implied that tamibarotene is more effective than ATRA as maintenance therapy in patients with high-risk APL [21]. In this JALSG APL204 study, newly diagnosed patients were treated during induction with ATRA, idarubicin, and Ara-C and during consolidation cycles with anthracyclines and Ara-C. Patients in molecular remission after consolidation were randomly assigned to ATRA ($n = 135$) (45 mg/m^2/day) or to tamibarotene ($n = 134$) (6 mg/m^2/day), for 14 days every 3 months (Fig. 11.3). The study showed a trend toward fewer relapses in the tamibarotene group (20 [15%] vs. 10 [7%]) and improved relapse-free survival (RFS) at 4 years (91% vs. 84%, $P = 0.095$), although neither difference was statistically significant. However, a subset analysis of 52 patients with high-risk APL showed significantly improved RFS in the tamibarotene group (87% vs. 52%, $P = 0.03$). These results suggest that tamibarotene has a potential role in frontline treatment and trials to evaluate concurrent treatment with tamibarotene, and ATO is warranted particularly in high-risk APL patients.

11.6 ATRA in the Treatment of AML Other than APL

Several clinical trials evaluated ATRA in combination with intensive chemotherapy for patients with AML subtypes other than APL [116, 117]. Among the German-Austrian AML Study Group (AMLSG) trial (AMLHD98B) in AML patients aged 61 years and older, ATRA was given at a dose of 45 mg/m^2 on day 3 through 5 and at 15 mg/m^2 on days 6 through 28 during induction [116]. During first consolidation, ATRA was given at 15 mg/m^2 on day 3 through 28. Patients randomized to the ATRA arm ($n = 242$) had a significantly higher 4-year RFS (20.9% vs. 4.8%, $P = 0.006$) and OS (10.8% vs. 5%, $P = 0.003$) rates compared with the no-ATRA arm ($n = 122$). In this study, patients with the genotype mutant *NPM1* without *FLT3*-ITD who had been randomized to ATRA ($n = 14$) had a significantly better outcome compared to patients with the same genotype who had not been randomized to ATRA ($n = 12$). However, the results of all other studies had been negative.

In the UK MRC AML12 trial, 1075 patients less than 60 years of age were randomized to receive ATRA at a dose of 45 mg/m^2 from days 1 to 60 or not during the first two courses of induction therapy [117]. Overall, there was no effect from the addition of ATRA with equal CR rates (83% with ATRA vs. 84% without ATRA) and OS (33% vs. 30%). Of 592 patients examined with *NPM1* and *FLT3*-ITD, *NPM1* mutations were present in 207 (35%) and *FLT3*-ITD in 137 (23%). Among patients with *NPM1* mutation and wild-type *FLT3*, 8-year OS was 56% in the ATRA group ($n = 66$) and 40% in the no-ATRA group ($n = 52$), but the difference was not statistically significant ($P = 0.2$).

The exact molecular mechanisms through which ATRA may exert its effects in AML with mutant *NPM1* remain elusive. In vitro studies suggest a link between NPM1 and ATRA-mediated transcriptional regulation under physiological conditions and in myeloid leukemogenesis. Recent studies also showed that ATRA and ATO synergistically induce proteasome-dependent degradation of NPM1 protein and apoptosis in *NPM1*-mutated AML cells [118, 119]. In addition, intracellular distribution of PML is altered in *NPM1*-mutated AML cells and reverted by treatment with ATRA and ATO. These findings may provide experimental evidence for further exploring ATRA and ATO in *NPM1*-mutated AML patients. Alternatively, overexpression of *EVI-1* occurs in approximately 10% of AML patients and is associated with very poor outcomes. Recent in vitro and in vivo experiment also showed that primary AML cells with enhanced *EVI-1* expression respond to ATRA by inducing differentiation, which implies that combination of ATRA with conventional chemotherapy might be a promising treatment strategy [120].

11.7 Conclusions

Advent of ATRA in the treatment of APL is the first example of successful molecular-targeted therapy. Since ATRA alone induces no molecular remission in most patients, chemotherapy is indispensable in the treatment of APL. While ATRA is quite effective and has only few side effects, DS is a serious adverse effect during induction therapy. In addition, point mutations in the LBD of PML-RARα induce resistance to ATRA in relapsed patients. Mutations in ATP-binding regions of BCR-ABL have also been found in patients with chronic myeloid leukemia refractory to tyrosine kinase inhibitors such as imatinib mesylate. This mechanism of resistance is an important problem in molecular-targeted agents. The experience of ATRA should be exploited in the treatment of other cancers. On the basis of further understanding of underlying mechanisms, drugs that specifically target pathogenic molecules should be developed for other tumors. The major causes of treatment failure in APL treated with ATRA and chemotherapy are early death such as hemorrhage and DS in induction, infection during consolidation, relapse, and therapy-related leukemia. Another agent targeted to APL cells, ATO, may lead to reduce NRM such as hemorrhage and infection in induction and consolidation because ATO is not myelosuppressive. Moreover, combination therapy with ATRA, chemotherapy, and

ATO may induce a durable CR in most APL patients by decreasing CIR because these agents possess different effects against APL cells.

Acknowledgments The author declares no potential conflicts of interest. This work was supported in part by Grants-in-Aid for Scientific Research from the Japanese Ministry of Education, Culture, Sport, Science, and Technology (JSPS KAKENHI Grant number 26461431); by the National Cancer Center Research and Development Fund (26-A-24); by Grants-in-Aid from the Cancer Research from the Japanese Ministry of Health, Labor and Welfare (Clinical Cancer Research 23-004); by the MHLW KAKENHI Grant Number H26-Kakushintekigan-Ippan-133; by Grants-in-Aid from the Project for Development of Innovative Research on Cancer Therapeutics (P-Direct); and by the Japan Leukaemia Research Fund.

References

1. Bennett JM, Catovsky D, Daniel MT, Flandrin G, Galton DA, Gralnick HR, et al. Proposals for the classification of the acute leukaemias. French-American-British (FAB) co-operative group. Br J Haematol. 1976;33:451–8.
2. Bennett JM, Catovsky D, Daniel MT, Flandrin G, Galton DA, Gralnick HR, et al. A variant form of hypergranular promyelocytic leukaemia (M3). Br J Haematol. 1980;44:169–70.
3. Tallman MS, Kwaan HC. Reassessing the hemostatic disorder associated with acute promyelocytic leukemia. Blood. 1992;79:543–53.
4. Breen KA, Grimwade D, Hunt BJ. The pathogenesis and management of the coagulopathy of acute promyelocytic leukaemia. Br J Haematol. 2012;156:24–36. doi:10.1111/j.1365-2141.2011.08922.x.
5. Rowley JD, Golomb HM, Dougherty C. 15/17 translocation, a consistent chromosomal change in acute promyelocytic leukaemia. Lancet. 1977;1(8010):549–50.
6. Grimwade D, Lo Coco F. Acute promyelocytic leukemia: a model for the role of molecular diagnosis and residual disease monitoring in directing treatment approach in acute myeloid leukemia. Leukemia. 2002;16:1959–73.
7. Borrow J, Goddard AD, Sheer D, Solomon E. Molecular analysis of acute promyelocytic leukemia breakpoint cluster region on chromosome 17. Science. 1990;249(4976):1577–80.
8. de Thé H, Chomienne C, Lanotte M, Degos L, Dejean A. The t(15;17) translocation of acute promyelocytic leukaemia fuses the retinoic acid receptor alpha gene to a novel transcribed locus. Nature. 1990;347(6293):558–61.
9. Kakizuka A, Miller Jr WH, Umesono K, Warrell Jr RP, Frankel SR, Murty VV, et al. Chromosomal translocation t(15;17) in human acute promyelocytic leukemia fuses RAR alpha with a novel putative transcription factor, PML. Cell. 1991;66:663–74.
10. Huang ME, Ye YC, Chen SR, Chai JR, Lu JX, Zhoa L, Gu LJ, Wang ZY. Use of all-trans retinoic acid in the treatment of acute promyelocytic leukemia. Blood. 1988;72:567–72.
11. Ohno R, Asou N, Ohnishi K. Treatment of acute promyelocytic leukemia: strategy toward further increase of cure rate. Leukemia. 2003;17:1454–63.
12. Asou N. All-trans retinoic acid in the treatment of acute promyelocytic leukemia. Intern Med. 2007;46:91–3.
13. Wang ZY, Chen Z. Acute promyelocytic leukemia: from highly fatal to highly curable. Blood. 2008;111:2505–15. doi:10.1182/blood-2007-07-102798.
14. Sanz MA, Grimwade D, Tallman MS, Lowenberg B, Fenaux P, Estey EH, et al. Management of acute promyelocytic leukemia: recommendations from an expert panel on behalf of the European LeukemiaNet. Blood. 2009;113:1875–91. doi:10.1182/blood-2008-04-150250.
15. Sanz MA, Lo-Coco F. Modern approaches to treating acute promyelocytic leukemia. J Clin Oncol. 2011;29:495–503. doi:10.1200/JCO.2010.32.1067.

16. Grignani F, De Matteis S, Nervi C, Tomassoni L, Gelmetti V, Cioce M, et al. Fusion proteins of the retinoic acid receptor-alpha recruit histone deacetylase in promyelocytic leukaemia. Nature. 1998;391(6669):815–8.
17. Lin RJ, Nagy L, Inoue S, Shao W, Miller Jr WH, Evans RM. Role of the histone deacetylase complex in acute promyelocytic leukaemia. Nature. 1998;391(6669):811–4.
18. He LZ, Guidez F, Tribioli C, Peruzzi D, Ruthardt M, Zelent A, et al. Distinct interactions of PML-RARalpha and PLZF-RARalpha with co-repressors determine differential responses to RA in APL. Nat Genet. 1998;18:126–35.
19. Tobita T, Takeshita A, Kitamura K, Ohnishi K, Yanagi M, Hiraoka A, et al. Treatment with a new synthetic retinoid, Am80, of acute promyelocytic leukemia relapsed from complete remission induced by all-trans retinoic acid. Blood. 1997;90:967–73.
20. Takeuchi M, Yano T, Omoto E, Takahashi K, Kibata M, Shudo K, et al. Relapsed acute promyelocytic leukemia previously treated with all-trans retinoic acid: clinical experience with a new synthetic retinoid, Am-80. Leuk Lymphoma. 1998;31:441–51.
21. Shinagawa K, Yanada M, Sakura T, Ueda Y, Sawa M, Miyatake J, et al. Tamibarotene as maintenance therapy for acute promyelocytic leukemia: results from a randomized controlled trial. J Clin Oncol. 2014;32:3729–35. doi:10.1200/JCO.2013.53.3570.
22. Sanford D, Lo-Coco F, Sanz MA, Di Bona E, Coutre S, Altman JK, et al. Tamibarotene in patients with acute promyelocytic leukaemia relapsing after treatment with all-trans retinoic acid and arsenic trioxide. Br J Haematol. 2015;171:471–7. doi:10.1111/bjh.13607.
23. de la Serna J, Montesinos P, Vellenga E, Rayón C, Parody R, León A, et al. Causes and prognostic factors of remission induction failure in patients with acute promyelocytic leukemia treated with all-trans retinoic acid and idarubicin. Blood. 2008;111:3395–402. doi:10.1182/blood-2007-07-100669.
24. Asou N, Adachi K, Tamura J, Kanamaru A, Kageyama S, Hiraoka A, et al. Analysis of prognostic factors in newly diagnosed acute promyelocytic leukemia treated with all-trans retinoic acid and chemotherapy. Japan Adult Leukemia Study Group. J Clin Oncol. 1998;16:78–85.
25. Guglielmi C, Martelli MP, Diverio D, Fenu S, Vegna ML, Cantù-Rajnoldi A, et al. Immunophenotype of adult and childhood acute promyelocytic leukaemia: correlation with morphology, type of PML gene breakpoint and clinical outcome. A cooperative Italian study on 196 cases. Br J Haematol. 1998;102:1035–41.
26. Foley R, Soamboonsrup P, Carter RF, Benger A, Meyer R, Walker I, et al. CD34-positive acute promyelocytic leukemia is associated with leukocytosis, microgranular/hypogranular morphology, expression of CD2 and bcr3 isoform. Am J Hematol. 2001;67:34–41.
27. Tallman MS, Kim HT, Montesinos P, Appelbaum FR, de la Serna J, Bennett JM, et al. Does microgranular variant morphology of acute promyelocytic leukemia independently predict a less favorable outcome compared with classical M3 APL? A joint study of the North American Intergroup and the PETHEMA Group. Blood. 2010;116:5650–9. doi:10.1182/blood-2010-06-288613.
28. Kiyoi H, Naoe T, Yokota S, Nakao M, Minami S, Kuriyama K, et al. Internal tandem duplication of FLT3 associated with leukocytosis in acute promyelocytic leukemia. Leukemia Study Group of the Ministry of Health and Welfare (Kohseisho). Leukemia. 1997;11(9):1447–52.
29. Callens C, Chevret S, Cayuela JM, Cassinat B, Raffoux E, de Botton S, Thomas X, et al. Prognostic implication of FLT3 and Ras gene mutations in patients with acute promyelocytic leukemia (APL): a retrospective study from the European APL Group. Leukemia. 2005;19:1153–60.
30. Melnick A, Licht JD. Deconstructing a disease: RARalpha, its fusion partners, and their roles in the pathogenesis of acute promyelocytic leukemia. Blood. 1999;93:3167–215.
31. Mistry AR, Pedersen EW, Solomon E, Grimwade D. The molecular pathogenesis of acute promyelocytic leukaemia: implications for the clinical management of the disease. Blood Rev. 2003;17:71–97.
32. de Thé H, Chen Z. Acute promyelocytic leukaemia: novel insights into the mechanisms of cure. Nat Rev Cancer. 2010;10:775–83. doi:10.1038/nrc2943.

33. de Thé H, Le Bras M, Lallemand-Breitenbach V. The cell biology of disease: acute promyelocytic leukemia, arsenic, and PML bodies. J Cell Biol. 2012;198:11–21. doi:10.1083/jcb.201112044.
34. Nasr R, de Thé H. Eradication of acute promyelocytic leukemia-initiating cells by PML/RARA-targeting. Int J Hematol. 2010;91:742–7. doi:10.1007/s12185-010-0582-0.
35. Grimwade D, Biondi A, Mozziconacci MJ, Hagemeijer A, Berger R, Neat M, et al. Characterization of acute promyelocytic leukemia cases lacking the classic t(15;17): results of the European Working Party. Groupe Français de Cytogénétique Hématologique, Groupe de Français d'Hematologie Cellulaire, UK Cancer Cytogenetics Group and BIOMED 1 European Community-Concerted Action "Molecular Cytogenetic Diagnosis in Haematological Malignancies". Blood. 2000;96:1297–308.
36. Redner RL. Variations on a theme: the alternate translocations in APL. Leukemia. 2002;16:1927–32.
37. Adams J, Nassiri M. Acute promyelocytic leukemia: a review and discussion of variant translocations. Arch Pathol Lab Med. 2015;139(10):1308–13. doi:10.5858/arpa.2013-0345-RS.
38. Iwanaga E, Nakamura M, Nanri T, Kawakita T, Horikawa K, Mitsuya H, et al. Acute promyelocytic leukemia harboring a STAT5B-RARA fusion gene and a G596V missense mutation in the STAT5B SH2 domain of the STAT5B-RARA. Eur J Haematol. 2009;83:499–501. doi:10.1111/j.1600-0609.2009.01324.x.
39. Welch JS, Ley TJ, Link DC, Miller CA, Larson DE, Koboldt DC, et al. The origin and evolution of mutations in acute myeloid leukemia. Cell. 2012;150:264–78. doi:10.1016/j.cell.2012.06.023.
40. Madan V, Shyamsunder P, Han L, Mayakonda A, Nagata Y, Sundaresan J, et al. Comprehensive mutational analysis of primary and relapse acute promyelocytic leukemia. Leukemia. 2016; doi:10.1038/leu.2016.69.
41. Brown D, Kogan S, Lagasse E, Weissman I, Alcalay M, Pelicci PG, et al. A PMLRARalpha transgene initiates murine acute promyelocytic leukemia. Proc Natl Acad Sci U S A. 1997;94:2551–6.
42. He LZ, Tribioli C, Rivi R, Peruzzi D, Pelicci PG, Soares V, et al. Acute leukemia with promyelocytic features in PML/RARalpha transgenic mice. Proc Natl Acad Sci U S A. 1997;94:5302–7.
43. Grisolano JL, Wesselschmidt RL, Pelicci PG, Ley TJ. Altered myeloid development and acute leukemia in transgenic mice expressing PML-RAR alpha under control of cathepsin G regulatory sequences. Blood. 1997;89(2):376–87.
44. Westervelt P, Lane AA, Pollock JL, Oldfather K, Holt MS, Zimonjic DB, et al. High-penetrance mouse model of acute promyelocytic leukemia with very low levels of PML-RARalpha expression. Blood. 2003;102:1857–65.
45. Collins SJ. The role of retinoids and retinoic acid receptors in normal hematopoiesis. Leukemia. 2002;16:1896–905.
46. Chen JD, Evans RM. A transcriptional co-repressor that interacts with nuclear hormone receptors. Nature. 1995;377(6548):454–7.
47. Hörlein AJ, Näär AM, Heinzel T, Torchia J, Gloss B, Kurokawa R, et al. Ligand-independent repression by the thyroid hormone receptor mediated by a nuclear receptor co-repressor. Nature. 1995;377(6548):397–404.
48. Chih DY, Chumakov AM, Park DJ, Silla AG, Koeffler HP. Modulation of mRNA expression of a novel human myeloid-selective CCAAT/enhancer binding protein gene (C/EBP epsilon). Blood. 1997;90:2987–94.
49. Daniel MT, Koken M, Romagné O, Barbey S, Bazarbachi A, Stadler M, et al. PML protein expression in hematopoietic and acute promyelocytic leukemia cells. Blood. 1993;82:1858–67.
50. Dyck JA, Maul GG, Miller Jr WH, Chen JD, Kakizuka A, Evans RM. A novel macromolecular structure is a target of the promyelocyte-retinoic acid receptor oncoprotein. Cell. 1994;76:333–43.

51. Koken MH, Puvion-Dutilleul F, Guillemin MC, Viron A, Linares-Cruz G, Stuurman N, et al. The t(15;17) translocation alters a nuclear body in a retinoic acid-reversible fashion. EMBO J. 1994;13:1073–83.
52. Ferbeyre G. PML a target of translocations in APL is a regulator of cellular senescence. Leukemia. 2002;16:1918–26.
53. Borden KL. Pondering the promyelocytic leukemia protein (PML) puzzle: possible functions for PML nuclear bodies. Mol Cell Biol. 2002;22:5259–69.
54. Ito K, Bernardi R, Morotti A, Matsuoka S, Saglio G, Ikeda Y, et al. PML targeting eradicates quiescent leukaemia-initiating cells. Nature. 2008;453(7198):1072–8. doi:10.1038/nature07016.
55. Perez A, Kastner P, Sethi S, Lutz Y, Reibel C, Chambon P. PMLRAR homodimers: distinct DNA binding properties and heteromeric interactions with RXR. EMBO J. 1993;12:3171–82.
56. Zhu J, Gianni M, Kopf E, Honoré N, Chelbi-Alix M, Koken M, et al. Retinoic acid induces proteasome-dependent degradation of retinoic acid receptor alpha (RARalpha) and oncogenic RARalpha fusion proteins. Proc Natl Acad Sci U S A. 1999;96:14807–12.
57. Zhu J, Zhou J, Peres L, Riaucoux F, Honoré N, Kogan S, et al. A sumoylation site in PML/RARA is essential for leukemic transformation. Cancer Cell. 2005;7:143–53.
58. Zhu J, Koken MH, Quignon F, Chelbi-Alix MK, Degos L, Wang ZY, et al. Arsenic-induced PML targeting onto nuclear bodies: implications for the treatment of acute promyelocytic leukemia. Proc Natl Acad Sci U S A. 1997;94:3978–83.
59. Zhang XW, Yan XJ, Zhou ZR, Yang FF, Wu ZY, Sun HB, et al. Arsenic trioxide controls the fate of the PML-RARalpha oncoprotein by directly binding PML. Science. 2010;328(5975):240–3. doi:10.1126/science.1183424.
60. Nasr R, Guillemin MC, Ferhi O, Soilihi H, Peres L, Berthier C, et al. Eradication of acute promyelocytic leukemia-initiating cells through PML-RARA degradation. Nat Med. 2008;14:1333–42. doi:10.1038/nm.1891.
61. Warrell Jr RP, Frankel SR, Miller Jr WH, Scheinberg DA, Itri LM, Hittelman WN, et al. Differentiation therapy of acute promyelocytic leukemia with tretinoin (all-trans-retinoic acid). N Engl J Med. 1991;324:1385–93.
62. Ohno R, Ohnishi K, Takeshita A, Tanimoto M, Murakami H, Kanamaru A, et al. All-trans retinoic acid therapy in relapsed/refractory or newly diagnosed acute promyelocytic leukemia (APL) in Japan. Leukemia. 1994;8(Suppl 3):S64–9.
63. Kanamaru A, Takemoto Y, Tanimoto M, Murakami H, Asou N, Kobayashi T, et al. All-trans retinoic acid for the treatment of newly diagnosed acute promyelocytic leukemia. Japan Adult Leukemia Study Group. Blood. 1995;85:1202–6.
64. Frankel SR, Eardley A, Lauwers G, Weiss M, Warrell Jr RP. The "retinoic acid syndrome" in acute promyelocytic leukemia. Ann Intern Med. 1992;117:292–6.
65. Tallman MS, Andersen JW, Schiffer CA, Appelbaum FR, Feusner JH, Ogden A, et al. All-trans retinoic acid in acute promyelocytic leukemia. N Engl J Med. 1997;337:1021–8.
66. Fenaux P, Le Deley MC, Castaigne S, Archimbaud E, Chomienne C, Link H, et al. Effect of all transretinoic acid in newly diagnosed acute promyelocytic leukemia. Results of a multicenter randomized trial. European APL 91 Group. Blood. 1993;82:3241.
67. Fenaux P, Chastang C, Chevret S, Sanz M, Dombret H, Archimbaud E, et al. A randomized comparison of all transretinoic acid (ATRA) followed by chemotherapy and ATRA plus chemotherapy and the role of maintenance therapy in newly diagnosed acute promyelocytic leukemia. The European APL Group. Blood. 1999;94:1192–200.
68. Adès L, Guerci A, Raffoux E, Sanz M, Chevallier P, Lapusan S, et al. Very long-term outcome of acute promyelocytic leukemia after treatment with all-trans retinoic acid and chemotherapy: the European APL Group experience. Blood. 2010;115:1690–6. doi:10.1182/blood-2009-07-233387.
69. Adès L, Chevret S, Raffoux E, de Botton S, Guerci A, Pigneux A, et al. Is cytarabine useful in the treatment of acute promyelocytic leukemia? Results of a randomized trial from the European Acute Promyelocytic Leukemia Group. J Clin Oncol. 2006;24:5703–10.

70. Adès L, Chevret S, Raffoux E, Guerci-Bresler A, Pigneux A, Vey N, et al. Long-term follow-up of European APL 2000 trial, evaluating the role of cytarabine combined with ATRA and Daunorubicin in the treatment of nonelderly APL patients. Am J Hematol. 2013;88:556–9. doi:10.1002/ajh.23451.
71. Avvisati G, Lo-Coco F, Paoloni FP, Petti MC, Diverio D, Vignetti M, et al. AIDA 0493 protocol for newly diagnosed acute promyelocytic leukemia: very long-term results and role of maintenance. Blood. 2011;117:4716–25. doi:10.1182/blood-2010-08-302950.
72. Lo-Coco F, Avvisati G, Vignetti M, Breccia M, Gallo E, Rambaldi A, et al. Front-line treatment of acute promyelocytic leukemia with AIDA induction followed by risk-adapted consolidation for adults younger than 61 years: results of the AIDA-2000 trial of the GIMEMA Group. Blood. 2010;116:3171–9. doi:10.1182/blood-2010-03-276196.
73. Sanz MA, Martín G, Rayón C, Esteve J, González M, Díaz-Mediavilla J, et al. A modified AIDA protocol with anthracycline-based consolidation results in high antileukemic efficacy and reduced toxicity in newly diagnosed PML/RARalpha-positive acute promyelocytic leukemia. PETHEMA group. Blood. 1999;94:3015–21.
74. Sanz MA, Martín G, González M, León A, Rayón C, Rivas C, et al. Risk-adapted treatment of acute promyelocytic leukemia with all-trans-retinoic acid and anthracycline monochemotherapy: a multicenter study by the PETHEMA group. Blood. 2004;103:1237–43.
75. Tallman MS, Andersen JW, Schiffer CA, Appelbaum FR, Feusner JH, Woods WG, et al. All-trans retinoic acid in acute promyelocytic leukemia: long-term outcome and prognostic factor analysis from the North American Intergroup protocol. Blood. 2002;100:4298–302.
76. Powell BL, Moser B, Stock W, Gallagher RE, Willman CL, Stone RM, et al. Arsenic trioxide improves event-free and overall survival for adults with acute promyelocytic leukemia: North American Leukemia Intergroup Study C9710. Blood. 2010;116:3751–7. doi:10.1182/blood-2010-02-269621.
77. Asou N, Kishimoto Y, Kiyoi H, Okada M, Kawai Y, Tsuzuki M, et al. A randomized study with or without intensified maintenance chemotherapy in patients with acute promyelocytic leukemia who have become negative for PML-RARalpha transcript after consolidation therapy: the Japan Adult Leukemia Study Group (JALSG) APL97 study. Blood. 2007;110:59–66.
78. Ono T, Takeshita A, Kishimoto Y, Kiyoi H, Okada M, Yamauchi T, et al. Long-term outcome and prognostic factors of elderly patients with acute promyelocytic leukemia. Cancer Sci. 2012;103:1974–8. doi:10.1111/j.1349-7006.2012.02390.x.
79. Sanz MA, Labopin M, Gorin NC, de la Rubia J, Arcese W, Meloni G, et al. Hematopoietic stem cell transplantation for adults with acute promyelocytic leukemia in the ATRA era: a survey of the European Cooperative Group for Blood and Marrow Transplantation. Bone Marrow Transplant. 2007;39:461–9.
80. Fujita H, Asou N, Iwanaga M, Hyo R, Nomura S, Kiyoi H, et al. Role of hematopoietic stem cell transplantation for relapsed acute promyelocytic leukemia: a retrospective analysis of JALSG-APL97. Cancer Sci. 2013;104:1339–45. doi:10.1111/cas.12230.
81. Sanz MA, Lo Coco F, Martín G, Avvisati G, Rayón C, Barbui T, et al. Definition of relapse risk and role of nonanthracycline drugs for consolidation in patients with acute promyelocytic leukemia: a joint study of the PETHEMA and GIMEMA cooperative groups. Blood. 2000;96:1247–53.
82. Adès L, Sanz MA, Chevret S, Montesinos P, Chevallier P, Raffoux E, et al. Treatment of newly diagnosed acute promyelocytic leukemia (APL): a comparison of French-Belgian-Swiss and PETHEMA results. Blood. 2008;111:1078–84.
83. Lehmann S, Ravn A, Carlsson L, Antunovic P, Deneberg S, Möllgård L, et al. Continuing high early death rate in acute promyelocytic leukemia: a population-based report from the Swedish Adult Acute Leukemia Registry. Leukemia. 2011;25:1128–34. doi:10.1038/leu.2011.78.
84. Lo-Coco F, Avvisati G, Vignetti M, Thiede C, Orlando SM, Iacobelli S, et al. Retinoic acid and arsenic trioxide for acute promyelocytic leukemia. N Engl J Med. 2013;369:111–21. doi:10.1056/NEJMoa1300874.

85. Burnett AK, Russell NH, Hills RK, Bowen D, Kell J, Knapper S, et al. Arsenic trioxide and all-trans retinoic acid treatment for acute promyelocytic leukaemia in all risk groups (AML17): results of a randomised, controlled, phase 3 trial. Lancet Oncol. 2015;16:1295–305. doi:10.1016/S1470-2045(15)00193-X.
86. Yanada M, Matsushita T, Asou N, Kishimoto Y, Tsuzuki M, Maeda Y, et al. Severe hemorrhagic complications during remission induction therapy for acute promyelocytic leukemia: incidence, risk factors, and influence on outcome. Eur J Haematol. 2007;78:213–9.
87. De Botton S, Dombret H, Sanz M, Miguel JS, Caillot D, Zittoun R, et al. Incidence, clinical features, and outcome of all trans-retinoic acid syndrome in 413 cases of newly diagnosed acute promyelocytic leukemia. The European APL Group. Blood. 1998;92:2712–8.
88. Tallman MS, Andersen JW, Schiffer CA, Appelbaum FR, Feusner JH, Ogden A, et al. Clinical description of 44 patients with acute promyelocytic leukemia who developed the retinoic acid syndrome. Blood. 2000;95:90–5.
89. Montesinos P, Bergua JM, Vellenga E, Rayón C, Parody R, de la Serna J, et al. Differentiation syndrome in patients with acute promyelocytic leukemia treated with all-trans retinoic acid and anthracycline chemotherapy: characteristics, outcome, and prognostic factors. Blood. 2009;113:775–83. doi:10.1182/blood-2008-07-168617.
90. Asou N. Arsenic trioxide in the treatment of relapsed and refractory acute promyelocytic leukemia. Intern Med. 2005;44:775–6.
91. Iland HJ, Bradstock K, Supple SG, Catalano A, Collins M, Hertzberg M, et al. All-trans-retinoic acid, idarubicin, and IV arsenic trioxide as initial therapy in acute promyelocytic leukemia (APML4). Blood. 2012;120:1570–80.
92. Specchia G, Lo Coco F, Vignetti M, Avvisati G, Fazi P, Albano F, et al. Extramedullary involvement at relapse in acute promyelocytic leukemia patients treated or not with all-trans retinoic acid: a report by the Gruppo Italiano Malattie Ematologiche dell'Adulto. J Clin Oncol. 2001;19:4023–8.
93. de Botton S, Sanz MA, Chevret S, Dombret H, Martin G, Thomas X, et al. Extramedullary relapse in acute promyelocytic leukemia treated with all-trans retinoic acid and chemotherapy. Leukemia. 2006;20:35–41.
94. Kelaidi C, Ades L, Chevret S, Sanz M, Guerci A, Thomas X, et al. Late first relapses in APL treated with all-trans-retinoic acid- and anthracycline- based chemotherapy: the European APL group experience (APL 91 and APL 93 trials). Leukemia. 2006;20:905–7.
95. Murray CK, Estey E, Paietta E, Howard RS, Edenfield WJ, Pierce S, et al. CD56 expression in acute promyelocytic leukemia: a possible indicator of poor treatment outcome? J Clin Oncol. 1999;17:293–7.
96. Ferrara F, Morabito F, Martino B, Specchia G, Liso V, Nobile F, et al. CD56 expression is an indicator of poor clinical outcome in patients with acute promyelocytic leukemia treated with simultaneous all-trans-retinoic acid and chemotherapy. J Clin Oncol. 2000;18:1295–300.
97. Montesinos P, Rayón C, Vellenga E, Brunet S, González J, González M, et al. Clinical significance of CD56 expression in patients with acute promyelocytic leukemia treated with all-trans retinoic acid and anthracycline-based regimens. Blood. 2011;117(6):1799–805. doi:10.1182/blood-2010-04-277434.
98. Ono T, Takeshita A, Kishimoto Y, Kiyoi H, Okada M, Yamauchi T, et al. Expression of CD56 is an unfavorable prognostic factor for acute promyelocytic leukemia with higher initial white blood cell counts. Cancer Sci. 2014;105:97–104. doi:10.1111/cas.12319.
99. Miller Jr WH, Kakizuka A, Frankel SR, Warrell Jr RP, DeBlasio A, Levine K, et al. Reverse transcription polymerase chain reaction for the rearranged retinoic acid receptor alpha clarifies diagnosis and detects minimal residual disease in acute promyelocytic leukemia. Proc Natl Acad Sci U S A. 1992;89:2694–8.
100. Lo Coco F, Diverio D, Avvisati G, Petti MC, Meloni G, Pogliani EM, et al. Therapy of molecular relapse in acute promyelocytic leukemia. Blood. 1999;94:2225.
101. Lo-Coco F, Cimino G, Breccia M, Noguera NI, Diverio D, Finolezzi E, et al. Gemtuzumab ozogamicin (Mylotarg) as a single agent for molecularly relapsed acute promyelocytic leukemia. Blood. 2004;104:1995–9.

102. Grimwade D, Jovanovic JV, Hills RK, Nugent EA, Patel Y, Flora R, et al. Prospective minimal residual disease monitoring to predict relapse of acute promyelocytic leukemia and to direct pre-emptive arsenic trioxide therapy. J Clin Oncol. 2009;27:3650–8. doi:10.1200/JCO.2008.20.1533.
103. Gallagher RE. Retinoic acid resistance in acute promyelocytic leukemia. Leukemia. 2002;16:1940–58.
104. Tomita A, Kiyoi H, Naoe T. Mechanisms of action and resistance to all-trans retinoic acid (ATRA) and arsenic trioxide (As2O 3) in acute promyelocytic leukemia. Int J Hematol. 2013;97:717–25. doi:10.1007/s12185-013-1354-4.
105. Marasca R, Zucchini P, Galimberti S, Leonardi G, Vaccari P, Donelli A, et al. Missense mutations in the PML/RARalpha ligand binding domain in ATRA-resistant As(2)O(3) sensitive relapsed acute promyelocytic leukemia. Haematologica. 1999;84:963–8.
106. Gallagher RE, Moser BK, Racevskis J, Poiré X, Bloomfield CD, Carroll AJ, et al. Treatment-influenced associations of PML-RARα mutations, FLT3 mutations, and additional chromosome abnormalities in relapsed acute promyelocytic leukemia. Blood. 2012;120:2098–108. doi:10.1182/blood-2012-01-407601.
107. de Botton S, Fawaz A, Chevret S, Dombret H, Thomas X, Sanz M, et al. Autologous and allogeneic stem-cell transplantation as salvage treatment of acute promyelocytic leukemia initially treated with all-trans-retinoic acid: a retrospective analysis of the European acute promyelocytic leukemia group. J Clin Oncol. 2005;23:120–6.
108. Yanada M, Tsuzuki M, Fujita H, Fujimaki K, Fujisawa S, Sunami K, et al. Phase 2 study of arsenic trioxide followed by autologous hematopoietic cell transplantation for relapsed acute promyelocytic leukemia. Blood. 2013;121:3095–102. doi:10.1182/blood-2012-11-466862.
109. Petti MC, Pinazzi MB, Diverio D, Romano A, Petrucci MT, De Santis S, et al. Prolonged molecular remission in advanced acute promyelocytic leukaemia after treatment with gemtuzumab ozogamicin (Mylotarg CMA-676). Br J Haematol. 2001;115:63–5.
110. Mandelli F, Latagliata R, Avvisati G, Fazi P, Rodeghiero F, Leoni F, et al. Treatment of elderly patients (> or =60 years) with newly diagnosed acute promyelocytic leukemia. Results of the Italian multicenter group GIMEMA with ATRA and idarubicin (AIDA) protocols. Leukemia. 2003;17:1085–90.
111. Sanz MA, Vellenga E, Rayón C, Díaz-Mediavilla J, Rivas C, Amutio E, et al. All-trans retinoic acid and anthracycline monochemotherapy for the treatment of elderly patients with acute promyelocytic leukemia. Blood. 2004;104:3490–3.
112. Ades L, Chevret S, De Botton S, Thomas X, Dombret H, Beve B, et al. Outcome of acute promyelocytic leukemia treated with all trans retinoic acid and chemotherapy in elderly patients: the European group experience. Leukemia. 2005;19:230–3.
113. Latagliata R, Petti MC, Fenu S, Mancini M, Spiriti MA, Breccia M, et al. Therapy-related myelodysplastic syndrome-acute myelogenous leukemia in patients treated for acute promyelocytic leukemia: an emerging problem. Blood. 2002;99:822–4.
114. Lobe I, Rigal-Huguet F, Vekhoff A, Desablens B, Bordessoule D, Mounier C, et al. Myelodysplastic syndrome after acute promyelocytic leukemia: the European APL group experience. Leukemia. 2003;17:1600–4.
115. Montesinos P, González JD, González J, Rayón C, de Lisa E, Amigo ML, et al. Therapy-related myeloid neoplasms in patients with acute promyelocytic leukemia treated with all-trans-retinoic acid and anthracycline-based chemotherapy. J Clin Oncol. 2010;28:3872–9. doi:10.1200/JCO.2010.29.2268.
116. Schlenk RF, Döhner K, Kneba M, Götze K, Hartmann F, Del Valle F, et al. Gene mutations and response to treatment with all-trans retinoic acid in elderly patients with acute myeloid leukemia. Results from the AMLSG Trial AML HD98B. Haematologica. 2009;94:54–60. doi:10.3324/haematol.13378.
117. Burnett AK, Hills RK, Green C, Jenkinson S, Koo K, Patel Y, et al. The impact on outcome of the addition of all-trans retinoic acid to intensive chemotherapy in younger patients with nonacute promyelocytic acute myeloid leukemia: overall results and results in genotypic sub-

groups defined by mutations in NPM1, FLT3, and CEBPA. Blood. 2010;115:948–56. doi:10.1182/blood-2009-08-236588.

118. El Hajj H, Dassouki Z, Berthier C, Raffoux E, Ades L, Legrand O, et al. Retinoic acid and arsenic trioxide trigger degradation of mutated NPM1, resulting in apoptosis of AML cells. Blood. 2015;125:3447–54. doi:10.1182/blood-2014-11-612416.
119. Martelli MP, Gionfriddo I, Mezzasoma F, Milano F, Pierangeli S, Mulas F, et al. Arsenic trioxide and all-trans retinoic acid target NPM1 mutant oncoprotein levels and induce apoptosis in NPM1-mutated AML cells. Blood. 2015;125:3455–65. doi:10.1182/blood-2014-11-611459.
120. Verhagen HJ, Smit MA, Rutten A, Denkers F, Poddighe PJ, Merle PA, et al. Primary acute myeloid leukemia cells with overexpression of EVI-1 are sensitive to all-trans retinoic acid. Blood. 2016;127:458–63. doi:10.1182/blood-2015-07-653840.

12 The Molecular Basis of Arsenic Trioxide Treatment for Acute Promyelocytic Leukemia (APL)

Masahiro Kizaki

Abstract

Arsenic trioxide (ATO) is a highly effective treatment for acute promyelocytic leukemia (APL). Early clinical studies conducted in China and the USA in the 1990s showed that ATO can induce sustained molecular remission when used as a single agent in patients who relapsed after treatment with all-*trans* retinoic acid (ATRA) with or without chemotherapy. ATO binds to the promyelocytic leukemia protein (PML) moiety of the PML-RARα oncoprotein, promoting the ubiquitination and degradation of the fusion protein by the ubiquitin-proteasome pathway. The degradation of PML-RARα removes the block to normal promyelocytic differentiation, leading ultimately to cell death of APL cells. Recent studies have shown that the combination of ATRA and ATO has synergistic effects in vitro and in vivo, and these findings have translated successfully to the clinic with great improved outcome for APL patients.

Keywords

Acute promyelocytic leukemia (APL) • Arsenic trioxide (ATO) • All-*trans* retinoic acid (ATRA) • PML-RARα

M. Kizaki (✉)
Department of Hematology, Saitama Medical Center, Saitama Medical University, 1981 Kamoda, Kawagoe, Saitama 350-8550, Japan
e-mail: makizaki@saitama-med.ac.jp

T. Ueda (ed.), *Chemotherapy for Leukemia*, DOI 10.1007/978-981-10-3332-2_12

12.1 Introduction

Acute promyelocytic leukemia (APL) is classified as the M3 subtype of acute myeloid leukemia (AML) according to the French-American-British leukemia classification scheme and is often associated with potentially life-threatening hemorrhagic complications due to disseminated intravascular coagulopathy (DIC).

Over the last decade, there have been significant advances both in the understanding of the molecular pathogenesis of APL and the development of more effective therapies for the disease.

APL is caused by a unique chromosomal translocation, t(15;17)(q22;q21), which results in the fusion of the *promyelocytic leukemia* (*PML*) gene on chromosome 15 with the *retinoic acid receptor* (*RARα*) gene on chromosome 17, to produce the *PML-RARα* chimeric gene and oncoprotein [1–3]. APL cells are blocked from differentiating into mature granulocytes because PML-RARα acts as a transcriptional repressor of genes involved in granulocytic differentiation [4].

The introduction of all-*trans* retinoic acid (ATRA) as a differentiation-inducing therapy in combination with conventional chemotherapy for patients with APL dramatically improved the outcome for this fatal disease, resulting in more than 90% complete remission (CR) and 70% event-free survival (EFS) [5]. Subsequently, the old drug arsenic trioxide (ATO), a drug that has been used to treat a broad spectrum of illnesses for the millennia, was introduced into the clinical setting as a new option for the treatment of relapsed/refractory patients with APL, with or without the addition of chemotherapy or ATRA [6]. Recent studies have shown that ATRA induces differentiation of APL cells to mature granulocytes by subverting epigenetic modifiers from corepressor complexes to coactivators on target genes by binding to the ligand-binding domain of RARα on the PML-RARα chimeric protein [7]. ATO binds to the PML moiety of the PML-RARα chimeric protein and enhances the conjugation of ubiquitin-like modifiers to PML-RARα resulting in ubiquitination and degradation of the chimeric oncoprotein [8–10]. Overall, ATRA and ATO act in concert to inhibit the capacity of *PML-RARα* chimeric gene products to activate oncogenic signaling pathways in APL, leading to a cure in the majority of cases.

12.2 Molecular Pathogenesis of APL

Most APL is caused by a t(15;17)(q22;q21) chromosomal translocation in a progenitor level of myeloid cells, resulting in the production of chimeric gene *PML-RARα* and its reciprocal *RARα−PML* chimeric genes [1–3]. PML-RARα, but not RARα−PML, is the main oncogenic driver of APL and can be transformed hematopoietic progenitors to leukemic cells. Disruption of normal myeloid differentiation by chimeric PML-RARα proteins is associated with maturation arrest of hematopoietic progenitor cells at the promyelocyte stage and subsequent leukemic transformation.

RARα is a member of the steroid receptor superfamily and binds to retinoic acid response elements (RAREs) as heterodimers with the retinoid X receptor (RXR)

[11–13]. In the absence of ligands, the binding of RAR/RXR heterodimers to DNA results in transcriptional repression, whereas in the presence of ligands, binding of the complex strongly induces transcriptional activation. RARα seems to be a particularly efficient repressor of transcription because of its strong interaction with transcriptional corepressors such as N-CoR/SMRT protein complexes, which contain histone deacetylases (HDACs) [14–16] and histone methyl transferases [17, 18]. PML-RARα oligomerizes with RXR or with other oncogenic transcription factors, and the protein complexes aberrantly recruit epigenetic modifying enzymes, such as HDACs and polycomb repressive complexes, which induce histone deacetylation and DNA methylation. The end result is transcriptional repression of downstream target genes essential for granulocytic differentiation, resulting in oncogenic transformation [7, 10, 19]. Ultimately, the *PML-RARα* chimeric gene disrupts myeloid differentiation programs mediated through the RARα signaling pathway and impairs the tumor suppressor activity of PML. Although PML-RARα rearrangement is present in most cases of APL, alternative partners of RARα have been identified including PLZF, NPM1, NuMA, PRKAR1A, FIPL1, STAT5b, and BCOR [20–26]. In addition, it has reported the new variant of APL with OBFC2A-RARα and IRF2BP-RARα fusion proteins [27, 28].

Murine models of APL indicate PML-RARα is necessary, but not sufficient for leukemogenesis, and additional genetic abnormalities are required to provide a proliferative signal. In 40–50% of patients with APL, that signal appears to be provided by constitutive activation of FMS-related tyrosine kinase 3 (FLT3) resulting from either an internal tandem duplication in the juxta-membrane domain (FLT3-ITD) or missense mutation primarily affecting aspartate-835 (FLT3-D835Y) in the kinase-II domain [29, 30]. The presence of *FLT3-ITD* is associated with APL patients with higher white blood cell counts, truncated forms of *PML-RARα* (short-form), and microgranular morphology [31, 32]. These recent findings provide important new insights into the molecular pathogenesis of APL and may ultimately translate into a major expansion of targeted therapy for APL. Further studies on the detail of molecular pathogenesis of APL should be performed.

12.3 ATO and APL

Arsenic was first used by the Greeks and the Chinese more than 2000 years ago as a panacea for the treatment of diseases ranging from infection to cancer. The antileukemic effect of Fowler's solution, essentially a dilute arsenic formulation, was first documented in 1878 for reducing white blood cells [9]. Subsequently, arsenic preparations were used for the treatment of leukemia until the introduction of modern chemotherapeutic agents [9]. The first treatment of APL with crude ATO was in 1973, and the details were published in 1981 before the introduction of ATRA for induction therapy [9]. The first documented use of ATO for the treatment of APL was in China in the 1990s, and high complete remission (CR) rate was achieved when used as a single agent [33, 34]. In more recent studies, ATO led to CR in approximately 70–85% of patients with APL and cure in about one third of patients who relapsed after treatment with ATRA and chemotherapy [35]. In the last few years, combination of ATRA and ATO therapy was shown to produce a higher CR rate and longer remission duration for low-/intermediate-risk APL [36, 37]. The potential of ATO as a chemotherapeutic agent is reflected by the many clinical trials using ATO as a single agent or in combination with other drugs for the treatment of leukemia and other malignancies.

12.4 Mechanisms of Action of ATO in APL

The mode of action of ATO has been investigated with molecular basis. ATO directly binds to the PML moiety of PML-RARα fusion protein, resulting in ubiquitination and degradation of the fusion protein. When this occurs, the nucleoplasmic PML-RARα fusion protein is sequestered within micro-speckled pattern into nuclear bodies (NBs) with a normal speckled pattern, and the subsequent degradation of PML-RARα fusion proteins contributes to both induction of differentiation and cell death of APL cells [38].

It has been shown that ATO has dose-dependent dual effects in APL in vitro, namely, relatively higher concentrations of ATO (0.5–2.0 μM) induce cell death, while lower concentrations of ATO (0.1–0.5 μM) induce partial differentiation of APL cells to mature granulocytes [39]. One possible additional molecular basis of ATO's mode of action in APL cells is induction of the SUMOylation of PML-RARα, followed by Lys 48-linked poly-ubiquitination and proteasome-dependent degradation [40–43]. ATO directly binds to PML at the C-C motif in its B2 domain, and subsequently, PML SUMOylation can be induced by enhancement of the SUMO-conjugating enzyme UBC9 binding at the PML RING domain [40]. SUMOylated PML recruits RING finger protein 4 (RNF4), ubiquitin, and proteasomes, which may integrate the SUMOylation, ubiquitination, and degradation pathways [44, 45]. Therefore, ATO induces PML oligomerization, which increases its interaction with the SUMO-conjugating enzyme UBC9, resulting in enhanced SUMOylation and degradation by the ubiquitin-proteasome pathway (Fig. 12.1). Ultimately, ATO treatment leads to the deactivation of the DNA-bound PML-RARα corepressor complex, which provides access to coactivator complexes and upregulation of target genes involved in driving induction of granulocytic differentiation and cell death of APL cells.

12.5 Resistance to ATO in APL

During the use of ATO as a front therapy for APL, it has demonstrated that some patients develop and acquire ATO resistance. However, the mechanisms underlying this phenomenon remain unknown compared with that of ATRA resistance in APL. As mentioned above, ATO binds directly to the cysteine motif (C212/C213) in the PML-B2 domain of the PML-RARα fusion protein, resulting in the SUMOylation, multimerization, and degradation [40]. This would suggest that the PML-B2 domain is a critical mediator ATO's chemotherapeutic effect, and mutations affecting this

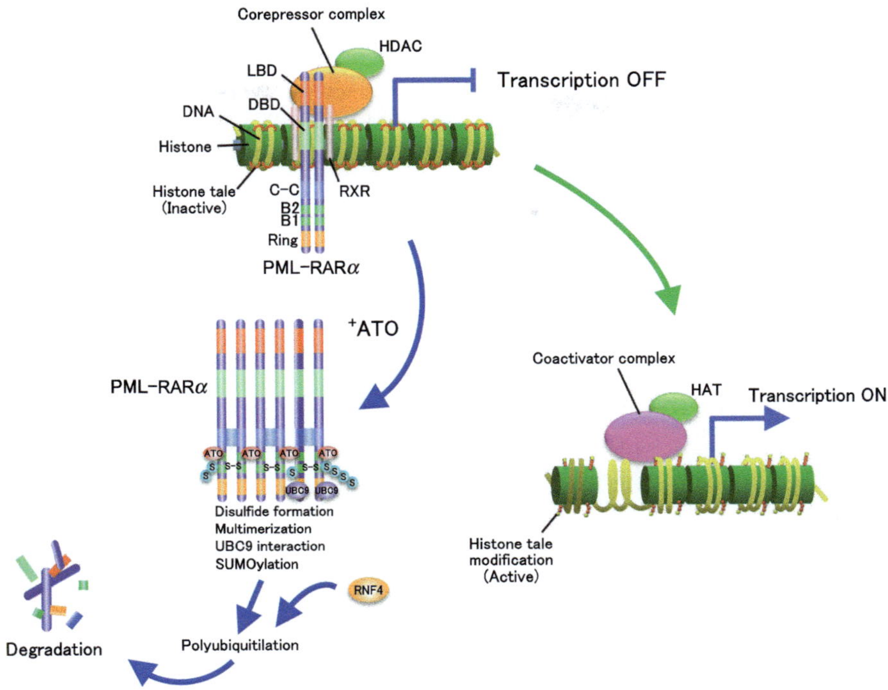

Fig. 12.1 The molecular mechanism of action of ATO in APL. ATO binds to the B2 domain of the PML moiety of the PML-RARα protein, inducing binding of UBC9 followed by multimerization and SUMOylation of PML. SUMOylated PML-RARα fusion protein is brought to the PML moiety and further poly-ubiquitinated, finally leading to degradation by the proteasome. ATO treatment leads to removal of the corepressor complex, in which PML-RARα binds to DNA. The coactivator complex then binds to DNA, and this event leads to granulocyte differentiation and cell death of APL cells

domain may contribute to the development of ATO-resistant APL. Indeed, mutations have been identified in the PML-B2 domain (A216V, L218P, S214L, A216T, S220G) in case of clinically acquired ATO-resistant APL, consistent with the existence of a mutational hotspot (S214-S220) within the PML-RARα fusion protein. Mutations within the putative hotspot resulted in the impairment of direct ATO binding to PML-RARα due to conformational changes in the ATO binding sites [46, 47]. These results suggest that the existence of a mutational hotspot (S214-S220) within the PML-RARα fusion protein in acquired ATO-resistant APL.

More recently, varying responses to ATO linked to different point mutations in the *PML* moiety of *PML-RARα* were reported [48]. Among these, the A216, S214L, and A216T mutations attenuated the negative regulation of PML-RARα by ATO, resulting in the retention of the fusion protein. In contrast, the L217F and S220G mutations functioned weakly in this context. Interestingly, high-dose ATO, or the combination of ATO and ATRA, can overcome the ATO resistance driven by the acquired point mutations. This may be relevant to the finding that the effects of ATO on APL cells are dose dependent with relatively higher concentrations inducing cell death, while lower concentrations induce partial differentiation of APL cells to mature granulocytes [39]. Ultimately, these data may contribute to improved prognostication and the development of more effective therapeutic strategies for the treatment of APL in the future.

12.6 Conclusion

APL exemplifies the great progress that has been made in the translation of basic research into effective molecularly targeted therapies for hematological malignancies.

Intensive research has addressed many important aspects of APL biology, including transcriptional regulation, nuclear organization, epigenetics, and the role of proteolysis in leukemogenesis, contributing to the development of new therapeutic strategies with significant clinical impact. APL is the first hematological malignancy to be cured using molecular-targeting therapy with ATRA and ATO, and the details of the molecular mechanisms underlying the curative effects of ATO, predominantly mediated by the degradation of the PML-RARα oncoprotein, are gradually being clarified. Future studies will aim to develop sophisticated new therapeutic strategies for the treatment of APL based on a more comprehensive understanding of the molecular mechanisms involved in the targeting and inhibition of PML-RARα by ATO.

References

1. de The H, Chomienne C, Lanotte M, Degos L, Dejean A. The t(15;17) translocation of acute promyelocytic leukemia fuses the retinoic acid receptor α gene to a novel transcribed locus. Nature. 1990;347:558–61.
2. Borrow J, Goddard AD, Sheer D, Solomon E. Molecular analysis of acute promyelocytic leukemia breakpoint cluster region on chromosome 17. Science. 1990;249:1577–80.
3. de The H, Lavau C, Marchio A, Chomienne C, Degos L, Dejean A. The PML-RARα fusion mRNA generated by the t(15;17) translocation in acute promyelocytic leukemia encodes a functionally altered RAR. Cell. 1991;66:675–84.
4. Lo-Coco F, Hasan SK. Understanding the molecular pathogenesis of acute promyelocytic leukemia. Best Pract Res Clin Haematol. 2014;27:3–9.
5. Coombs CC, Tavakkoli M, Tallman. Acute promyelocytic leukemia: where did we start, where are we now, and the future. Blood Cancer J. 2015;5:e304. doi:10.1038/ bcj.2015.25.
6. Zhu J, Chen Z, Lallemand-Breitenbach V, de The H. How acute promyelocytic leukemia revived arsenic. Nat Rev Cancer. 2002;2:1–9.
7. Arteaga MF, Mikesch J-H, Fung T-K, So CWE. Epigenetics in acute promyelocytic leukaemia pathogenesis and treatment response: a transition to targeted therapies. Br J Cancer. 2015;112:413–8.
8. Miller Jr WH, Schipper HM, Lee JS, Singer J, Waxman S. Mechanisms of arsenic trioxide. Cancer Res. 2001;62:3893–903.
9. Iland HJ, Seymour JF. Role of arsenic trioxide in acute promyelocytic leukemia. Curr Treat Option Oncol. 2013;14:179–84.
10. Nitto T, Sawaki K. Molecular mechanisms of the antileukemia activities of retinoid and arsenic. J Pharmacol Sci. 2014;126:179–85.

11. Giguere V, Ong ES, Segui P, Evans RM. Identification of a receptor for the morphogen retinoic acid. Nature. 1987;330:624–9.
12. Zechel C, Shen XQ, Chambon P, Gronemeyer H. Dimerization interfaces formed between the DNA binding domains determine the cooperative binding RXR/RAR and RXR/TR heterodimers to DR5 and DR4 elements. EMBO J. 1994;13:1414–24.
13. Kurokawa R, DiRenzo J, Boehm M, Sugarman J, Gloss B, Rosenfeld MG, et al. Regulation of retinoid signaling by receptor polarity and allosteric control of ligand binding. Nature. 1994;371:528–31.
14. Grignani F, De Matteis S, Nervi C, Tomassoni L, Gelmetti V, Cioce M, et al. Fusion proteins of the retinoic acid receptor-α recruit histone deacetylase in promyelocytic leukaemia. Nature. 1998;391:815–8.
15. He LZ, Guidez F, Tribioli C, Peruzzi D, Ruthardt M, Zelent A, et al. Distinct interactions of PML-RARα and PLZF-RARα with co-repressors determine differential responses to RA in APL. Nat Genet. 1998;18:126–35.
16. Tomita A, Buchholz DR, Obata K, Shi YB. Fusion protein of retinoic acid receptor α with promyelocytic leukemia protein or promyelocytic leukemia zinc finger protein recruits N-CoR-TBLR1 corepressor complex to repress transcription in vivo. J Biol Chem. 2003;278:30788–95.
17. Carbone R, Bortugno OA, Ronzoni S, Insinga A, Di Croce L, Pelicci PG, et al. Recruitment of the histone methyltransferase SUV39H1 and its role in the oncogenic properties of the leukemia-associated PML-retinoic acid receptor fusion protein. Mol Cell Biol. 2006;26:1288–96.
18. Villa R, Pasini D, Gutierrez A, Morey L, Occhionorelli M, Vire E, et al. Role of the polycomb repressive complex 2 in acute promyelocytic leukemia. Cancer Cell. 2007;11:513–25.
19. Tomita A, Kiyoi H, Naoe T. Mechanisms of action and resistance to all-*trans* retinoic acid (ATRA) and arsenic trioxide (As_2O_3) in acute promyelocytic leukemia. Int J Hematol. 2013;97:717–25.
20. Chen Z, Brand NJ, Chen A, Chen SJ, Tong JH, Wang ZY, et al. Fusion between a novel kruppel-like zinc finger gene and the retinoic acid receptor-a locus due to a variant t(11;17) translocation associated with acute promyelocytic leukemia. EMBO J. 1993;12:1161–7.
21. Redner RL, Rush EA, Faas S, Rudert WA, Corey SJ. The t(5;17) variant of acute promyelocytic leukemia expresses a nucleophosmin-retinoic acid receptor fusion. Blood. 1996;87:882–6.
22. Wells RA, Catzavelos C, Kamel-Reid S. Fusion of retinoic acid receptor α to NuMA, the nuclear mitotic apparatus protein, by a variant translocation in acute promyelocytic leukaemia. Nat Genet. 1997;17:109–13.
23. Arnould C, Philippe C, Bourdon V, Grégoire MJ, Berger R, Jonveaux P. The signal transducer and activator of transcription STAT5b gene is a new partner of retinoic acid receptor α in acute promyelocytic-like leukaemia. Hum Mol Genet. 1999;8:1741–9.
24. Catalano A, Dawson MA, Somana K, Opat S, Schwarer A, Campbell LJ, et al. The PRKAR1A gene is fused to RARA in a new variant acute promyelocytic leukemia. Blood. 2007;110:4073–6.
25. Kondo T, Mori A, Darmanin S, Hashino S, Tanaka J, Asaka M. The seventh pathogenic fusion gene FIP1L1-RARA was isolated from a t(4;17)-positive acute promyelocytic leukemia. Haematologica. 2008;93:1414–6.
26. Yamamoto Y, Tsuzuki S, Tsuzuki M, Handa K, Inaguma Y, Emi N. BCOR as a novel fusion partner of retinoic acid receptor α in a t(X;17)(p11;q12) variant of acute promyelocytic leukemia. Blood. 2010;116:4247–83.
27. Won D, Shin SY, Park CJ, Jang S, Chi H-S, Lee K-H, et al. OBFC2A/RARA: a novel fusion gene in variant acute promyelocytic leukemia. Blood. 2013;121:1432–5.
28. Yin CC, Jain N, Mehrotra M, Zhagn J, Protopopov A, Zuo Z, et al. Identification of a novel fusion gene, IRF2BP2-RARA, in acute promyelocytic leukemia. J Natl Compr Netw. 2015;13:19–22.

29. Kelly LM, Kutok JL, Williams IR, Boulton CL, Amaral SM, Curley DP, et al. PML/RARα and FLT3-ITD induce an APL-like disease in a mouse model. Proc Natl Acad Sci U S A. 2002;99:8283–8.
30. Kiyoi H, Naoe T. Biology, clinical relevance, and molecularly targeted therapy in acute leukemia with FLT3 mutation. Int J Hematol. 2006;83:301–8.
31. Meshinchi S, Appelbaum FR. Structural and functional alterations of FLT3 in acute myeloid leukemia. Clin Cancer Res. 2009;15:8283–8.
32. Beitinjaneh A, Jang S, Roukoz H, Majhail NS. Prognostic significance of FLT3 internal tandem duplication and tyrosine kinase domain mutations in acute promyelocytic leukemia: a systematic review. Leuk Res. 2010;34:831–6.
33. Zang P, Wang SY, Hu LH. Arsenic trioxide treated 72 cases of acute promyelocytic leukemia. Chin J Hematol. 1996;17:58–62.
34. Shen ZX, Chen GQ, Ni JH, Li XS, Xiong SM, Qiu QY, et al. Use of arsenic trioxide (As_2O_3) in the treatment of acute promyelocytic leukemia (APL): II. Clinical efficacy and pharmacokinetics in relapsed patients. Blood. 1997;89:3354–60.
35. Tallman MS, Altman JK. How I treat acute promyelocytic leukemia. Blood. 2009;114:5126–35.
36. Lo-Coco F, Avvisati G, Vignetti M, Thiede C, Orlando SM, Iacobelli S, et al. Retinoic acid and arsenic trioxide for acute promyelocytic leukemia. N Engl J Med. 2013;369:111–21.
37. Burnett AK, Russell NH, Hills RK, Bowen D, Kell J, Knapper S, et al. Arsenic trioxide and all-trans retinoic acid treatment for acute promyelocytic leukemia in all risk groups (AML17): results of a randomized, controlled, phase 3 trial. Lancet Oncol. 2015;16:1295–305.
38. Muller S, Matunis MJ, Dejean A. Conjugation with the ubiquitin-related modifier SUMO-1 regulates the partitioning of PML within the nucleus. EMBO J. 1998;17:61–70.
39. Chen GQ, Shi XG, Tang W, Xiong SM, Zhu J, Cai X, et al. Use of arsenic trioxide (As_2O_3) in the treatment of acute promyelocytic leukemia (APL): I. As_2O_3 exerts dose-dependent dual effects on APL cells. Blood. 1997;89:3345–53.
40. Lallemand-Breitenbach V, Zhu J, Puvion F, Koken M, Honore N, Doubeikovsky A, et al. Role of promyelocytic leukemia (PML) sumolation in nuclear body formation, 11S proteasome recruitment, and As_2O_3-induced PML or PML/retinoic acid receptor α degradation. J Exp Med. 2001;193:1361–71.
41. Zhang XW, Yan XJ, Zhou ZR, Yang FF, Wu ZY, Sun HB, et al. Arsenic trioxide controls the fate of the PML-RARα oncoprotein by directly binding PML. Science. 2010;328:240–3.
42. Jeanne M, Lallemand-Breitenbach V, Ferhi O, Koken M, Le Bras M, Duffort S, et al. PML/RARA oxidation and arsenic binding initiate the antileukemia response of As_2O_3. Cancer Cell. 2010;18:88–98.
43. Lang E, Grudic A, Pankiv S, Bruserud D, Simonsen A, Bjerkvig R, et al. The arsenic-based cure of acute promyelocytic leukemia promotes cytoplasmic sequestration of PML and PML/RARA through inhibition of PML body recycling. Blood. 2012;120:847–57.
44. Lallemand-Breitenbach V, Jeanne M, Benhenda S, Nasr R, Lei M, Peres L, et al. Arsenic degrades PML or PML-RARα through a SUMO-triggered RNF/ubiquitin-mediated pathway. Nat Cell Biol. 2008;10:547–55.
45. Maroui MA, Kheddache-Atmane S, El Asmi F, Dianoux L, Aubry M, Chelbi-Alix MK. Requirement of PML SUMO interacting motif for RNF4- or arsenic trioxide-induced degradation of nuclear PML isoforms. PLoS ONE. 2012;7:e44949.
46. Goto E, Tomita A, Hayakawa F, Atsumi A, Kiyoi H, Naoe T. Missense mutations in PML-RARA are critical for the lack of responsiveness to arsenic trioxide treatment. Blood. 2011;118:1600–9.
47. Zhu HH, Qin YZ, Huang XJ. Resistance to arsenic therapy in acute promyelocytic leukemia. N Engl J Med. 2014;370:1864–6.
48. Liu J, Zhu HH, Jiang H, Jiang Q, Huang X-J. Varying responses of PML-RARA with different genetic mutations to arsenic trioxide. Blood. 2016;127:243–50.

Arsenic Trioxide: Clinical Pharmacology and Therapeutic Results

13

Nobuhiko Emi

Abstract

Treatment with arsenic trioxide (ATO) has been shown to result in high CR rates for a majority of patients with acute promyelocytic leukemia (APL). First, it was demonstrated that ATO is effective against refractory and relapsed cases of APL. Many trials have been conducted to determine the optimal schedule for ATO as a single agent or in combination with other drugs. It has been suggested that administration of ATO in the earlier stages of a therapy course is most beneficial. However, the potential toxicity of ATO has been a matter of concern because of the toxicity profile from people with long exposure through natural contamination. In this chapter, the pharmacokinetics and results of clinical trials of treatment of APL are presented. In addition, the toxicity and side effects of ATO occurring during treatment are considered.

Keywords

Arsenic trioxide • Acute promyelocytic leukemia • Pharmacokinetics

13.1 History of Arsenic Compounds

Arsenic compounds have been used for over 2000 years, both as a medicine and as a poison. History has it that Hippocrates used sulfur derivatives of arsenic to treat skin lesions. In the eighteenth century, Fowler's solution (1% potassium arsenite) was used in the treatment of dermatological diseases. It was even used for chronic myelogenous leukemia by traditional Chinese medicine [1].

N. Emi (✉)
Department of Hematology, Fujita Health University School of Medicine,
Dengakugakubo 1-98, Kutsukake, Toyoake, Aichi 470-1192, Japan
e-mail: nemi@fujita-hu.ac.jp

T. Ueda (ed.), *Chemotherapy for Leukemia*, DOI 10.1007/978-981-10-3332-2_13

However, chronic arsenic exposure through occupational exposure and natural contamination of drinking water can be a public health problem because of its association with bladder, lung, and skin cancers [2, 3]. Arsenic contamination of sugar used in making beer caused 70 deaths among 6000 people affected in Northern England in 1903, and in France 40,000 people were poisoned when wine and bread were contaminated with arsenic in 1928 [4]. Between June and August 1955 in the Western areas of Japan, 12,131 newborn babies were poisoned because arsenic had been mixed in during production of the powdered milk used for their feeding formulas [5]. These incidents have created an unfavorable reputation for arsenic compounds.

However, an arsenic compound was reintroduced into new medicine as a result of Chinese studies on relapse after treatment of acute promyelocytic leukemia (APL) [6]. Historically, ATO was introduced into the treatment of APL following the findings of Chinese investigators at Harbin Medical University, who systematically studied the function and performance of an arsenic-based traditional Chinese compound called "Ailing I" [7]. Two subsequent Chinese studies confirmed the benefits of this agent for APL. Subsequently, clinical trials with ATO, initiated at Shanghai Second Medical University in 1994, confirmed the efficacy of ATO for patients with APL who had undergone relapse after treatment with all-trans retinoic acid (ATRA) plus chemotherapy [8].

At that time, Western authorities were concerned about the presence of mercury and ATO in Chinese traditional medicines. However, after the Chinese results had been rapidly validated in clinical trials performed in Japan, Europe, and the United States [9, 10], ATO is now used worldwide to treat patients with APL who have suffered relapse after their primary therapy. The drug has been licensed in Japan, Europe, and the United States for the treatment of relapsed and refractory APL. It can induce complete remission when used for remission induction with or without the addition of chemotherapy or ATRA, and recently ATO and ATRA combination therapy has been shown to be highly efficient and has low toxic effects [11, 12]. Figure 13.1 shows the timeline for the history of arsenic use.

13.2 Dosage, Schedule, and Pharmacokinetics of Arsenic Trioxide

13.2.1 Dosage and Administration

For remission induction, ATO is administered by a 2-h infusion at a daily dose of 0.15 mg/kg until a complete hematological remission (CR) or a maximum of 60 days. One vial contains 10 mg of ATO in a 10 ml solution. ATO must be dissolved in 100–200 ml of 5% glucose solution or 0.9% saline solution immediately after it has been removed from the vial. The solution should be infused for 2–4 h after it has been prepared. If vasomotor reactions occur, the infusion should take place over 4 h [8, 13]. Consolidation treatment is initiated 2–4 weeks after completion of induction therapy. For an additional consolidation courses, it is

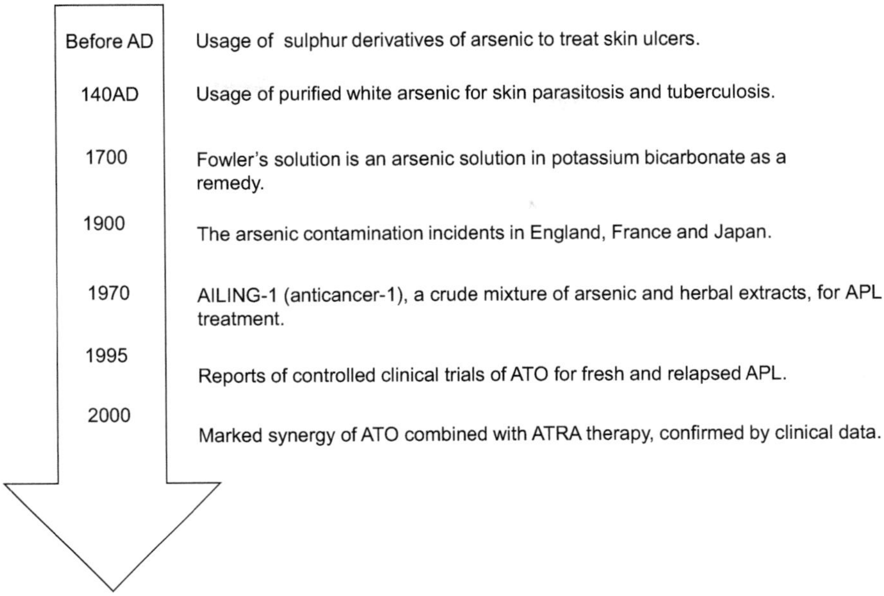

Fig. 13.1 Timeline of the use of arsenic

recommended for ATO to be administered intravenously at a dose of 0.15 mg/kg daily for 25 doses over a period up to 5 weeks. It is important to note that this dosing is based on the use of ATO for native Chinese medicine and not in a phase I study. Treatment with ATRA or chemotherapy or a combination thereof should follow each protocol.

13.2.2 Pharmacokinetics of ATO

Only a few studies have described the pharmacokinetics of ATO, and in one of these, a Chinese pharmacokinetic study, it was analyzed on the first day of ATO administration for eight relapsed APL patients and it was found that MMN peak plasma levels of 6.85 μ moles/L (range: 5.54–7.30) were attained. The plasma half-life was 12.13 ± 3.31 h and these parameters did not change with continuous administration [8]. In an unpublished study of ours, the trough levels of arsenic were analyzed during the administration of ATO. Figure 13.2 shows the trough levels gradually increased from 1 to 2 μ moles during treatment.

Fukai et al. [14] found that urinary excretion is the major elimination route for ATO. Other findings for daily urinary excretion reported in the literature vary from between 1% and 8% to 32% and 65% of the daily dose administered [8]. ATO is excreted in the urine unchanged in the form of AsIII.

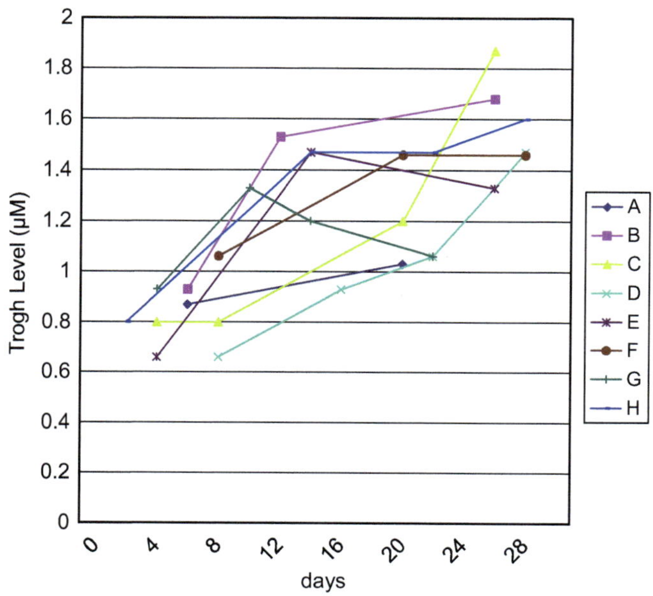

Fig. 13.2 Plasma trough levels of arsenic

13.2.3 Arsenic Monitoring in the Hair of APL Patients

The hair has widely been used to assess content of a broad range of substances; organic and inorganic, as well endogenous, metabolites; or exogenous contaminants. For assessing the content of arsenic, the hairs of two patients and control individuals were measured in our study. The hair of the patients contained 1108–7900 ppm, which is more than ten times higher than the reference value.

Nicolis et al. [15] reported the results of their analysis of hair of patients receiving ATO. A unique property of hair is that incorporated elements remain in place during its growth. Since human hair grows at an average rate of 1.1 cm per month, analysis of 1 cm of hair yields the history of approximately 1 month of past exposure. According to the results obtained with clinical materials, arsenic content rapidly returns to normal levels after the end of administration [8].

13.2.4 Arsenic Metabolism

Arsenic is the 33rd element in the periodic table and exists ubiquitously in either inorganic or organic forms. It has long been accepted that arsenic is metabolized via a succession of oxidative methylation and reduction steps leading from inorganic trivalent arsenic to pentavalent dimethylarsinic acid. When the inorganic, lyophilized form of arsenic trioxide is placed into solution, it immediately forms the hydrolysis product arsenious acid (AsIII), which is the pharmacologically active species of arsenic trioxide. In addition to arsenic acid (AsV), a product of AsIII oxidation, monomethylarsonic acid (MMAV) and dimethylarsinic acid (DMAV) are the main pentavalent metabolites formed during metabolism [16].

The pharmacokinetics of arsenical species (AsIII, AsV, MMAV, DMAV) were determined in a study of six APL patients following once daily doses of 0.15 mg/kg for 5 days per week. For a total single-dose range of 7–22 mg (administered at 0.15 mg/kg), systemic exposure (AUC) appears to be linear. Peak plasma concentrations of arsenious acid (AsIII), the primary active arsenical species, were reached at the end of infusion (2 h). Plasma concentrations of AsIII then declined in a biphasic manner with a mean elimination half-life of 10–14 h and were characterized by an initial rapid distribution phase followed by a slower terminal elimination phase. The daily exposure to AsIII (mean AUC0-24) was 194 ng·h/mL ($n = 5$) on day 1 of cycle 1 and 332 ng·h/mL ($n = 6$) on day 25 of cycle 1, which represents an approximate twofold accumulation. The primary pentavalent metabolites, MMAV and DMAV, were slow to appear in plasma (approximately 10–24 h after the first administration of arsenic trioxide), but, due to their longer half-life, had accumulated more than AsIII following multiple dosing. The mean estimated terminal elimination half-lives of the metabolites MMAV and DMAV were determined as 32 and 72 h, respectively. AsV was detected in plasma only at relatively low levels [13].

13.2.5 Drug Interactions

No formal assessments of pharmacokinetic drug-drug interactions between ATO and other drugs have been conducted. However, it is known that the methyltransferases responsible for metabolizing arsenic trioxide are not members of the cytochrome P450 family of isoenzymes [13, 17]. Moreover, in vitro incubation of arsenic trioxide with human liver microsomes showed no inhibitory activity on substrates of the major cytochrome P450 (CYP) enzymes such as 1A2, 2A6, 2B6, 2C8, 2C9, 2C19, 2D6, 2E1, 3A4/5, and 4A9/11. The pharmacokinetics of drugs that are substrates for these CYP enzymes can therefore be assumed not to be affected by concomitant treatment with ATO.

13.3 Clinical Results for the Use of ATO in the Treatment of APL

13.3.1 ATO for Relapsed and Refractory APL

The introduction of ATO into the treatment of patients with APL was prompted by the findings from two studies in China in the early 1990s and resulted in a high complete remission (CR) rate with relatively long-term remissions when ATO was used as a single agent. Initial studies at Harbin Medical University in 1992 found that ATO induced CR in 72% of patients [7]. This was followed by a clinical trial at the Shanghai Institute of Hematology in 1997, which documented a 90% CR rate achieved with the use of ATO alone for patients with relapsed and newly diagnosed

APL. The duration of ATO administration needed to attain such a high CR rate was between 28 and 44 days [8]. These results showed that ATO is effective for cases relapsed after ATRA and chemotherapy treatments.

An American study for single ATO conducted in 1998 showed a 91.7% CR rate for 12 patients [10]. Additional study showed an 85% CR rate for 40 relapsed patients. The rate of molecular remissions after an induction cycle with ATO was 50% and after consolidation with a further ATO cycle increased to 83%. The 3-year overall survival (OS) rate was 50%. A subgroup analysis 4.2 years after the induction cycle showed a relapse-free survival (RFS) of 22% if ATO monotherapy was used for induction and consolidation and of 86% if ATO monotherapy was followed by an autologous or allogeneic transplant [18].

We studied the effect of ATO on 35 relapsed APL cases. The median age of the patients was 46 years and the median white blood cell (WBC) count at presentation was 2600/mm^3 (500–18,100). ATO was infused at 0.15 mg/kg/day for 2 h until abnormal cells had disappeared from the bone marrow. Complete remission was attained for 81% of those with hematologic relapse, and most patients became negative for PML-RARA after the first ATO consolidation course with only four patients remaining positive [19]. Table 13.1 summarizes the results of ATO induction therapy for relapsed and refractory APL. These studies clearly showed that ATO re-induction therapy is highly effective in these settings. European LeukemiaNet (ELN) registry data confirmed the efficacy of ATO for re-induction of remission, since of the 115 patients with hematological or extramedullary relapse, 91% attained CR and only 2% showed ATO-resistant leukemia [20].

Table 13.1 Summary of studies using ATO induction therapy for relapse or front-line APL

Reference	Patients	Pt no.	Regimen (RI/Post-RI)	CR (%)	OS
Shen et al. [8]	Relapsed	15	ATO	93	85% 1-year OS
Soignet et al. [10]	Relapsed	12	ATO/ATO	91.7	63% 2-year OS
Soignet et al. [18]	Relapsed	40	ATO/ATO	85	66% 1.5-year OS
Niu et al. [21]	Fresh/relapsed	11/47	ATO/ATO or CHT	72.7/85.1	50% 2-year OS
Ghavamzadeh et al. [22]	Fresh	197	ATO/ATO	85.8	64% 5-year OS
Mathews et al. [23]	Fresh	72	ATO/ATO	86.1	74% 5-year OS
Shigeno et al. [9]	Relapsed	34	ATO/ATO	91	56% 2-year OS
Yanada et al. [19]	Relapsed	35	ATO/ATO/auto-HCT	81	77% 5-year OS

13.3.2 ATO in Frontline Therapy

The first report of the use of ATO for de novo APL cases came from China. Niu et al. [21], for remission induction in 11 new cases of APL, observed a 72.7% CR rate, but hepatotoxicity was observed in seven patients. Three large-scale studies using ATO in frontline therapy have been conducted. Ghavamzadeh et al. [22] used ATO alone for remission induction and consolidation in APL patients. The remission rate was 85.8% and the 5-year disease-free survival (DFS) rate was 66.7% (132 out of 197 patients). Between January 1998 and December 2004, 72 newly diagnosed cases of APL were treated with a regimen of single-agent ATO at the single Indian center [23]. CR was achieved for 62 patients (86.1%), and 13 patients relapsed. The 5-year Kaplan-Meier estimates of event-free survival (EFS), DFS, and overall survival (OS) after a median follow-up of 60 months were 69% ± 5.5%, 80% ± 5.2%, and 74.2% ± 5.2%, respectively.

The C9710 Study [24] was the first multicenter and randomized trial to emphasize the importance of ATO in consolidation therapy. This study randomized 481 patients (age >15 years) with untreated APL to either a standard induction regimen of tretinoin, cytarabine, and daunorubicin, followed by two courses of consolidation therapy with tretinoin plus daunorubicin, or to the same induction and consolidation regimen plus two 25-day courses of ATO consolidation immediately after induction. EFS at 3 years was 80% for the latter versus 63% for the former regimen. ATO consolidation provided significant benefits both to patients with low/intermediate risk and to those with high-risk APL. Lou et al. [25] also reached the conclusion that with the involvement of ATO in the post-CR period improved the long-term outcome. At a median follow-up of 49 months, the Kaplan-Meier estimates of 5-year relapse-free survival were significantly better for patients in the ATO group than in the non-ATO group, 94.4% vs. 54.8%, and the 5-year overall survival rate was 95.7% vs. 64.1%, in the two groups.

13.3.3 ATO Combined with ATRA as a Synergistic Therapy

Treatment outcomes for APL have improved dramatically since the advent of all-trans retinoic acid (ATRA). While ATO is effective as induction therapy with a relatively high CR rate, ATRA is believed to allow for better control over hemorrhagic events in the early stages of APL. Preclinical models demonstrated synergism of the combination of ATRA and ATO in inducing differentiation and apoptosis [26]. This synergism between ATRA and ATO has been confirmed through specific binding of the PML/RAR-α oncoprotein [27]. Investigators at the Shanghai Institute of Hematology performed a randomized clinical trial in which patients received ATRA, ATO, or the combination of ATRA plus ATO as induction therapy. Similar CR rates (between 90% and 95.2%) were observed for the three groups, but the patients receiving the combination ATRA+ATO therapy showed a statistically significant improvement in the time until achievement of CR, the time needed for platelet recovery, and decrease in the rate of relapse [28]. The long-term follow-up showed that the CR, 5-year EFS, and OS rates for the combination therapy were 94.1%, 89.2%, and 91.7%, respectively [29].

The Australasian Leukaemia and Lymphoma Group (ALLG) performed a phase 2, single-armed study (APML4), reporting the outcome of 124 patients with newly diagnosed APL treated with triple induction with ATRA, ATO, and idarubicin, followed by two courses of consolidation with ATRA and ATO and 2 years of maintenance with ATRA, methotrexate, and 6-MP. Outcomes were compared with historical controls from the APML3 study that used ATRA plus idarubicin (AIDA) for induction and consolidation without ATO. With a median follow-up of 4.2 years, the 5-year OS and EFS rates were 94% and 90%, respectively. Compared with results for APML3, this trial demonstrated a statistically significant improvement in EFS and OS [30]. This regimen thus appears to be very promising, although, given its phase 2 nature and comparison with historical controls, it may be premature to suggest it is superior.

Investigators at the MD Anderson Cancer Center demonstrated that the combination treatment of ATRA and ATO is an effective treatment for untreated APL with a high CR rate of 92%. However, high-risk patients (WBC: >10,000/μl at presentation) showed an inferior CR rate of 81% because of early treatment failure due to fatal hemorrhage and differentiation syndrome despite the addition of either gemtuzumab ozogamicin during induction to control elevated WBC counts. The estimated 3-year survival rate was 85%. The main advantage of this regimen was in patients who are unlikely to tolerate cytotoxic chemotherapy (e.g., older patients or patients with cardiac dysfunction or multiple comorbidities) [31].

Lo-Coco et al. [32, 33] compared the two approaches in a randomized trial involving patients with non-high-risk APL (white cell count: $\leq 10 \times 10^9$ per liter). With a median follow-up of 53 months, the event-free survival rate at 50 months for the 156 patients whose data were used for the intention-to-treat analysis was 96% for the ATRA+ATO group and 81% for the ATRA+chemotherapy group ($P = 0.003$) with corresponding overall survival rates of 99% and 88%.

To summarize, these studies suggest that the combination of ATRA and ATO, particularly for patients with low-risk disease, is promising. For patients with high WBC, however, the combined use of cytotoxic agents such as anthracyclines in induction appears to be important to prevent rapid development of leukocytosis, APL differentiation syndrome, and relapse. Table 13.2 shows a summary of the studies using combination therapy with ATO and ATRA for de novo APL patients.

13.3.4 ATO for Post-Induction Therapy

The role of ATO in post-induction therapy for newly diagnosed APL patients has been explored not only to enhance CR with the aim to minimize or even eliminate chemotherapy but also to bolster standard ATRA+chemotherapy regimens. Results of the four studies using ATO for induction and post-remission therapy demonstrated the strong antileukemic activity of this agent.

Table 13.2 Summary of studies using ATO and ATRA combined therapy in fresh APL patients

Reference	Pt no.	Regimen (RI/consolidation/maintenance)	CR (%)	Outcome/OS
Shen et al. [28]	21	ATRA+ATO/CHT/ATRA+ATO+CHT	95.2	No relapsed in 20 months
	20	ATRA/CHT/ATRA+CHT	95	26.3% relapsed in 13 months
	20	ATO/CHT/ATO+CHT	90	11.1% relapsed in 12 months
Hu et al. [29]	85	ATRA+ATO ±CHT/CHT/ATRA+ATO+CHT	94.1	91.7% 5-year OS
Ravandi et al. [31, 49]	82	ATRA+ATO±GO/ATRA+ATO/ –	92	85% 3-year OS
Powell et al. [24]	244	ATRA+CHT/ATRA+ATO+CHT/ATRA±CHT	90	86% 3-year OS
	237	ATRA+CHT/ATRA+CHT/ATRA±CHT		81% 3-year OS
Lou et al. [25]	109	ATRA+CHT/ATRA+ATO/ATRA+ATO+CHT	96.3	95.7% 5-year OS
		ATRA+CHT/ATRA/ATRA+CHT		64.1% 5-year OS
Iland et al. [30]	124	ATRA+ATO+CHT/ATRA+ATO/ATRA+CHT	95	94% 5-year OS
Lo-Coco et al. [32, 33]	77	ATRA+ATO/ATRA+ATO/ –	100	99% 4-year OS
	79	ATRA+CHT/ATRA+CHT/ATRA+CHT	95	88% 4-year OS

A European registry of relapsed APL recently reported its results [20]. The therapies administered for hematological relapse were ATO monotherapy (61%), ATO+ATRA (22%), and systemic chemotherapy (17%). This publication is also important for a better understanding of the status of transplantation. After ATO±ATRA induction and consolidation treatment, the patients (n = 148) underwent autologous transplantation (n = 60) and allogeneic transplantation (n = 33) or received other treatments (n = 55). For autologous transplantation, the stem cell source was the peripheral blood in almost all cases. The preferred conditioning regimen was busulfan combined with cyclophosphamide or melphalan. Approximately 80% of the conditioning regimens before allogeneic transplantation were myeloablative and 20% were of the reduced intensity type. The 3-year OS rates for autologous transplantation, allogeneic transplantation, and no transplantation were 77%, 79%, and 59%, respectively. However, these analyses of relapsed APL have been retrospective and their results are heterogeneous. The results indicate that transplantation may enhance survival when compared with no transplantation during second CR. It should be emphasized, however, that the validity of the comparison of the three patient groups is limited.

13.3.5 Kinetics of PML-RARA Transcript Levels

Minimal residual disease (MRD) is the most important prognostic factor for APL treated with different protocols. The rate of MRD detection is based on the method used for the MRD assay and the sensitivity of the test [34]. Continuous positive results for MRD after therapy are predictive of the extent of relapse. Several results concerning MRD after ATO therapy have been reported. For patients treated with ATO, almost half remain MDR positive after remission induction, but their status changes to MRD negative after the consolidation phase of treatment.

Our results for the serial reverse transcription polymerase chain reaction (RT-PCR) tests during the ATO treatment can be summarized as follows. The negativity of molecular remission after an induction cycle with ATO was 9 out of 31 (29%), but after consolidation with another ATO cycle, it increased to 24/28 (86%), with four patients remaining positive for PML-RARA at that time. The PCR results became negative for one patient, each after the second and third consolidation, respectively. Of the two patients who remained positive for PML-RARA after the third consolidation, one showed positive and the other negative PCR test results for PBSCs [19].

These results indicate that continuous detection of MRD in APL patients treated with several courses of ATO therapy can show the need to alter the treatment strategy such as by changing to another medicine or allogeneic transplantation.

13.3.6 Mechanisms of Resistance to ATO

Although the CR rate is high even for relapsed patients, resistance to ATO treatment has been recognized as a clinically critical problem. Information on ATO resistance remains limited compared with that on ATRA resistance. Two cases have been reported of clinical ATO resistance after treatment with ATRA/chemotherapy. These cases exhibited missense mutations leading to substitution of amino acids in the promyelocytic leukemia protein (PML)-B2 domain in PML-retinoic acid receptor α (RARA). The presence of an M3 variant expressing PML (RARA-LBD mutation) was confirmed in leukemia cells harvested from one patient at the terminal stage. These results suggest that genetic mutations identified in ATO-resistant patients resulting in substitution of A216V and L218P may contribute to ATO resistance through impairment of direct ATO binding to PML-RARA due to conformational changes in ATO-binding sites [35].

Some rare genetic variants have been detected in APL cases with the aid of cytogenetics, which is potentially useful for the characterization of cases lacking the PML-RARA fusion. It may also facilitate identification of rarer molecular subtypes of APL including those with t(11;17)(q23;q21), t(11;17)(q13;q21), t(X;11)(p11;q21), and t(5;17)(q35;q21), which lead to PLZF-RARA [36], NuMA-RARA [37], BCOR-RARA [38], and NPM1-RARA [39] fusions, respectively. PLZR-RARA is relatively resistant, while the other three are known to be ATRA sensitive. As for sensitivity to ATO, PLZF-RARA- and BCOA-RARA-positive APLs have been shown to be resistant and NPM1-RARA to be sensitive [40]. Findings for other genetic variants have not been documented.

13.4 Toxicity Profile of Arsenic Trioxide

13.4.1 APL Differentiation Syndrome and Hyperleukocytosis

The major toxicity associated with ATO treatment during remission induction is APL differentiation syndrome. It is characterized by fever, peripheral edema, pulmonary opacities, hypoxemia, respiratory distress, hypotension, renal and hepatic dysfunction, skin rash, and serositis resulting in pleural and pericardial effusions. This complication has been observed in about 5–30% of patients. APL differentiation syndrome is the major cause of remission induction failure and occurs in patients with high or low initial WBC counts. Management of the syndrome has not been fully investigated, but high-dose steroids have been used at the first suspicion of the emergence of APL differentiation syndrome and appear to mitigate signs and symptoms [34, 41]. Such suspicion, based on the detection of signs that could suggest the presence of the syndrome [unexplained fever, dyspnea and/or weight gain, abnormal chest auscultatory findings, or radiographic abnormalities (Fig. 13.3)], should generate the immediate initiation of the administration of high-dose steroids (dexamethasone 10 mg intravenously BID) irrespective of the leukocyte count, which should be continued for at least 3 days or longer until signs and symptoms have abated. Termination of the ATO therapy is recommended during treatment of the APL differentiation syndrome.

Development of hyperleukocytosis (≥10,000/μl) was observed in 10–20% of patients treated. There was no relationship between baseline WBC counts and

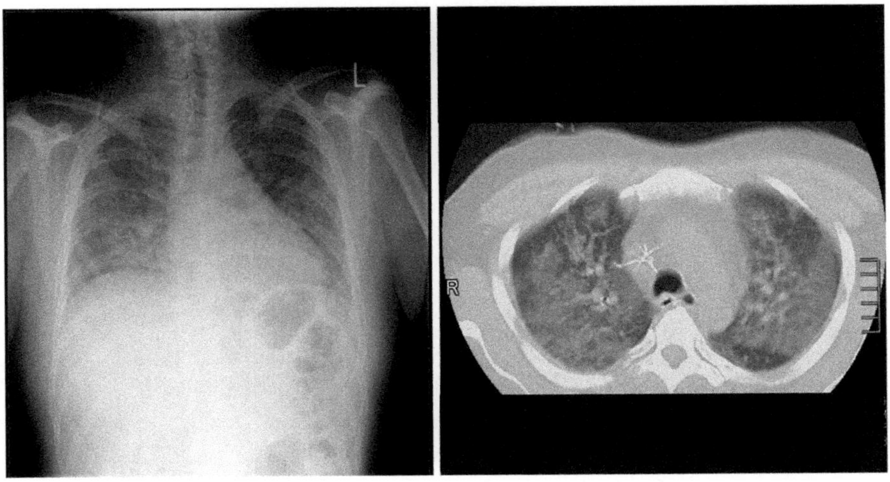

Fig. 13.3 Chest X-ray and CT performed on the 12th day of arsenic therapy. Interstitial infiltrates (septal lines and ground glass opacity) are shown

development of hyperleukocytosis nor between baseline WBC counts and peak WBC counts. Hyperleukocytosis accompanied by disseminated intravascular coagulation (DIC) should be treated with additional chemotherapy consisting of 12 mg/ m^2 of idarubicin (IDA) [34].

13.4.2 Hypereosinophilia

During induction therapy with ATO, significant amounts of eosinophils were detected in the peripheral blood, with 20–40% of WBC that were identified as eosinophils on days 30–40. In our experience, about 10% of patients with ATO induction therapy developed eosinophilia, and these patients did not present any eosinophilia-related symptoms such as fever, rash, or dyspnea [42]. An increase in eosinophils was not observed during the first induction therapy with ATRA and chemotherapy or during the consolidation therapy with ATO. Evidence from clinical observations and in vitro data suggest that APL cells differentiated into an eosinophilic granulocytic line.

13.4.3 Abnormalities on Electrocardiograms and Hepatotoxicity

Another major complication reported is QTc prolongation and sometimes torsade de pointes (TdP) arrhythmia, which can cause sudden cardiac-related death [43]. Prior to initiating ATO therapy, a 12-lead electrocardiograph (ECG) and echocardiogram should be used for the assessment of cardiac function. Serum electrolytes (potassium, calcium, and magnesium) and creatinine should be assessed. Patients with preexisting heart disease may have a higher risk of cardiac toxicity secondary to the treatment with ATO. The risk of TdP is related to the extent of QTc-interval prolongation, history of TdP, preexisting QTc-interval prolongation, and the presence of congestive heart failure. Several drugs, such as diuretics and amphotericin B, cause imbalance of serum electrolytes resulting in hypokalemia and hypomagnesemia which induce QTc-interval prolongation. If feasible, drugs that are known to prolong the QTc interval should be discontinued. Even if a high rate of cardiac arrhythmia is not observed, it is suggested QTc should be monitored during the treatment. If the QTc interval is prolonged, close monitoring of the ECGs and of the electrolytes is necessary. Depending on the individual risk/benefit ratio, an interruption of ATO is indicated until the QTc interval is less than 460 ms, which may take several days. In the case of renal insufficiency, the longer time needed for elimination of ATO must be taken into account [34, 43].

Hepatotoxicity has been widely observed in most clinical trials with incidence rates ranging from 33% to 75%. In several of these trials, the incidence of grade 3/4 hepatotoxicity was as high as 10% for the ATO group. In comparison, the increase in liver enzymes was mostly mild and reversible. The onset rate of hepatotoxicity occurred in induction is 65.5%, during consolidation is 10.3%, and during maintenance is 20.7% [44]. For the patients with grade 3/4 hepatotoxicity, ATO was withheld till the liver function tests had returned to a level below grade 3.

13.4.4 Other Complications

Other toxicities associated with arsenic trioxide include nephrotoxicity, neurotoxicity, metabolic disturbance (hyperglycemia, hypomagnesemia, and hypokalemia), fluid retention, skin discoloration and eruption (Fig. 13.4), and conjunctivitis. Table 13.3 shows the main adverse events for patients with APL who received ATO remission induction therapy [13]. During the consolidation phase, however, the occurrence of these complications was very rare, and in most cases, the toxic effects were eliminated with temporary discontinuation of ATO. Furthermore, an adequate supply of vitamins should be ensured, as development of severe neurological disorders (neuropathy, cramps) has been reported due to thiamine deficiency during ATO administration [45]. N-Acetylcysteine (NAC) should not be administered as a concomitant medication, as in vitro study results have shown it has led to an increase in glutathione concentration, which reduces the effect of ATO [46].

The following points should be stressed:

1. Depending on the specific circumstances, with any toxicity of WHO grade ≥3, ATO treatment must either be stopped altogether or interrupted.
2. If ATO is used again, the dosage should only be 50% of the initial dose.
3. For clinical signs of overdose, dimercaprol or dimercaptosuccinic acid may be administered [47, 48].

Patients should be closely monitored to detect any of the following:

1. Cardiac insufficiency NYHA stages III and IV
2. Refractory kidney function disorder (serum creatinine ≥2 mg/100 ml)
3. Severe liver function disorder (bilirubin ≥2 mg/100 ml, alanine aminotransferase/aspartate aminotransferase (ALAT/ASAT) ≥3 times normal)

A B

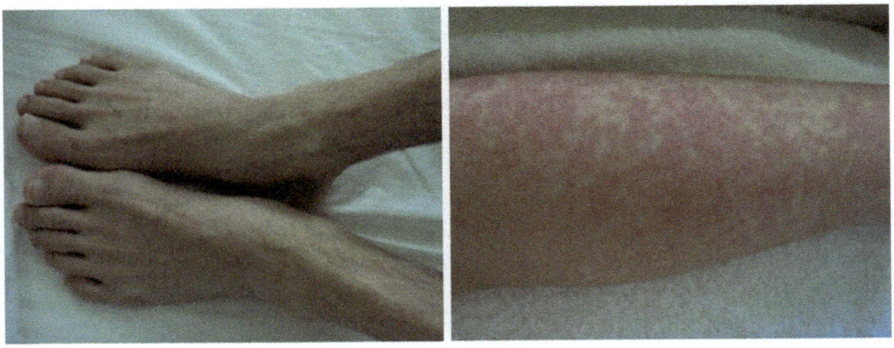

Fig. 13.4 Skin eruption after ATO therapy. **a** Erythema on the tenth day of ATO administration. **b** Erythema on the 14th day of ATO administration

Table 13.3 Main adverse events for APL patients treated with ATO therapy

Adverse event	Any grade (%)	Grade 3/4 events (%)
General disorders		
Fatigue	63	5
Fever	63	5
APL differentiation syndrome	24 [9]	6 [9], 14 [30], 16 [31]
Gastrointestinal disorders		
Nausea	75	
Anorexia	23	
Metabolism		
Hypokalemia	50	13
Hypomagnesemia	45	13
Nervous system disorders		
Headache	60	3
Paresthesia	33	5
Skin disorders		
Urticaria	8	
Eruption	13, 24 [21]	
Cardiac disorders		
ECG QT prolongation	40, 74 [9]	18 [9],
Tachycardia	55	
Liver and renal disorders		
ALT/AST increased	33, 35 [9]	8, 6 [9], 3.4 [21]
Renal failure	8	3
Hematologic disorders		
Leukocytosis	50, 58 [21]	3
Thrombocytopenia	18	13
Neutropenia	10	10

13.5 Conclusion

In the early 1970s, a group of medical researchers from Harbin Medical University in China were studying about compounds of the Chinese medications. Such research was focused on which among the Chinese medications used in rural areas were effective for cancer treatment. Finally, they discovered a remedy which is the arsenic stone powder, used by a family practicing traditional medicine. This was the first stage of the development of ATO. The intensive study of this compound by Dr. Wang's group led to the worldwide publication of their exceptional results. Although at first many researchers did not trust the robustness of these findings, hematologists began to take a closer look at this compound after follow-up studies in Europe, the United States, and Japan confirmed the effectiveness of ATO therapy.

Many clinical trials using ATO have been launched in the last two decades, and some important results of these studies are introduced in this chapter. These findings have led to the suggestion that ATO combined therapy may be a suitable first-line agent. However, in order to achieve more favorable outcome in conjunction with minimized toxicity, risk-adapted optimization of the use of ATO is needed.

References

1. Zhu J, Chen Z, Lallemand-Breitenbach V, de Thé H. How acute promyelocytic leukaemia revived arsenic. Nat Rev Cancer. 2002;2(9):705–13.
2. Rahman MM, Ng JC, Naidu R. Chronic exposure of arsenic via drinking water and its adverse health impacts on humans. Environ Geochem Health. 2009 Apr 4;31(S1):189–200. Available from: http://link.springer.com/10.1007/s10653-008-9235-0
3. Wojeck GA, Nigg HN, Braman RS, Stamper JH, Rouseff RL. Worker exposure to arsenic in Florida grapefruit spray operations. Arch Environ Contam Toxicol. 1982 Nov;11(6):661–7. Available from: http://link.springer.com/10.1007/BF01059152
4. Kiburn KH. Neurobehavioral impairment from long-term residential arsenic exposure. In: Abernathy CO, Calderson RL, Chappell WR, editors. Arsen Expo Heal Eff London, Chapman Hall. Dordrecht: Springer Netherlands; 1997;159–75. Available from: http://www.springerlink.com/index/10.1007/978-94-011-5864-0_14
5. Dakeishi M, Murata K, Grandjean P. Long-term consequences of arsenic poisoning during infancy due to contaminated milk powder. Environ Health.. BioMed Central; 2006;5(1):31. Available from: http://www.ehjournal.net/content/5/1/31
6. Zhang TD, Chen GQ, Wang ZG, Wang ZY, Chen SJ, Chen Z. Arsenic trioxide, a therapeutic agent for APL. Oncogene. 2001;20(49):7146–53.
7. Sun H, Ma L, Hu X, Zhang T. Ai-Lin I treated 32 cases of APL. Chin J Intgr Chin West Med. 1992;12:170–2.
8. Shen ZX, Chen GQ, Ni JH, Li XS, Xiong SM, Qiu QY, et al. Use of arsenic trioxide (As_2O_3) in the treatment of acute promyelocytic leukemia (AFL): II. Clinical efficacy and pharmacokinetics in relapsed patients. Blood. 1997;89(9):3354–60. Available from: http://www.ncbi.nlm.nih.gov/pubmed/9129042
9. Shigeno K, Naito K, Sahara N, Kobayashi M, Nakamura S, Fujisawa S, et al. Arsenic trioxide therapy in relapsed or refractory Japanese patients with acute promyelocytic leukemia: updated outcomes of the phase II study and postremission therapies. Int J Hematol. 2005 Oct;82(3):224–9. Available from: http://www.ncbi.nlm.nih.gov/pubmed/16207595
10. Soignet SL, Maslak P, Wang Z-G, Jhanwar S, Calleja E, Dardashti LJ, et al. Complete remission after treatment of acute promyelocytic leukemia with arsenic trioxide. N Engl J Med. 1998;339(19):1341–8.
11. Chen S, Zhou G, Zhang X, Mao J, de The H, Chen Z, et al. Underlying the therapeutic effects of arsenic in fighting leukemia from an old remedy to a magic bullet: molecular mechanisms underlying the therapeutic effects of arsenic in fighting leukemia. Blood. 2012;117(24):6425–37.
12. Li J, Zhu H, Hu J, Mi J, Chen S, Chen Z, et al. Progress in the treatment of acute promyelocytic leukemia: optimization and obstruction. Int J Hematol. 2014;100(1):38–50.
13. Drug Information of "TRISENOX". (n.d.). Available from: http://www.rxlist.com/trisenox-drug.htm
14. Fukai Y, Hirata M, Ueno M, Ichikawa N, Kobayashi H, Saitoh H, et al. Clinical pharmacokinetic study of arsenic trioxide in an acute promyelocytic leukemia (APL) patient: speciation of arsenic metabolites in serum and urine. Biol Pharm Bull. 2006;29(5):1022–7.
15. Nicolis I, Curis E, Deschamps P, Bénazeth S. Arsenite medicinal use, metabolism, pharmacokinetics and monitoring in human hair. Biochimie. 2009;91(10):1260–7.
16. Fujisawa S, Ohno R, Shigeno K, Sahara N, Nakamura S, Naito K, et al. Pharmacokinetics of arsenic species in Japanese patients with relapsed or refractory acute promyelocytic leukemia

treated with arsenic trioxide. Cancer Chemother Pharmacol. 2007 Mar;59(4):485–93. Available from: http://www.ncbi.nlm.nih.gov/pubmed/16937107
17. Thomas DJ, Waters SB, Styblo M. Elucidating the pathway for arsenic methylation. Toxicol Appl Pharmacol. 2004;198(3):319–26.
18. Soignet S, Frankel S, Douer D, Tallman MS, Kantarjian H, Calleja E, et al. United States multicenter study of arsenic trioxide in relapsed acute promyelocytic leukemia. J Clin Oncol. 2001;19(18):3852–60. Available from: http://jco.ascopubs.org/content/19/18/3852.short
19. Yanada M, Tsuzuki M, Fujita H, Fujimaki K, Fujisawa S, Sunami K, et al. Phase 2 study of arsenic trioxide followed by autologous hematopoietic cell transplantation for relapsed acute promyelocytic leukemia. Blood. 2013;121(16):3095–102.
20. Lengfelder E, Lo-Coco F, Ades L, Montesinos P, Grimwade D, Kishore B, et al. Arsenic trioxide-based therapy of relapsed acute promyelocytic leukemia: registry results from the European LeukemiaNet. Leukemia. 2015;29(5):1084–91. Available from: http://www.nature.com/doifinder/10.1038/leu.2015.12
21. Niu C, Yan H, Yu T, Sun HP, Liu JX, Li XS, et al. Studies on treatment of acute promyelocytic leukemia with arsenic trioxide: remission induction, follow-up, and molecular monitoring in 11 newly diagnosed and 47 relapsed acute promyelocytic leukemia patients. Blood. 1999;94(10):3315–24. Available from: http://www.bloodjournal.org/content/94/10/3315.short
22. Ghavamzadeh A, Alimoghaddam K, Rostami S, Ghaffari SH, Jahani M, Iravani M, et al. Phase II study of single-agent arsenic trioxide for the front-line therapy of acute promyelocytic leukemia. J Clin Oncol. 2011;29(20):2753–7. Available from: http://jco.ascopubs.org/content/29/20/2753.short
23. Mathews V, Chendamarai E, George B, Viswabandya A, Srivastava A. Treatment of acute promyelocytic leukemia with single-agent arsenic trioxide. Mediterr J Hematol Infect Dis. 2011;3(1):e2011056.
24. Powell BL, Moser B, Stock W, Gallagher RE, Willman CL, Stone RM, et al. Arsenic trioxide improves event-free and overall survival for adults with acute promyelocytic leukemia: North American Leukemia Intergroup Study C9710. Blood. 2010;116(19):3751–7.
25. Lou Y, Qian W, Meng H, Mai W, Tong H, Tong Y, et al. Long-term efficacy of low-dose all-trans retinoic acid plus minimal chemotherapy induction followed by the addition of intravenous arsenic trioxide post-remission therapy in newly diagnosed acute promyelocytic leukaemia. Hematol Oncol. 2014 Mar;32(1):40–6. Available from: http://www.ncbi.nlm.nih.gov/pubmed/23963734
26. Mathieu J, Besancon F. Arsenic trioxide represses NF-kB activation and increases apoptosis in ATRA-treated APL cells. In: Annals of the New York Academy of Sciences. 2006. p. 203–8. Available from: http://onlinelibrary.wiley.com/doi/10.1196/annals.1378.022/full
27. Lallemand-Breitenbach V, Guillemin MC, Janin A, Daniel MT, Degos L, Kogan SC, et al. Retinoic acid and arsenic synergize to eradicate leukemic cells in a mouse model of acute promyelocytic leukemia. J Exp Med. 1999;189(7):1043–52. Available from: http://jem.rupress.org/content/189/7/1043.abstract
28. Shen Z-X, Shi Z-Z, Fang J, Gu B-W, Li J-M, Zhu Y-M, et al. All-trans retinoic acid/As2O3 combination yields a high quality remission and survival in newly diagnosed acute promyelocytic leukemia. Proc Natl Acad Sci U S A. 2004;101(15):5328–35. Available from: https://www.ncbi.nlm.nih.gov/pmc/articles/PMC397380/?tool=pmcentrez
29. Hu J, Liu YF, Wu CF, Xu F, Shen ZX, Zhu YM, et al. Long-term efficacy and safety of all-trans retinoic acid/arsenic trioxide-based therapy in newly diagnosed acute promyelocytic leukemia. Proc Natl Acad Sci U S A. 2009;106(9):3342–7. Available from: http://www.pnas.org/content/106/9/3342.short
30. Iland HJ, Collins M, Bradstock K, Supple SG, Catalano A, Hertzberg M, et al. Use of arsenic trioxide in remission induction and consolidation therapy for acute promyelocytic leukaemia in the Australasian Leukaemia and Lymphoma Group (ALLG) APML4 study: a non-randomised phase 2 trial. Lancet Haematol. 2015 Sep;2(9):e357–66. Available from: http://dx.doi.org/10.1016/S2352-3026(15)00115-5

31. Ravandi F, Estey E, Jones D, Faderl S, O'Brien S, Fiorentino J, et al. Effective treatment of acute promyelocytic leukemia with all-trans-retinoic acid, arsenic trioxide, and gemtuzumab ozogamicin. J Clin Oncol. 2009 Feb 1;27(4):504–10. Available from: http://www.ncbi.nlm.nih.gov/pubmed/19075265
32. Lo-Coco F, Avvisati G, Vignetti M, Thiede C, Orlando SM, Iacobelli S, et al. Retinoic acid and arsenic trioxide for acute promyelocytic leukemia – supplementary appendix. N Engl J Med. 2013;369(2):111–21. Available from: http://www.nejm.org/doi/pdf/10.1056/NEJMoa1300874
33. Lo-Coco F, Di Donato L, Schlenk RF, for GIMEMA, German–Austrian Acute Myeloid Leukemia Study Group and Study Alliance Leukemia. Targeted therapy alone for acute promyelocytic leukemia. N Engl J Med. 2016 Mar 24;374(12):1197–8. Available from: http://www.ncbi.nlm.nih.gov/pubmed/27007970
34. Sanz MA, Grimwade D, Tallman MS, Lowenberg B, Fenaux P, Estey EH, et al. Management of acute promyelocytic leukemia: recommendations from an expert panel on behalf of the European LeukemiaNet. Blood. 2009;113(9):1875–91.
35. Tomita A, Kiyoi H, Naoe T. Mechanisms of action and resistance to all-trans retinoic acid (ATRA) and arsenic trioxide (As_2O_3) in acute promyelocytic leukemia. Int J Hematol. 2013;97(6):717–25.
36. Rohr SS, Pelloso LAF, Borgo A, De Nadai LC, Yamamoto M, Rego EM, et al. Acute promyelocytic leukemia associated with the PLZF-RARA fusion gene: two additional cases with clinical and laboratorial peculiar presentations. Med Oncol. 2012 Dec;29(4):2345–7. Available from: http://www.ncbi.nlm.nih.gov/pubmed/22205181
37. Hummel JL, Zhang T, Wells RA, Kamel-Reid S. The retinoic acid receptor alpha (RARalpha) chimeric proteins PML-, PLZF-, NPM-, and NuMA-RARalpha have distinct intracellular localization patterns. Cell Growth Differ. 2002 Apr;13(4):173–83. Available from: http://www.ncbi.nlm.nih.gov/pubmed/11971817
38. Yamamoto Y, Tsuzuki S, Tsuzuki M, Handa K, Inaguma Y, Emi N. BCOR as a novel fusion partner of retinoic acid receptor alpha in a t(X;17)(p11;q12) variant of acute promyelocytic leukemia. Blood. 2010;116(20):4274–83.
39. Pandolfi PP. PML, PLZF and NPM genes in the molecular pathogenesis of acute promyelocytic leukemia. Haematologica. 1996;81(5):472–82. Available from: http://www.ncbi.nlm.nih.gov/pubmed/8952164
40. Chen Y, Gu L, Zhou C, Wu X, Gao J, Li Q, et al. Relapsed APL patient with variant NPM-RARa fusion responded to arsenic trioxide-based therapy and achieved long-term survival. Int J Hematol. Springer Japan; 2010 May 20;91(4):708–10. Available from: http://link.springer.com/10.1007/s12185-010-0553-5
41. Camacho L, Soignet S, Chanel S, Ho R, Heller G, Scheinberg DA, et al. Leukocytosis and the retinoic acid syndrome in patients with acute promyelocytic leukemia treated with arsenic trioxide. J Clin Oncol. 2000;18(13):2620–5. Available from: http://jco.ascopubs.org/content/18/13/2620.short
42. Yamamoto K, Emi N, Kajiguchi T, Yamamori S, Ono Y, Naoe T. Eosinophils derived from acute promyelocytic leukemia cells after arsenic trioxide treatment. Int J Hematol. 2007;85(5):456–7.
43. Naito K, Kobayashi M, Sahara N, Shigeno K, Nakamura S, Shinjo K, et al. Two cases of acute promyelocytic leukemia complicated by torsade de pointes during arsenic trioxide therapy. Int J Hematol. 2006;83(4):318–23. Available from: http://www.ncbi.nlm.nih.gov/pubmed/16757431
44. Mathews V, Desire S, George B, Lakshmi KM, Rao JG, Viswabandya A, et al. Hepatotoxicity profile of single agent arsenic trioxide in the treatment of newly diagnosed acute promyelocytic leukemia, its impact on clinical outcome and the effect of genetic polymorphisms on the incidence of hepatotoxicity. Leukemia. 2006 May;20(5):881–3. Available from: http://www.ncbi.nlm.nih.gov/pubmed/16525498
45. Yip SF, Yeung YM, Tsui EYK. Severe neurotoxicity following arsenic therapy for acute promyelocytic leukemia: potentiation by thiamine deficiency. Blood. 2002;99:3481–2.

46. Flora SJS. Arsenic-induced oxidative stress and its reversibility following combined administration of N-acetylcysteine and meso 2,3-dimercaptosuccinic acid in rats. Clin Exp Pharmacol Physiol. Blackwell Science Pty; 1999 Nov 4;26(11):865–9. Available from: http://doi.wiley.com/10.1046/j.1440-1681.1999.03157.x
47. Chan K-M, Matthews WS. Acute arsenic overdose. Lab Med. The Oxford University Press; 1990 Oct 1;21(10):649–52. Available from: http://labmed.oxfordjournals.org/lookup/doi/10.1093/labmed/21.10.649
48. Isbister GK, Dawson AH, Whyte IM. Arsenic trioxide poisoning: a description of two acute overdoses. Hum Exp Toxicol. 2004 Jul 1;23(7):359–64. Available from: http://het.sagepub.com/cgi/doi/10.1191/0960327104ht459cr
49. Estey E, Garcia-Manero G, Ferrajoli A, Faderl S, Verstovsek S, Jones D, et al. Use of all-trans retinoic acid plus arsenic trioxide as an alternative to chemotherapy in untreated acute promyelocytic leukemia. Blood. 2006;107(9):3469–73. Available from: http://www.bloodjournal.org/content/107/9/3469.short

Part V

New Chemotherapeutic Agents Including Antimetabolite

Nelarabine

14

Takahiro Yamauchi and Takanori Ueda

Abstract

Nelarabine (2-amino-9-β-D-arabinofuranosyl-6-methoxy-9*H*-purine) is a water-soluble prodrug of 9-β-D-arabinofuranosylguanine (ara-G). Nelarabine is demethoxylated to ara-G by adenosine deaminase in the blood. The ara-G is subsequently transported into cancer cells via nucleoside transporters. Inside the cells, ara-G is phosphorylated by either deoxycytidine kinase to cytosolic ara-G monophosphate or by deoxyguanosine kinase to mitochondrial ara-G monophosphate; these are further phosphorylated to ara-G triphosphate, an intracellular active metabolite, by nucleotide kinases. Ara-G triphosphate is incorporated into DNA strands, thereby inhibiting DNA synthesis and eventually inducing apoptosis. Nelarabine is approved as a treatment for relapsed/refractory T-cell acute lymphoblastic leukemia/T-cell lymphoblastic lymphoma. The recommended dose of the drug in adult patients is 1500 mg/m^2 by intravenous (IV) infusion given over 2 h on days 1, 3, and 5 and repeated every 21 days. In pediatric patients, the recommended dose is 650 mg/m^2 IV given over 1 h for five consecutive days and repeated every 21 days. In a large phase II study conducted by the German Multicenter Study Group for Adult Acute Lymphoblastic Leukemia, nelarabine at 1500 mg/m^2 was administered on days 1, 3, and 5 in patients with relapsed or refractory T-cell acute lymphoblastic leukemia or T-cell lymphoblastic lymphoma. Thirty-six percent of the patients achieved a complete remission, and 10% achieved a partial remission.

Keywords

Nelarabine • Ara-G • Ara-GTP • T-cell lymphoid malignancies

T. Yamauchi (✉)
Department of Hematology and Oncology, University of Fukui,
23-3 Shimoaizuki, Matsuoka, Eiheiji, Fukui 910-1193, Japan
e-mail: tyamauch@u-fukui.ac.jp

T. Ueda
Vice-President, University of Fukui, 3-9-1 Bunkyo, Fukui 910-8507, Japan

T. Ueda (ed.), *Chemotherapy for Leukemia*, DOI 10.1007/978-981-10-3332-2_14

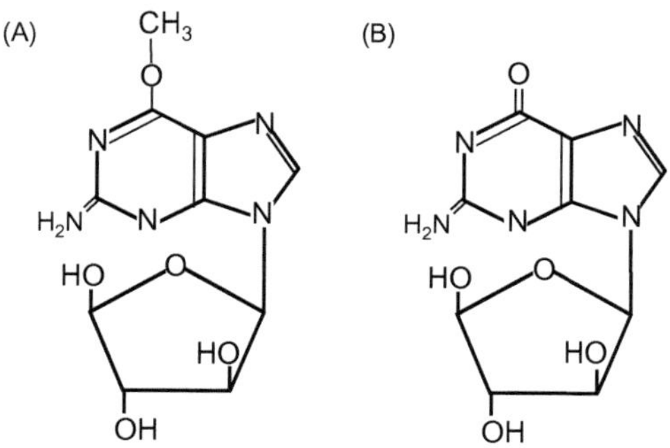

Fig. 14.1 The chemical structures of nelarabine and ara-G. (**a**) Nelarabine. (**b**) Ara-G

14.1 Introduction

Purine nucleoside phosphorylase (PNP) is a key enzyme in the purine-salvage metabolic pathway. PNP catalyzes the phosphorolysis of the N-ribosidic bonds of both purine nucleosides and deoxyribonucleosides (inosine, guanosine, and 2′-deoxyguanosine), splitting the substrates into purine bases and ribose monophosphates/deoxyribose monophosphates. 9-(β-D-Arabinofuranosyl)guanine (ara-G) is a deoxyguanosine derivative that is resistant to degradation by endogenous PNP and is toxic to T lymphoblasts [1, 2]. Inside cells, ara-G is phosphorylated by deoxycytidine kinase or deoxyguanosine kinase into ara-G triphosphate [2–4]. The resultant accumulation of intracellular ara-G triphosphate inhibits DNA synthesis [5]. Similar to deoxyguanosine, ara-G exhibits antileukemic activities in T-cell malignancies through the T-cell-specific accumulation of ara-G triphosphate in the cells [6, 7].

Nelarabine (2-amino-9-β-D-arabinofuranosyl-6-methoxy-9*H*-purine) is a water-soluble prodrug of ara-G (Fig. 14.1). It belongs to a group of guanosine analogues in which the hydrogen of the hydroxide group at the 6-position of the guanine ring is substituted by a methoxy group. In 2005, nelarabine received European Medicines Agency orphan drug status. The agent was also approved by the US Food and Drug Administration for the treatment of relapsed/refractory T-cell acute lymphoblastic leukemia/T-cell lymphoblastic lymphoma [8–12]. Nelarabine has been shown to be cytotoxic to T-cell malignancies, including T-cell acute lymphoblastic leukemia and T-cell lymphoblastic lymphoma [13].

14.2 Mechanisms of Action

14.2.1 Mechanisms of Action (Fig. 14.2)

In the blood, nelarabine is rapidly demethoxylated to ara-G by adenosine deaminase. The ara-G is subsequently transported into cancer cells via p-nitrobenzylthioinosine-sensitive and p-nitrobenzylthioinosine-insensitive transporters, including human equilibrative nucleoside transporters [14]. Ara-G is phosphorylated by either deoxycytidine kinase to cytosolic ara-G monophosphate or by

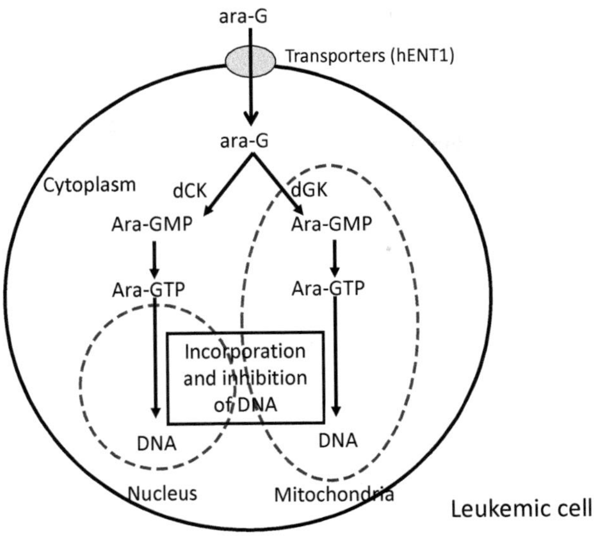

Fig. 14.2 The intracellular activation and the mechanism of action of ara-G. *dCK* deoxycytidine kinase, *dGK* deoxyguanosine kinase, *ara-GMP* ara-G monophosphate, *ara-GTP* ara-G triphosphate

deoxyguanosine kinase to mitochondrial ara-G monophosphate [4]. These nucleotides are further phosphorylated to ara-G triphosphate, an intracellular active metabolite, by nucleotide kinases. Nucleosides are degraded by adenosine deaminase, nucleotidase, or PNP [4]. Ara-G triphosphate competes with intrinsic deoxyribonucleotides as a substrate for incorporation into DNA by DNA polymerases. DNA-incorporated ara-G monophosphate inhibits DNA synthesis and consequently induces apoptosis [13].

14.2.2 Mechanisms of Drug Resistance

We developed a novel ara-G-resistant variant of the human T-lymphoblastic leukemia cell line CCRF-CEM, and we investigated the mechanisms behind its resistance to ara-G [15]. The CEM-resistant variant cells were 70-fold more ara-G resistant than the control CEM cells. The transcription level of human equilibrative nucleoside transporter 1 and the protein levels of deoxycytidine kinase and deoxyguanosine kinase were decreased in the resistant cells when compared to the control CEM cells. The production of intracellular ara-G triphosphate was one-fourth that of the control CEM cells. The level of antiapoptotic Bcl-xL was increased, and those of proapoptotic Bax and Bad were decreased in the resistant cells when compared to the control CEM cells. It was concluded that the reduction of drug incorporation into nuclear DNA and the inhibition of apoptosis were the crucial mechanisms behind the ara-G resistance in this cell line.

14.2.3 Adult T-Cell Leukemia/Lymphoma

Adult T-cell leukemia/lymphoma is an aggressive malignancy of mature activated CD4+ T cells that is associated with human T-cell leukemia virus 1 infection. Adult T-cell leukemia/lymphoma is difficult to treat, and the therapeutic outcomes of chemotherapy and allogeneic stem cell transplantation are still unsatisfactory [16]. The cytotoxicity of ara-G was evaluated using 12 cultured adult T-cell leukemia/lymphoma cell lines (ATL-43T, KOB, SO4, M8166, MT-2, MT-4, ED-40515 (+), ED-40515 (−), ST-1-dependent, ST-1-independent, KK1-dependent, and KK1-independent) in vitro [17]. The production of intracellular ara-G triphosphate in these cell lines was less than one-fourth of that in the CEM cell line. Moreover, the majority of the 50% inhibitory concentration values of these cell lines was higher than 1 mM. Thus, ara-G was not cytotoxic to adult T-cell leukemia/lymphoma cells.

14.3 Pharmacokinetics

The pharmacokinetics of nelarabine has been evaluated in patients with hematologic malignancies.

Gandhi et al. conducted a phase I multicenter trial of nelarabine in 26 patients with hematologic malignancies [6]. In their study, nelarabine (20–60 mg/kg) was administered for 5 days. The serum level of nelarabine increased over the duration of the intravenous (IV) infusion, reaching a peak (190 μmol/L) at the end of the infusion (dose of 30 mg/kg); the half-life of nelarabine was 16 min. The peak concentration of ara-G was 115 μmol/L, and it had a half-life of 3.4 h. The median peak intracellular ara-G triphosphate concentrations after the administration of 20, 30, 40, and 60 mg/kg of nelarabine were 23, 42, 85, and 93 pmol/L, respectively. Blasts from patients with T-cell acute lymphoblastic leukemia or T-cell lymphoid blast crisis of chronic myeloid leukemia accumulated relatively greater levels of ara-G triphosphate when compared to other lineages.

Kisor et al. evaluated the pharmacokinetics of nelarabine and ara-G in pediatric and adult patients with refractory hematologic malignancies [18]. Seventy-one patients with leukemia (acute lymphoblastic leukemia, chronic lymphocytic leukemia, acute myeloid leukemia, or chronic myeloid leukemia) or lymphoma (non-Hodgkin lymphoma) were evaluated in this study. The patients received 0.75–2 h IV infusions of nelarabine at 5–75 mg/kg for 5 consecutive days. The maximum concentration of nelarabine occurred at the end of the drug infusion. The harmonic mean half-lives of nelarabine were 14.1 and 16.5 min in the pediatric patients and adult patients, respectively. The maximum concentrations of ara-G, ranging between 11.6 and 308.7 μmol/L, occurred at or near the end of the nelarabine infusion.

Gandhi et al. also performed a phase I trial of nelarabine in 35 patients with relapsed/refractory indolent leukemias [19]. Patients were treated with nelarabine at 20, 30, 40, or 60 mg/kg by IV infusion for 1 h daily for 5 days, with nelarabine at a dose range between 1500 and 2900 mg/m^2 on days 1, 3, and 5, or with nelarabine at 1200 mg/m^2 on days 1, 3, and 5 combined with 30 mg/m^2 of fludarabine on days 3 and 5. Pharmacokinetic data demonstrated that the dose-adjusted plasma nelarabine area under the concentration-time curve from baseline to infinity value was 59 μmol/L·h, and the half-life was 23 min. The maximum concentration of ara-G occurred at or near the end of the nelarabine infusion. The ara-G concentration increased with increasing doses of nelarabine. The dose-adjusted area under the concentration-time curve for ara-G was 521 μmol/L·h (range, 315–1177 μmol/L·h), and the half-life of ara-G was 3.7 h (range, 2.4–7.2 h). Leukemic cells isolated from the patients receiving nelarabine were analyzed for the intracellular production of ara-G triphosphate. The median peak concentration of ara-G triphosphate was 89 μmol/L (range, 22–1438 μmol/L), and the dose-adjusted median value was 65 μmol/L (range, 17–1438 μmol/L).

In a Japanese phase I study, 13 patients with relapsed/refractory T-cell acute lymphoblastic leukemia/T-cell lymphoblastic lymphoma were treated with nelarabine [20]. The maximum serum concentration of nelarabine on day 1 was 28.3 μM with the administration of 1000 mg/m^2 nelarabine and 26.3 μM with the administration of 1500 mg/m^2 nelarabine in adults; the half-life of nelarabine was 0.2–0.3 h. The area under the concentration-time curve of nelarabine from zero to infinity was 36.3 μM·h with the administration of 1000 mg/m^2 nelarabine and 33.0 μM·h with the administration of 1500 mg/m^2 nelarabine. The maximum serum concentration of ara-G on day 1 was 87.0 μM with the administration of 1000 mg/m^2 nelarabine and 131.8 μM with the administration of 1500 mg/m^2 nelarabine; the half-life of ara-G was 3.0–3.5 h. The area under the concentration-time curve of ara-G from zero to infinity was 440.7 μM·h with the administration of 1000 mg/m^2 nelarabine and 622.5 μM·h with the administration of 1500 mg/m^2 nelarabine. In children-administered 400 or 650 mg/m^2 nelarabine, the maximum concentrations of nelarabine at the end of the infusions were 16.1 and 34.6 μM, respectively, and the half-lives of nelarabine were 0.2 and 0.2–0.3 h, respectively. The maximum concentrations of ara-G at the end of the 400 and 650 mg/m^2 nelarabine infusions were 41.0 and 63.8 μM, respectively, and the half-life of ara-G was 1.5–2.0 h.

14.4 The Method of Administration

The recommended dose of nelarabine in adults is 1500 mg/m^2 IV given over 2 h on days 1, 3, and 5 and repeated every 21 days. In pediatric patients, the recommended dose is 650 mg/m^2 IV given over 1 h for five consecutive days and repeated every 21 days [11, 21].

14.5 Toxicities

Kurtzberg et al. conducted a phase I study of nelarabine administered for five consecutive days in 93 patients with refractory hematologic malignancies [22]. The maximum tolerated dose was 60 mg/kg daily, and the dose-limiting toxicity was neurologic events. Neurotoxicity was observed in 72% of the patients; this occurred typically within 12 days of the start of drug administration in the first treatment course. The most frequent symptoms included transient somnolence, malaise, confusion, fatigue, and gait disorder, particularly in adult patients. Both central and peripheral neurotoxicities were observed. Other toxicities included nausea, vomiting, diarrhea, fever, and anorexia. As hematologic toxicities, grade 1 and 2 neutropenia and thrombocytopenia were observed.

A phase I trial of nelarabine was performed by Gandhi et al. in 35 patients with indolent leukemia, including B-cell chronic lymphocytic lymphoma and T-cell prolymphocytic leukemia [19]. The patients were treated with 20, 30, 40, or 60 mg/kg of nelarabine daily for 5 days, with 1500–2900 mg/m^2 nelarabine on days 1, 3, and 5 or with 1200 mg/m^2 nelarabine combined with fludarabine. Hematologic toxicity was modest. Grade 4 neutropenia and thrombocytopenia occurred in <15% of the patients. Neurotoxicities, including weakness, tiredness, drowsiness, ataxia, myalgia, and confusion, were noted, but they were transient and self-limiting. Symmetric sensorimotor peripheral neuropathy complications occurred in 21% of the patients.

Gökbuget et al. conducted a single-arm phase II study of nelarabine in 126 patients with T-cell acute lymphoblastic leukemia/T-cell lymphoblastic lymphoma [23]. Nelarabine was administered as a 2 h infusion at 1500 mg/m^2/day on days 1, 3, and 5. Toxicity was evaluated in 201 cycles administered to 126 patients. As hematologic toxicities, grade 3–4 leukopenia, granulocytopenia, and thrombocytopenia were observed after 41%, 37%, and 17% of the cycles, respectively. Increases in the levels of transaminases and bilirubin were observed after 6–8% and 3% of the cycles, respectively. Neurologic toxicities were found in 20 patients (16%); the majority was grade 1–2 neurologic toxicities. Seven percent of the patients presented with grade 3–4 neurotoxicities, among which dizziness and mood alterations were the most frequent. Other toxicities included cognitive disturbance, confusion, memory impairment, and neuropathy.

A Japanese phase I study evaluated the administration of nelarabine in patients with relapsed/refractory T-cell acute lymphoblastic leukemia/T-cell lymphoblastic lymphoma [20]. A total of 13 patients (7 adults, 6 children) were studied. The most frequently encountered events were somnolence and nausea in the adults and leukocytopenia and lymphopenia in the children. Neurotoxicities, including somnolence and headache, were observed in all of the 7 adults and in 2 children.

14.6 Clinical Studies (Table 14.1)

14.6.1 Phase I Studies

Kurtzberg et al. reported the clinical efficacy of nelarabine in a phase I study of 93 patients with refractory hematologic malignancies, including T-cell acute lymphoblastic leukemia and T-cell non-Hodgkin lymphoma [22]. Nelarabine at seven dose levels between 5 and 75 mg/kg/day was administered for 5 days in 198 cycles to 93 patients (59 adults, 34 children). Nine complete remissions (23%) and 12 partial responses (31%) were attained in 39 patients with T-cell acute lymphoblastic

Table 14.1 Clinical studies of nelarabine in patients with hematologic malignancies

Study	Disease	Patient number	Dose of nelarabine	Results
Phase 1 study by Kurtzberg (2005)	Hematologic malignancies including T-ALL, T-LBL	93	Intravenous infusion 5 and 75 mg/kg, 5 days	Nine CR, 12 PR in T-ALL and T-LBL
Phase 1 study by Horibe (2011)	T-ALL, T-LBL	13	1000 or 1500 mg/m^2 (1,3,5) 400 or 650 mg/m^2, 5 days	Three CR, 2 SD
Phase 2 study by DeAngelo (2007)	T-ALL, T-LBL	39	1500 mg/m^2 (1,3,5)	CR (31%), overall response (41%)
Phase 2 study by Gökbuget (2011)	T-ALL, T-LBL	126	1500 mg/m^2 (1,3,5)	CR (36%), PR (10%)
Combination by Commander (2010)	T-ALL, T-LBL	7	Etoposide (100 mg/m^2/5 days)+ Cyclophosphamide (440 mg/m^2/5 days)+ Nelarabine (650 mg/m^2/5 days)	Five CR

T-ALL T-cell acute lymphoblastic leukemia, *T-LBL* T-cell lymphoblastic lymphoma, *CR* complete remission, *PR* partial response, *SD* stable disease

leukemia and T-cell lymphoblastic lymphoma. One additional response was attained in a patient with lymphoid blast crisis of chronic myeloid leukemia.

A Japanese phase I study was performed for evaluating the clinical efficacy of nelarabine in 13 patients with relapsed/refractory T-cell acute lymphoblastic leukemia/T-cell lymphoblastic lymphoma [20]. Nelarabine at 1000 or 1500 mg/m^2 was used as an IV infusion on days 1, 3, and 5 in the adults. In the children, the agent was administered at 400 or 650 mg/m^2 for 5 days. One complete remission and two stable diseases were reported in the seven adults, and two complete remissions were attained in the four children.

14.6.2 Phase II Studies

DeAngelo et al. treated 26 patients with T-cell acute lymphoblastic leukemia and 13 patients with T-cell lymphoblastic lymphoma in a phase II open-label multicenter clinical trial to evaluate the efficacy and safety of nelarabine as a single agent (Cancer and Leukemia Group B study 19801) [24]. A dose of 1.5 g/m^2/day was administered on days 1, 3, and 5 to decrease the potential risk of neurological toxicities. Complete remission was attained in 31% of the patients, and the overall response rate was 41%. The median disease-free survival was 20 weeks, and the median overall survival was 20 weeks.

The German Multicenter Study Group for Adult Acute Lymphoblastic Leukemia conducted a prospective phase II study with nelarabine as a single agent in patients with relapsed or refractory T-cell acute lymphoblastic leukemia or T-cell lymphoblastic lymphoma [23]. Nelarabine at 1500 mg/m^2 was administered on days 1, 3, and 5. Thirty-six percent of the patients achieved a complete remission (45 of 126 evaluable patients), and 10% achieved a partial remission (12 patients). The probability of survival after 1 and 3 years was 24% and 12%, respectively, and the median survival was 6 months. The 3-year survival rate of patients with failure to respond or a partial response was 4%, while that of those with a complete remission was 28%.

14.6.3 Nelarabine Combined with Other Anticancer Agents

Commander et al. investigated the therapeutic efficacy of nelarabine combined with etoposide and cyclophosphamide as salvage therapy in seven children (2–19 years old) with relapsed/refractory T-cell leukemia/lymphoma [25]. Etoposide (100 mg/m^2/day) + cyclophosphamide (440 mg/m^2/day) was administered from day 1 to 5, followed by nelarabine (650 mg/m^2/day) for 5 days. Four patients obtained a complete remission after one course of the therapy, and one patient attained a complete remission after two courses of the therapy.

Luskin et al. reported the administration of nelarabine + etoposide + cyclophosphamide as salvage therapy for five adult patients (50–63 years old) with relapsed T-cell leukemia/lymphoma [26]. Nelarabine (650 mg/m^2) was administered on days 1–5, followed by the administration of etoposide (100 mg/m^2) + cyclophosphamide (440 mg/m^2) on days 7–11, or the reverse order. Three patients achieved a complete remission. The remaining two patients died from toxicity prior to disease reassessment. Luskin et al. concluded that the results provide a rationale for chemotherapy with nelarabine in combination with other anticancer agents as a method of inducing remission in adults in the salvage setting to prepare for stem cell transplantation.

References

1. Cohen A, Gudas LJ, Ammann AJ, Staal GE, Martin Jr DW. Deoxyguanosine triphosphate as a possible toxic metabolite in the immunodeficiency associated with purine nucleoside phosphorylase deficiency. J Clin Invest. 1978;61:1405–9.
2. Rodriguez Jr CO, Stellrecht CM, Gandhi V. Mechanisms for T-cell selective cytotoxicity of arabinosylguanine. Blood. 2003;102:1842–8.
3. Ullman B, Martin Jr DW. Specific cytotoxicity of arabinosylguanine toward cultured T lymphoblasts. J Clin Invest. 1984;74:951–5.
4. Rodriguez Jr CO, Mitchell BS, Ayres M, Eriksson S, Gandhi V. Arabinosylguanine is phosphorylated by both cytoplasmic deoxycytidine kinase and mitochondrial deoxyguanosine kinase. Cancer Res. 2002;62:3100–5.
5. Cohen A, Lee JW, Gelfand EW. Selective toxicity of deoxyguanosine and arabinosyl guanine for T-leukemic cells. Blood. 1983;61:660–6.
6. Gandhi V, Plunkett W, Rodriguez Jr CO, Nowak BJ, Du M, Ayres M, Kisor DF, Mitchell BS, Kurtzberg J, Keating MJ. Compound GW506U78 in refractory hematologic malignancies:

relationship between cellular pharmacokinetics and clinical response. J Clin Oncol. 1998;16:3607–15.
7. Gandhi V, Plunkett W, Weller S, Du M, Ayres M, Rodriguez Jr CO, Ramakrishna P, Rosner GL, Hodge JP, O'Brien S, Keating MJ. Evaluation of the combination of nelarabine, fludarabine in leukemias: clinical response, pharmacokinetics and pharmacodynamics in leukemia cells. J Clin Oncol. 2001;19:2142–52.
8. Lambe CU, Averett DR, Paff MT, Reardon JE, Wilson JG, Krenitsky TA. 2-Amino-6-methoxypurine arabinoside: an agent for T-cell malignancies. Cancer Res. 1995;55:3352–6.
9. Roecker AM, Allison JC, Kisor DF. Nelarabine: efficacy in the treatment of clinical malignancies. Future Oncol. 2006;2:441–8.
10. Buie LW, Epstein SS, Lindley CM. Nelarabine: a novel purine antimetabolite antineoplastic agent. Clin Ther. 2007;29:1887–99.
11. Cohen MH, Johnson JR, Massie T, Sridhara R, McGuinn Jr WD, Abraham S, Booth BP, Goheer MA, Morse D, Chen XH, Chidambaram N, Kenna L, Gobburu JV, Justice R, Pazdur R. Approval summary: nelarabine for the treatment of T-cell lymphoblastic leukemia/lymphoma. Clin Cancer Res. 2006;12:5329–35.
12. Cohen MH, Johnson JR, Justice R, Pazdur R. FDA drug approval summary: nelarabine (Arranon) for the treatment of T-cell lymphoblastic leukemia/lymphoma. Oncologist. 2008;13:709–14.
13. Gandhi V, Plunkett W. Clofarabine and nelarabine: two new purine nucleoside analogs. Curr Opin Oncol. 2006;18:584–90.
14. Prus KL, Averett DR, Zimmerman TP. Transport and metabolism of 9-beta-Darabinofuranosylguanine in a human T-lymphoblastoid cell line nitrobenzylthioinosine-sensitive and -insensitive influx. Cancer Res. 1990;50:1817–21.
15. Yamauchi T, Uzui K, Nishi R, Shigemi H, Ueda T. Reduced drug incorporation into DNA and antiapoptosis as the crucial mechanisms of resistance in a novel nelarabine-resistant cell line. BMC Cancer. 2014;14:547.
16. Kato K, Akashi K. Recent advances in therapeutic approaches for adult T-cell leukemia/lymphoma. Viruses. 2015;7:6604–12.
17. Yamauchi T, Nishi R, Kitazumi K, Nakano T, Ueda T. A new high-performance liquid chromatography method determines low production of 9-beta-D-arabinofuranosylguanine triphosphate, an active metabolite of nelarabine, in adult T-cell leukemia cells. Oncol Rep. 2010;23:499–504.
18. Kisor DF, Plunkett W, Kurtzberg J, Mitchell B, Hodge JP, Ernst T, Keating MJ, Gandhi V. Pharmacokinetics of nelarabine and 9-beta-D-arabinofuranosyl guanine in pediatric and adult patients during a phase I study of nelarabine for the treatment of refractory hematologic malignancies. J Clin Oncol. 2000;18:995–1003.
19. Gandhi V, Tam C, O'Brien S, Jewell RC, Rodriguez Jr CO, Lerner S, Plunkett W, Keating MJ. Phase I trial of nelarabine in indolent leukemias. J Clin Oncol. 2008;26:1098–105.
20. Horibe K, Takimoto T, Yokozawa T, Makimoto A, Kobayashi Y, Ogawa C, Ohno R, Koh N, Katsura K, Tobinai K. Phase I study of nelarabine in patients with relapsed or refractory T-ALL/T-LBL. Rinsho Ketsueki. 2011;52:406–15.
21. Berg SL, Blaney SM, Devidas M, Lampkin TA, Murgo A, Bernstein M, Billett A, Kurtzberg J, Reaman G, Gaynon P, Whitlock J, Krailo M, Harris MB, Children's Oncology Group. Phase II study of nelarabine (compound 506U78) in children and young adults with refractory T-cell malignancies: a report from the Children's Oncology Group. J Clin Oncol. 2005;23:3376–82.
22. Kurtzberg J, Ernst TJ, Keating MJ, Gandhi V, Hodge JP, Kisor DF, Lager JJ, Stephens C, Levin J, Krenitsky T, Elion G, Mitchell BS. Phase I study of 506U78 administered on a consecutive 5-day schedule in children and adults with refractory hematologic malignancies. J Clin Oncol. 2005;23:3396–403.
23. Gökbuget N, Basara N, Baurmann H, Beck J, Brüggemann M, Diedrich H, Güldenzoph B, Hartung G, Horst HA, Hüttmann A, Kobbe G, Naumann R, Ratei R, Reichle A, Serve H, Stelljes M, Viardot A, Wattad M, Hoelzer D. High single-drug activity of nelarabine in relapsed

T-lymphoblastic leukemia/lymphoma offers curative option with subsequent stem cell transplantation. Blood. 2011;118:3504–11.
24. DeAngelo DJ, Yu D, Johnson JL, Coutre SE, Stone RM, Stopeck AT, Gockerman JP, Mitchell BS, Appelbaum FR, Larson RA. Nelarabine induces complete remissions in adults with relapsed or refractory T-lineage acute lymphoblastic leukemia or lymphoblastic lymphoma: cancer and leukemia group B study 19801. Blood. 2007;109:5136–42.
25. Commander LA, Seif AE, Insogna IG, Rheingold SR. Salvage therapy with nelarabine, etoposide, and cyclophosphamide in relapsed/refractory paediatric T-cell lymphoblastic leukaemia and lymphoma. Br J Haematol. 2010;150:345–51.
26. Luskin MR, Ganetsky A, Landsburg DJ, Loren AW, Porter DL, Nasta SD, Svoboda J, Luger SM, Frey NV. Nelarabine, cyclophosphamide and etoposide for adults with relapsed T-cell acute lymphoblastic leukaemia and lymphoma. Br J Haematol. In press.

Forodesine

15

Takahiro Yamauchi and Takanori Ueda

Abstract

Purine nucleoside phosphorylase (PNP) is a key enzyme in the purine-salvage metabolic pathway. A deficiency in PNP is associated with significant T-cell depletion and immune deficiency. Forodesine is a potent PNP inhibitor that was designed based on the transition-state structure stabilized by the enzyme. When PNP is inhibited by forodesine, 2′-deoxyguanosine remains unmetabolized and is transported into cancer cells via nucleoside transporters. Inside the cells, 2′-deoxyguanosine is phosphorylated to deoxyguanosine monophosphate by deoxycytidine kinase and then to deoxyguanosine triphosphate by other kinases. The intracellular deoxyguanosine triphosphate inhibits ribonucleotide reductase, induces deoxyribonucleotide pool imbalance, and inhibits DNA synthesis and repair. In early clinical trials, forodesine demonstrated modest anticancer efficacies. Drug-related adverse events, including lymphocytopenia and neutropenia, were generally tolerable. Forodesine is now being investigated for its clinical efficacy against T-cell malignancies, such as T-cell leukemia and cutaneous T-cell lymphoma.

Keywords

Forodesine • Purine nucleoside phosphorylase • 2′-deoxyguanosine • Deoxyguanosine triphosphate • T-cell malignancies

T. Yamauchi (✉)
Department of Hematology and Oncology, University of Fukui,
23-3 Shimoaizuki, Matsuoka, Eiheiji, Fukui 910-1193, Japan
e-mail: tyamauch@u-fukui.ac.jp

T. Ueda
Vice-President, University of Fukui, 3-9-1 Bunkyo, Fukui 910-8507, Japan

T. Ueda (ed.), *Chemotherapy for Leukemia*, DOI 10.1007/978-981-10-3332-2_15

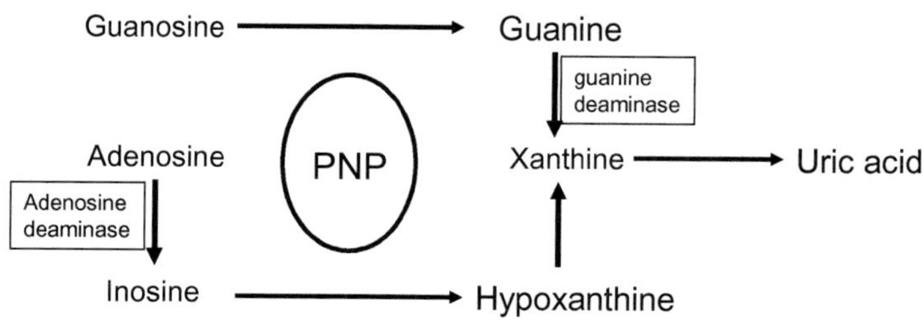

Fig. 15.1 Metabolism of purine nucleotides

15.1 Purine Nucleoside Phosphorylase

Purine nucleoside phosphorylase (PNP) is an enzyme that catalyzes the phosphorolysis of N-ribosidic bonds of both purine nucleosides and deoxyribonucleosides (inosine, guanosine, and 2′-deoxyguanosine) and splits the substrates into purine bases and ribose monophosphates/deoxyribose monophosphates (Fig. 15.1) [1, 2]. Congenital defects in PNP result in severe immunodeficiency syndromes, and PNP inhibition has been shown to selectively deplete T cells [3–6]. Giblett et al. reported that a 5-year-old girl with a history of recurrent infection and anemia had no measurable PNP activity in her red blood cells [3]. Her serum immunoglobulin levels were normal; however, she had severe lymphocytopenia, a lack of lymphocyte response to mitogenic and allogeneic cell stimuli, and decreased T-cell rosette formation. They concluded that the PNP inactivity was responsible for her syndrome. Subsequent studies have shown that T-cell deficiency is attributable to an altered purine metabolism pathway in the absence of PNP, that is, the accumulation of plasma 2′-deoxyguanosine and intracellular deoxyguanosine triphosphate. In the case of PNP deficiency, 2′-deoxyguanosine accumulates in the blood and is thereby incorporated into blood cells. Inside the cells, deoxyguanosine is phosphorylated to deoxyguanosine triphosphate, which induces a nucleotide imbalance and consequently cellular damage [7–9]. Therefore, the inhibition of PNP was soon identified as a target for treating malignant T cells, including T-cell leukemia and lymphoma [10, 11].

15.2 Forodesine

Forodesine [BCX-1777, immucillin-H, 7-[(2S,3S,4R,5R)-3,4-dihydroxy-5-hydroxymethyl-2-pyrrolidinyl]-1,5-dihydro-4H-pyrrolo-[3,2-d]-pyrimidin-4-one, monohydrochloride] is a transition-state analog that potently inhibits PNP enzyme activity (Fig. 15.2) [12–15]. Forodesine has shown anticancer effects against several types of cancer cells in preclinical studies and is now being investigated for its clinical efficacy against T-cell malignancies, including T-cell leukemia and cutaneous T-cell lymphoma [12, 16, 17].

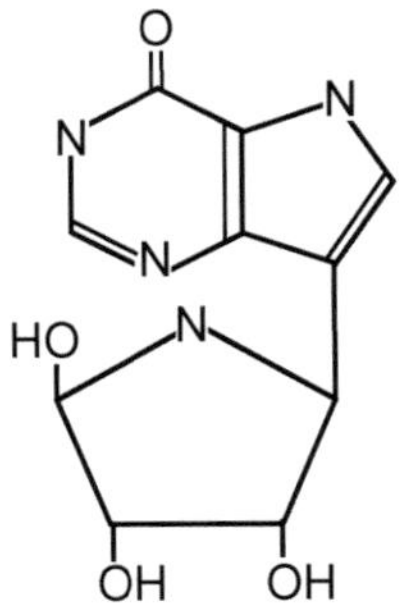

Fig. 15.2 The structure of forodesine

15.3 Mechanisms of Action

15.3.1 Mechanisms of Action of the Usual Nucleoside Analogs

The mechanisms of action of forodesine are different from those of the usual nucleoside analogs. After exposure to patients, these conventional nucleoside analogs are transported into cancer cells via nucleoside transporters and are then phosphorylated to their corresponding triphosphates. These analog triphosphates are subsequently incorporated into DNA by DNA polymerases, thereby inducing the termination of DNA synthesis and consequently inducing apoptosis [18–20]. In contrast to these nucleoside analogs, forodesine itself is not phosphorylated to its triphosphate form, nor is it incorporated into DNA strands.

15.3.2 Mechanisms of Action of Forodesine

In the blood, 2′-deoxyguanosine is converted to guanine and deoxyribose monophosphate via phosphorolysis in the presence of PNP. The guanine is then deaminated to xanthine, and the xanthine is subsequently metabolized to uric acid by xanthine oxidase (Fig. 15.3). If PNP is inhibited by forodesine, 2′-deoxyguanosine remains unmetabolized and is transported into cancer cells via nucleoside transporters. Inside the cells, 2′-deoxyguanosine is phosphorylated to deoxyguanosine monophosphate by deoxycytidine kinase and then to deoxyguanosine triphosphate by other kinases. The intracellular deoxyguanosine triphosphate inhibits ribonucleotide reductase, induces deoxyribonucleotide pool imbalance, and inhibits DNA synthesis and repair [15, 21–23]. Forodesine selectively inhibits the in vitro growth of malignant T-cell lines in the presence of 2′-deoxyguanosine. It is preferentially cytotoxic to T cells, because T cells possess a relatively high level of kinase activity and a relatively low level of nucleotidase activity [8].

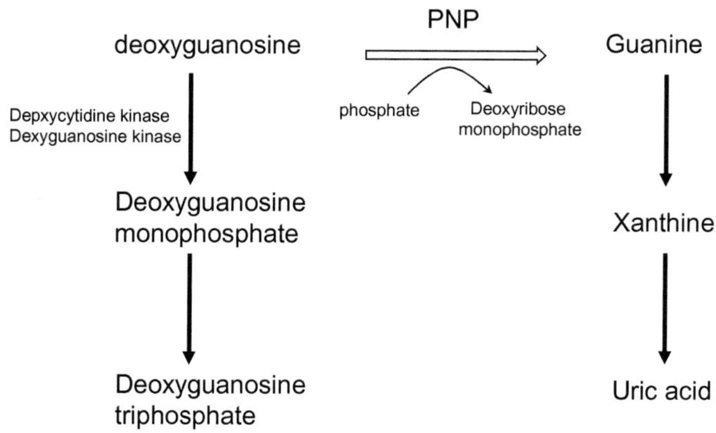

Fig. 15.3 Inhibition of purine nucleoside phosphorylase. *PNP* purine nucleoside phosphorylase

15.3.3 The Role of p53 in the Cytotoxic Activity of Forodesine

Balakrishnan et al. reported that when chronic lymphocytic leukemia lymphocytes were treated with forodesine and 2′-deoxyguanosine, intracellular deoxyguanosine triphosphate accumulated in the cells. This accumulation was associated with DNA damage-induced p53 stabilization, phosphorylation of p53 at Ser15, and activation of p21 [24]. In another study, Alonso et al. demonstrated that forodesine was highly cytotoxic as a single agent or in combination with bendamustine and rituximab in primary chronic lymphocytic leukemia cells. This cytotoxicity was independent of CD38/ZAP-70 expression and p53 or ATM deletion [25].

15.3.4 The Cytotoxicity of Forodesine in Combination with Nelarabine

We investigated the cytotoxicity of forodesine in combination with nelarabine in vitro using the human T-lymphoblastic leukemia cell line CCRF-CEM, because both agents are cytotoxic to T-cell malignancies [26]. Nelarabine is a purine nucleoside analog with anticancer properties that is used for treating refractory or relapsed T-cell acute lymphoblastic leukemia and T-cell lymphoblastic lymphoma. When the CCRF-CEM cells were treated with forodesine in the presence of 2′-deoxyguanosine, the forodesine was active and inhibited cell growth. However, the addition of 9-β-D-arabinofuranosylguanine, an active compound of nelarabine, to the forodesine and 2′-deoxyguanosine did not enhance the growth inhibition effect of forodesine. The combination index revealed antagonism between forodesine and 9-β-D-arabinofuranosylguanine. The intracellular production of 9-β-D-arabinofuranosylguanine triphosphate was reduced in the presence of forodesine. A CEM subclone resistant to 9-β-D-arabinofuranosylguanine was cross-resistant to forodesine. Thus, the combination of forodesine and nelarabine would not be an effective regimen for treating patients with T-cell malignancies.

15.4 Pharmacokinetics

15.4.1 Phase I Studies

A phase I clinical trial was conducted by Gandhi et al. in five patients with previously treated T-cell malignancies, such as T-cell lymphoblastic lymphoma, T-cell acute lymphoblastic leukemia, and T-cell prolymphocytic leukemia, as the first study of forodesine in humans [11]. Forodesine (40 mg/m^2) was infused over 30 min on the first day. Plasma and cellular pharmacokinetics and pharmacodynamics were investigated. The median plasma peak level of forodesine (5.4 μM; range, 4.9–7.8 μM) occurred at the end of the infusion. The half-life of plasma forodesine was between 6 and 17 h. The plasma 2′-deoxyguanosine concentration after eight intravenous infusions of forodesine reached a maximum of 20 μM (range, 2.6–36.8 μM). The intracellular deoxyguanosine triphosphate concentrations were also determined in leukemic cells. After the administration of forodesine on day 1, deoxyguanosine triphosphate concentrations increased by five- to tenfold within the first 8 h and by 10- to 20-fold within the first 24 h after the start of therapy [11].

A phase I study was conducted in 13 Japanese patients with relapsed or refractory peripheral T/natural killer-cell malignancies [27]. Forodesine was administered orally once daily at 100, 200, or 300 mg. The mean maximum concentrations of plasma forodesine were 139.2 ng/mL (day 1) and 216.5 ng/mL (day 5) at 100 mg, 335.3 ng/mL (day 1) and 499.0 ng/mL (day 5) at 200 mg, and 328.0 ng/mL (day 1) and 421.6 ng/mL (day 5) at 300 mg. The area under the plasma concentration-time curve values at the doses of 100, 200, and 300 mg were 1948 ng·h/mL (day 1) and 2730 ng·h/mL (day 5), 4608 ng·h/mL (day 1) and 6303 ng·h/mL (day 5), and 4596 ng·h/mL (day 1) and 5587 ng·h/mL (day 5), respectively. As for the pharmacodynamics, the mean maximum concentrations of plasma 2′-deoxyguanosine were 270.4 ng/mL (day 1) and 315.5 ng/mL (day 15) at 100 mg, 348.7 ng/mL (day 1) and 410.7 ng/mL (day 15) at 200 mg, and 374.4 ng/mL (day 1) and 515.8 ng/mL (day 15) at 300 mg. The area under the plasma concentration-time curve values of 2′-deoxyguanosine at the doses of 100, 200, and 300 mg were 4023 ng·h/mL (day 1) and 5384 ng·h/mL (day 15), 5705 ng·h/mL (day 1) and 7696 ng·h/mL (day 15), and 6074 ng·h/mL (day 1) and 9533 ng·h/mL (day 15), respectively.

15.4.2 A Phase II Study

In a phase II study by Balakrishnan et al., 200 mg of forodesine was administered orally in eight patients with chronic lymphocytic leukemia [28]. On day 1, a plasma forodesine level of 300 nM was achieved (range, 126–600 nM). Overall, the plasma forodesine levels on days 2, 3, 4, and 5 ranged between 200 and 1300 nM. The level of 2′-deoxyguanosine in pretreated samples was below the level of detection. On day 1, the plasma concentration of 2′-deoxyguanosine reached a median of 1.2 μM (range, 0.57–2.2 μM), and on day 27, it was between 1.1 and 2.3 μM.

15.5 The Method of Administration

Clinical studies of forodesine are underway. In such studies, forodesine is mainly administered orally once a day at 200–600 mg. The bioavailability of forodesine after oral administration was 40–59% in humans [29].

15.6 Toxicities

15.6.1 Phase I Studies

In the phase I study performed by Gandhi et al., the most common toxicity observed was grade 3–4 neutropenia associated with infection. Other grade 3–4 toxicities included dyspnea, renal failure, depression, and hypoxemia. The grade 1–2 toxicities observed during the period of forodesine infusion were hyperbilirubinemia, hypotension, headache, hypocalcemia, tremors, constipation, and nausea/vomiting [11]. Hematologic toxicities other than neutropenia were inevaluable owing to baseline cytopenias.

In the Japanese phase I study, the grade 3–4 adverse events included lymphocytopenia, anemia, leukocytopenia, and pyrexia. Laboratory test results showed no remarkable changes, and vital signs and body weight showed no consistent changes during the study treatment period. None of the patients showed any new, clinically significant abnormal findings on 12-lead electrocardiograms, and none of them developed any dose-limiting toxicities due to the treatment with forodesine at the designated dose range of 100–300 mg [27].

15.6.2 Phase II Studies

The phase II trial reported by Balakrishnan et al. demonstrated mild adverse events in patients with chronic lymphocytic leukemia treated with oral forodesine [28]. The adverse events were fatigue, bronchitis/pneumonia, diarrhea, fever, neutropenia, and thrombocytopenia.

In the phase II study by Dummer et al., the most commonly reported adverse events were peripheral edema, fatigue, insomnia, pruritus, diarrhea, headache, and nausea [30]. Severe adverse events included anemia, lymphocytopenia, arterial fibrillation, fatigue, edema, Herpes zoster, skin infection, CD4 lymphocyte depletion, depression, pruritus, and rash.

Apart from these reports, serum uric acid level decreases have also been reported as a consequence of PNP inhibition (Fig. 15.1).

Table 15.1 Clinical studies of forodesine in patients with hematological malignancies

Study	Disease	Patient number	Dose of forodesine	Results
Phase 1 study by Gandhi (2005)	T-ALL, T-PLL	5	IV inf 30 min 5 days, 40–90 mg	Three SD patients, 2 PD patients
Phase 2 study by Balakrishnan (2010)	CLL	8	200 mg orally, daily	Two patients had transient decrease in lymphocyte count to normal. Progressed in 5 patients
Phase 1 study by Ogura (2012)	Peripheral T/natural killer-cell malignancies	13	100–300 mg orally, daily	One CR patient, 2 PR patients, 3 SD patients
Phase 2 study by Dummer (2014)	Cutaneous T-cell lymphomas (Mycosis fungoides, Sézary syndrome)	144	200 mg orally, daily	Among 101 patients, 11 PR patients, 50 SD patients

T-ALL T-cell acute lymphoblastic leukemia, *T-PLL* T-cell prolymphocytic leukemia, *CLL* Chronic lymphocytic leukemia, *CR* complete remission, *PR* partial response, *SD* stable disease, *PD* progressive disease

15.7 Clinical Studies (Table 15.1)

15.7.1 Phase I Studies

The first-ever clinical study of forodesine was performed by Gandhi et al. [11]. Five patients (three T-cell acute lymphoblastic leukemias, two T-cell prolymphocytic leukemias) were treated with an intravenous infusion of forodesine (40 mg/m^2) on day 1; treatment continued on day 2, and thereafter, forodesine was administered every 12 h for an additional eight doses. The dose of forodesine was increased to 90 mg in the subsequent courses in one patient. Overall, no objective responses were observed. Three patients had stable disease after one course of forodesine. The disease progressed in two patients.

In Japan, a phase I multicenter, open-label, dose escalation study was conducted in patients with peripheral T/natural killer-cell malignancies (peripheral T-cell lymphoma, not otherwise specified; anaplastic large cell lymphoma; anaplastic lymphoma kinase-negative lymphoma; primary cutaneous anaplastic large cell lymphoma; and mycosis fungoides) [27]. Forodesine as a single agent was administered orally at an escalating dose from 100 to 300 mg. A total of 13 patients were enrolled; five patients received 100 mg once daily, three patients received 200 mg once daily, and five patients received 300 mg once daily. In the overall response assessment, there was a complete response in one patient (anaplastic lymphoma kinase-negative lymphoma) and partial responses in two patients (mycosis fungoides). Three patients had stable diseases. The researchers concluded that the forodesine treatment was well tolerated, showing preliminary evidence of its therapeutic activity that warranted further investigation.

15.7.2 Phase II Studies

Balakrishnan et al. conducted a phase II study of oral forodesine in patients with chronic lymphocytic leukemia acquiring fludarabine resistance. Forodesine was administered at a dose of 200 mg orally once daily for 4 weeks to complete one cycle of therapy, with the intent of administering forodesine continuously without interruptions between cycles, up to a maximum of six cycles in eight patients. Among the evaluable seven patients, the median number of cycles of forodesine received was two (range, 1–4 cycles), and the median duration of therapy was 8.7 weeks (range, 4–20 weeks). Only two patients showed a decrease in the peripheral blood absolute lymphocyte count to normal levels after the first cycle, but this was short-lasting and the counts increased thereafter. In the other five patients, the white blood cell counts increased progressively, and in three patients, there was also progression in the lymph nodes [28].

Dummer et al. conducted an open-label, single-arm, multicenter phase II study of oral forodesine at 200 mg daily in relapsed or refractory advanced cutaneous T-cell lymphomas. The response rate, safety, and tolerability were evaluated. A total of 144 patients with a performance status of 0–2 were included. The median number of prior therapies received was four. None of the patients achieved a complete remission. Eleven percent (11/101) of the patients achieved a partial remission, and 50% (51/101) of the patients had stable diseases. The median time to the therapeutic response was 56 days, and the median duration of the response was 191 days. The authors concluded that oral forodesine at a dose of 200 mg daily was feasible and that it showed partial efficacy and induced relatively long-lasting responses in this highly selected cutaneous T-cell lymphoma population.

References

1. Schramm VL. Enzymatic transition states and transition state analog design. Annu Rev Biochem. 1998;67:693–720.
2. de Azevedo Jr WF, Canduri F, Dos Santos DM, Pereira JH, Bertacine Dias MV, Silva RG, Mendes MA, Basso LA, Palma MS, Santos DS. Crystal structure of human PNP complexed with guanine. Biochem Biophys Res Commun. 2003;312:767–72.
3. Giblett ER, Ammann AJ, Wara DW, Sandman R, Diamond LK. Nucleoside-phosphorylase deficiency in a child with severely defective T-cell immunity and normal B-cell immunity. Lancet. 1975;1:1010–3.
4. Cohen A, Gudas LJ, Ammann AJ, Staal GE, Martin Jr DW. Deoxyguanosine triphosphate as a possible toxic metabolite in the immunodeficiency associated with purine nucleoside phosphorylase deficiency. J Clin Invest. 1978;61:1405–9.
5. Bantia S, Ananth SL, Parker CD, Horn LL, Upshaw R. Mechanism of inhibition of T-acute lymphoblastic leukemia cells by PNP inhibitor – BCX-1777. Int Immunopharmacol. 2003;3:879–87.

6. Markert ML. Purine nucleoside phosphorylase deficiency. Immunodefic Rev. 1991;3:45–81.
7. Krenitsky TA, Tuttle JV, Koszalka GW, Chen IS, Beacham 3rd LM, Rideout JL, Elion GB. Deoxycytidine kinase from calf thymus. Substrate and inhibitor specificity. J Biol Chem. 1976;251:4055–61.
8. Carson DA, Kaye J, Seegmiller JE. Lymphospecific toxicity in adenosine deaminase deficiency and purine nucleoside phosphorylase deficiency: possible role of nucleoside kinase(s). Proc Natl Acad Sci U S A. 1977;74:5677–81.
9. Ullman B, Gudas LJ, Clift SM, Martin Jr DW. Isolation and characterization of purine-nucleoside phosphorylase-deficient T-lymphoma cells and secondary mutants with altered ribonucleotide reductase: genetic model for immunodeficiency disease. Proc Natl Acad Sci U S A. 1979;76:1074–8.
10. Ealick SE, Babu YS, Bugg CE, Erion MD, Guida WC, Montgomery JA, Secrist 3rd JA. Application of crystallographic and modeling methods in the design of purine nucleoside phosphorylase inhibitors. Proc Natl Acad Sci U S A. 1991;88:11540–4.
11. Gandhi V, Kilpatrick JM, Plunkett W, Ayres M, Harman L, Du M, Bantia S, Davisson J, Wierda WG, Faderl S, Kantarjian H, Thomas D. A proof-of-principle pharmacokinetic, pharmacodynamic, and clinical study with purine nucleoside phosphorylase inhibitor immucillin-H (BCX-1777, forodesine). Blood. 2005;106:4253–60.
12. Miles RW, Tyler PC, Furneaux RH, Bagdassarian CK, Schramm VL. One-third-the-sites transition-state inhibitors for purine nucleoside phosphorylase. Biochemistry. 1998;37:8615–21.
13. Kline PC, Schramm VL. Purine nucleoside phosphorylase. Catalytic mechanism and transition-state analysis of the arsenolysis reaction. Biochemistry. 1993;32:13212–9.
14. Kline PC, Schramm VL. Pre-steady-state transition-state analysis of the hydrolytic reaction catalyzed by purine nucleoside phosphorylase. Biochemistry. 1995;34:1153–62.
15. Kicska GA, Long L, Hörig H, Fairchild C, Tyler PC, Furneaux RH, Schramm VL, Kaufman HL. Immucillin H, a powerful transition-state analog inhibitor of purine nucleoside phosphorylase, selectively inhibits human T lymphocytes. Proc Natl Acad Sci U S A. 2001;98:4593–8.
16. Evans GB, Furneaux RH, Lewandowicz A, Schramm VL, Tyler PC. Synthesis of second-generation transition state analogues of human purine nucleoside phosphorylase. J Med Chem. 2003;46:5271–6.
17. Clinch K, Evans GB, Fleet GW, Furneaux RH, Johnson SW, Lenz DH, Mee SP, Rands PR, Schramm VL, Taylor Ringia EA, Tyler PC. Synthesis and bio-activities of Lenantiomers of two potent transition state analogue inhibitor of purine nucleoside phosphorylases. Org Biomol Chem. 2006;4:1131–9.
18. Yamauchi T, Ueda T, Nakamura T. A new sensitive method for determination of intracellular 1-β-D-arabinofuranosylcytosine 5′-triphosphate content in human materials in vivo. Cancer Res. 1996;56:1800–4.
19. Shigemi H, Yamauchi T, Tanaka Y, Ueda T. Novel leukemic cell lines resistant to clofarabine by mechanisms of decreased active metabolite and increased antiapoptosis. Cancer Sci. 2013;104:732–9.
20. Yamauchi T, Uzui K, Nishi R, Shigemi H, Ueda T. Reduced drug incorporation into DNA and antiapoptosis as the crucial mechanisms of resistance in a novel nelarabine-resistant cell line. BMC Cancer. 2014;14:547.
21. Mitchell BS, Mejias E, Daddona PE, Kelley WN. Purinogenic immunodeficiency diseases: selective toxicity of deoxyribonucleosides for T cells. Proc Natl Acad Sci U S A. 1978;75:5011–4.
22. Bantia S, Miller PJ, Parker CD, Ananth SL, Horn LL, Kilpatrick JM, Morris PE, Hutchison TL, Montgomery JA, Sandhu JS. Purine nucleoside phosphorylase inhibitor BCX-1777 (Immucillin-H) – a novel potent and orally active immunosuppressive agent. Int Immunopharmacol. 2001;1:1199–210.
23. Bantia S, Kilpatrick JM. Purine nucleoside phosphorylase inhibitors in T-cell malignancies. Curr Opin Drug Discov Devel. 2004;7:243–7.

24. Balakrishnan K, Nimmanapalli R, Ravandi F, Keating MJ, Gandhi V. Forodesine, an inhibitor of purine nucleoside phosphorylase, induces apoptosis in chronic lymphocytic leukemia cells. Blood. 2006;108:2392–8.
25. Alonso R, López-Guerra M, Upshaw R, Bantia S, Smal C, Bontemps F, Manz C, Mehrling T, Villamor N, Campo E, Montserrat E, Colomer D. Forodesine has high antitumor activity in chronic lymphocytic leukemia and activates p53-independent mitochondrial apoptosis by induction of p73 and BIM. Blood. 2009;114:1563–75.
26. Yamauchi T, Uzui K, Nishi R, Tasaki T, Ueda T. A nelarabine-resistant T-lymphoblastic leukemia CCRF-CEM variant cell line is cross-resistant to the purine nucleoside phosphorylase inhibitor forodesine. Anticancer Res. 2014;34:4885–92.
27. Ogura M, Tsukasaki K, Nagai H, et al. Phase I study of BCX1777 (forodesine) in patients with relapsed or refractory peripheral T/natural killer-cell malignancies. Cancer Sci. 2012;103:1290–5.
28. Balakrishnan K, Verma D, O'Brien S, Kilpatrick JM, Chen Y, Tyler BF, Bickel S, Bantia S, Keating MJ, Kantarjian H, Gandhi V, Ravandi F. Phase 2 and pharmacodynamic study of oral forodesine in patients with advanced, fludarabine-treated chronic lymphocytic leukemia. Blood. 2010;116:886–92.
29. Kezar 3rd HS, Kilpatrick JM, Phillips D, Kellogg D, Zhang J, Morris Jr PE. Synthesis and pharmacokinetic and pharmacodynamic evaluation of the forodesine HCl analog BCX-3040. Nucleosides Nucleotides Nucleic Acids. 2005;24:1817–30.
30. Dummer R, Duvic M, Scarisbrick J, Olsen EA, Rozati S, Eggmann N, Goldinger SM, Hutchinson K, Geskin L, Illidge TM, Giuliano E, Elder J, Kim YH. Final results of a multicenter phase II study of the purine nucleoside phosphorylase (PNP) inhibitor forodesine in patients with advanced cutaneous T-cell lymphomas (CTCL) (Mycosis fungoides and Sézary syndrome). Ann Oncol. 2014;25:1807–12.

Clofarabine: Structure, Mechanism of Action, and Clinical Pharmacology

16

William B. Parker and Varsha Gandhi

Abstract

Similar to fludarabine and cladribine, clofarabine (2-chloro-2′-fluoro-2′-deoxyarabinosyladenine) is resistant to deamination by adenosine deaminase due to the presence of a halogen group at the two position of the base. However, unlike other 2′-deoxyadenosine analogs, clofarabine also has a halogen in the sugar that prevents cleavage of the glycosidic bond by purine nucleoside phosphorylase. The cytotoxic activity of clofarabine is due to both its inhibition of ribonucleotide reductase and its efficient incorporation in DNA, where it inhibits DNA synthesis. While some activity has been observed in lymphoid malignancies, clinical efficacy has primarily been observed in acute leukemias. The recommended dose of clofarabine for adult acute leukemia (40 $mg/m^2/day \times 5$ days) results in plasma levels of around 1 μM. The accumulation of clofarabine triphosphate in circulating leukemia cells is dose dependent, with a long half-life. This is particularly the case in responders, resulting in incremental increases in clofarabine triphosphate with every daily infusion of the drug. The actions of clofarabine triphosphate on ribonucleotide reductase and incorporation in the DNA repair patch suggest that a mechanism-based combination with arabinosylcytosine and DNA-damaging agents would be effective. Combination clinical trials have been conducted, while new trials are underway.

Keywords

Acute leukemia • Clofarabine • Chloro-fluoro-arabinosyladenine • Clofarabine triphosphate • Pharmacology

W.B. Parker
PNP Therapeutics, Inc., Birmingham, AL, USA

V. Gandhi (✉)
Department of Experimental Therapeutics and Leukemia, The University of Texas MD Anderson Cancer Center, P.O. Box 301429, 1515 Holcombe Blvd, Houston, TX 77230-1429, USA
e-mail: vgandhi@mdanderson.org

T. Ueda (ed.), *Chemotherapy for Leukemia*, DOI 10.1007/978-981-10-3332-2_16

16.1 Introduction

The natural nucleobases and nucleosides, such as adenine and adenosine, are important molecules in cells because they are components of DNA, RNA, and various intracellular nucleotides, such as cAMP, ATP, CTP, GTP, and UTP as well as their corresponding deoxynucleotides. Nucleotides are synthesized de novo in human cells, and nucleobases and nucleosides are usually only present in cells at low concentrations. However, if available, these compounds are salvaged from the environment and used for the synthesis of DNA, RNA, and nucleotide triphosphates, a process that involves many enzymes. Analogs of these compounds are a major class of drugs (referred to as antimetabolites) that are important in the treatment of viral infections and cancer. The FDA has approved over 25 nucleoside analogs for use in the treatment of viral infections [1] and 14 antimetabolites for the treatment of cancer [2].

Nucleobase and nucleoside analogs are structurally similar to the natural compounds and are used by many of the anabolic enzymes in a manner similar to that of the natural compounds, usually without interfering with the activity of the enzyme. For the most part, the analog and its metabolites must appear to the cell as the natural compound. However, because of the small structural difference in these molecules, one of its metabolites eventually interacts with an enzyme in a negative way, resulting in its inhibition, and the resulting disruption of nucleic acid synthesis or function results in the death of the cancer cell or virus. The structural modifications must be small so that the anabolic enzymes recognize them as substrates and convert them to a metabolite that eventually disrupts a vital enzyme in nucleotide metabolism. However, it is important to realize that small structural differences in nucleoside analogs can have a major impact on their mechanism of action and their clinical activity. As we illustrate in this chapter, clofarabine (abbreviated in the literature as CAFDA, chloro-fluoro-ara-A, and Cl-F-ara-A) or 9-β-D-[2-deoxy-2-fluoro-arabinofuranosyl]-2-chloroadenine (Fig. 16.1) is an excellent example of this principle. The drug is sold as Clolar in the USA and Evoltra in Europe. The only structural difference between clofarabine and cladribine is the replacement of a hydrogen atom at the 2′ position with a fluorine atom. However, this small difference endows clofarabine with biochemical activities that are sufficiently different from cladribine as to result in different clinical activities.

The basis of selectivity with antiviral agents usually involves selective activation by an enzyme expressed by the virus or selective inhibition of an enzyme important to the synthesis of the viral genetic material. With anticancer analogs, the basis for selectivity is much less clear because the enzymes involved in activation and activity in cancer cells are identical to those found in normal cells. However, the antitumor selectivity of nucleoside analogs can be attributed to enhanced metabolism in cancer cells or inhibition of DNA synthesis or function. The goal of cancer drugs is to prevent replication of the cancer cell because it is this replication that leads to the death of the patient. Since most host cells in humans are not replicating and therefore are not sensitive to agents that inhibit DNA synthesis, inhibition of DNA synthesis in cancer cells affords modest selectivity. However, some tissues have cells

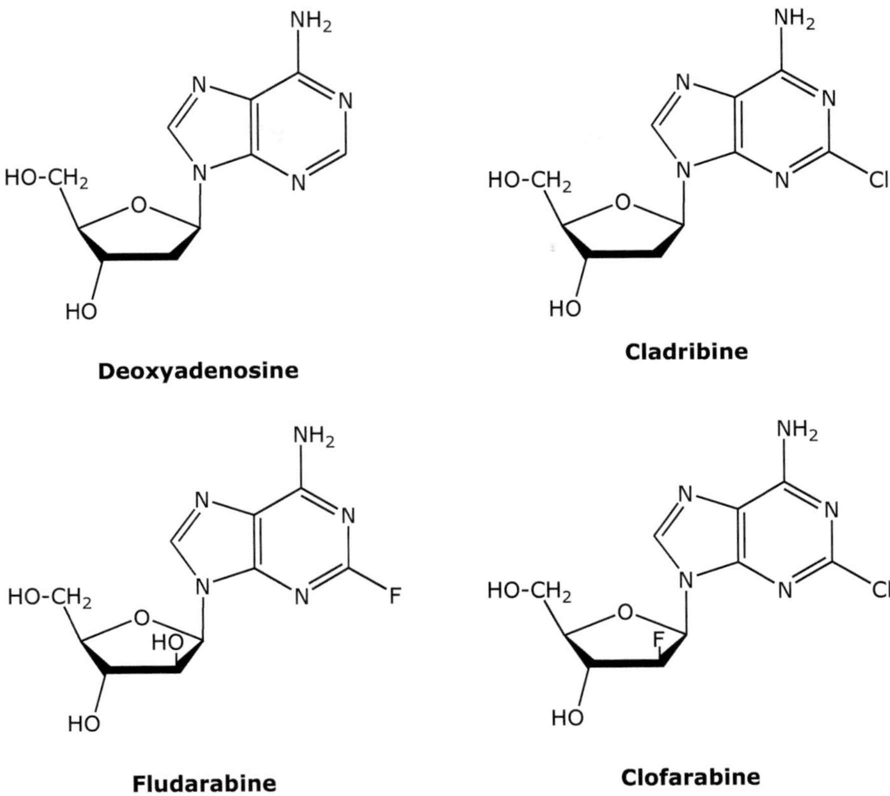

Fig. 16.1 Structures of deoxyadenosine, cladribine, fludarabine, and clofarabine

with rapid turnover (bone marrow, gastrointestinal tract, and hair follicles), and toxicity in these tissues due to the inhibition of DNA synthesis limits the amount of drug that can be administered.

Because clofarabine is an analog of 2′-deoxyadenosine (dAdo), the metabolism of dAdo in human cells, summarized in Fig. 16.2, introduces the enzymes that are important in the activation and antitumor activity of clofarabine. Adenosine deaminase is expressed in the plasma; therefore, the primary metabolic route for dAdo that is injected into animals is deamination by adenosine deaminase to deoxyinosine, which is rapidly cleaved by purine nucleoside phosphorylase (PNP) to hypoxanthine. Hypoxanthine can be reused by hypoxanthine/guanine phosphoribosyl transferase (HGPRT) for the generation of purine nucleotides, although it is more likely to be converted by xanthine oxidase to xanthine and uric acid, which is eventually excreted. Adenine-containing nucleosides are extremely poor substrates for mammalian PNP [3]; therefore, little, if any, dAdo that is administered intravenously is cleaved to adenine in mammalian systems. However, dAdo is a good substrate for bacterial PNP [4] and would be readily cleaved in the gastrointestinal tract. A small amount of dAdo administered to animals is phosphorylated to dAMP,

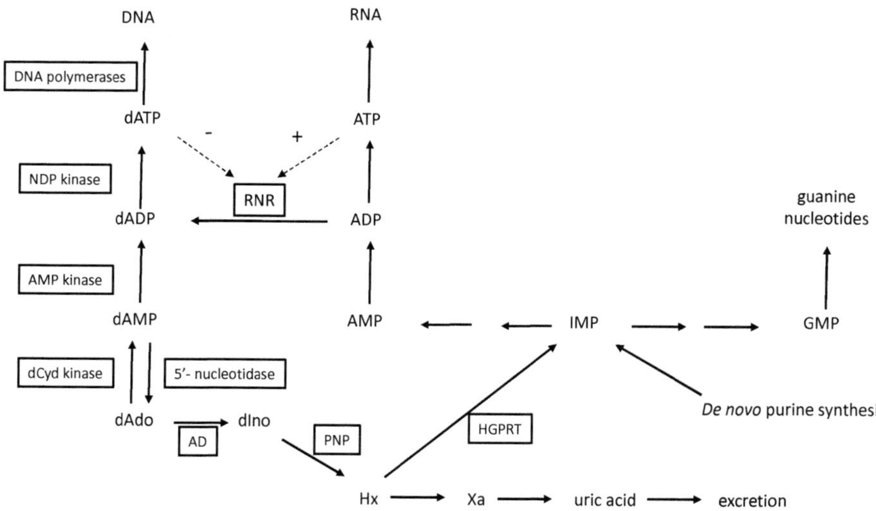

Fig. 16.2 Schema depicting the metabolism of deoxyadenosine. Enzymes are *boxed in rectangles*. *Abbreviations*: *NDP* nucleoside diphosphate, *dCyd* 2′-deoxycytidine, *dAdo* 2′-deoxyadenosine, *dIno* 2′-deoxyinosine, *Hx* hypoxanthine, *Xa* xanthine, *AD* adenosine deaminase, *PNP* purine nucleoside phosphorylase, *HGPRT* hypoxanthine-guanine phosphoribosyl transferase, *RNR* ribonucleotide reductase, *IMP* inosine 5′-monophosphate, *GMP* guanosine 5′-monophosphate, *AMP* adenosine 5′-monophosphate

primarily by deoxycytidine kinase (dCyd kinase), which is further phosphorylated to dADP and dATP. dATP is the primary acid-soluble intracellular metabolite of dAdo, and it is used as a substrate for the synthesis of DNA. An important enzyme in the generation of deoxynucleotides for DNA synthesis is ribonucleotide reductase. The activity of this enzyme is controlled by the natural NTPs and dNTPs to maintain the proper balance of nucleotides for DNA synthesis. As can be seen in Fig. 16.2, dATP represses ribonucleotide reductase activity, whereas ATP stimulates its activity.

16.2 Rationale for the Synthesis of Clofarabine

Numerous enzymes are involved in the activation and activity of nucleoside analogs, which is a primary reason why drug discovery within this class of compounds is a very empirical process. It is difficult, if not impossible, to design a compound that will behave as needed with each of the enzymes that must be involved in its activity. Therefore, the rational drug discovery strategy with these molecules is to generate numerous analogs that are based on a thorough understanding of the biological activity of the many synthesized compounds and then evaluate them in appropriate model systems to identify the agents with the desired activities.

A thorough explanation of the rationale for the synthesis of clofarabine can be found in a review by Secrist et al. [5]. In brief, nucleosides with halogens at the two position of the adenine base are known to be very poor substrates for adenosine deaminase [6] and therefore are known to be stable in plasma. These compounds (2-halo-2′-deoxyadenosine analogs) potently inhibit tumor cell growth. In addition, 2′-flouro nucleosides have been synthesized and are known to have biological activity [7]. 2′-Halogens on nucleoside analogs are also resistant to cleavage by acid and purine nucleoside phosphorylases, another feature that would contribute to their in vivo stability. Therefore, in a search for new anticancer agents, numerous 2′-halo (F, Cl, or Br) and 2-halo (F, Cl, or Br) dAdo analogs have been synthesized and evaluated for biological activity in both in vitro and in vivo tumor models [8]. Clofarabine was the most potent compound in in vitro cell-killing assays and demonstrated excellent activity against numerous human tumor xenografts in mice [9, 10].

16.3 Transport

Human cells will salvage natural nucleosides, if available, for nucleic acid synthesis in place of de novo synthesis, and cells express numerous transporters to aid the entry of these compounds. Both equilibrative transporters (hENT1, hENT2, and hENT3) and concentrative transporters (hCNT1, hCNT2, and hCNT3) are expressed on most human cells [11]. Because of the abundance of these transporters, natural nucleosides in the cell culture will equilibrate across the cell membrane in just a few seconds. To be active, all nucleoside analogs (with the possible exceptions of deoxycoformycin and forodesine) must be able to cross cellular membranes to interact with their cellular targets. Most nucleoside analogs that are useful in the treatment of various diseases are recognized by these transporters; therefore, they also equilibrate across cell membranes very quickly. Precise transport studies have been conducted with clofarabine, and it has been shown that it is transported into cells by both human equilibrative and concentrative nucleoside transporters [12]. Cells producing hENT1 exhibited the highest uptake of clofarabine (0.14 pmole/μl), followed by hCNT2 (0.025 pmole/μl), whereas uptake in cells producing hENT2 or hCNT1 was not higher than that in cells that were nucleoside transport deficient. In oocytes expressing recombinant transporters, the efficiency of transport by hCNT3 (1.3) was much greater than that of hENT1, hENT2, or hCNT2 (0.11, 0.20, or 0.15). Although not entirely consistent, these results indicate that clofarabine can enter cells by all known transporters except hCNT1, which is selective for pyrimidine nucleosides. In addition, at high concentrations, diffusion of clofarabine directly through the membrane is also possible [12].

Comparative studies have shown [12] that cladribine had the highest efficiency of transport with hENT1, with a V_{max}/K_m value of 1.8 versus 0.7 for clofarabine and 0.8 for fludarabine (9-β-D-[arabinofuranosyl]-2-F-adenine). The uptake and flux of clofarabine, cladribine, and fludarabine were very similar in human renal proximal tubule cells, which express equilibrative hENT1, hENT2, and hCNT3 [13]. These results indicate that although there are some differences in transport, all of these compounds are readily transported across human membranes.

Some studies have evaluated the importance of ABCG2 to the activity of clofarabine. This ABC transporter is known as the breast cancer resistance protein and transports various metabolites, including nucleoside monophosphates, out of cells. Cells transfected with DNA constructs, resulting in overexpression of human or mouse ABCG2, had significantly reduced transport of both clofarabine and cladribine metabolites [14]. These results were correlated with decreased levels of cellular metabolites of cladribine in ABCG2-expressing cells, which were much less sensitive to clofarabine and cladribine. In these studies, the ABCG2 transporter transported both cladribine monophosphate and cladribine itself. The results of a study by Nagai et al. [15] supported these conclusions and showed that ABCG2 primarily transports clofarabine. Their results indicate that the metabolism of clofarabine and its cytotoxicity are strongly determined by the interplay between dCyd kinase and ABCG2, and they suggest that inhibition of ABCG2 will improve antitumor activity in tumors in which dCyd kinase levels are low. The role of ABC transporters in nucleoside analog metabolism and activity has recently been reviewed [16].

16.4 Metabolism

The metabolism of clofarabine is schematically presented in Fig. 16.3. Once inside the cell, clofarabine is converted to clofarabine triphosphate [17]. Xie and Plunkett [18] showed that at low concentrations, the primary intracellular metabolite was clofarabine monophosphate, which was approximately twice the level of clofarabine triphosphate. At high concentrations of clofarabine, the monophosphate and triphosphate levels were similar. Clofarabine diphosphate levels were very low, indicating that phosphorylation of the monophosphate of clofarabine is the rate-limiting step in its activation to the triphosphate. This characteristic is similar to that of cladribine [19] and indicates that the monophosphate kinase does not prefer molecules with substitutions at the two position of a purine nucleoside as large as a Cl atom. In the case of most other deoxynucleoside analogs used for the treatment of cancer, the nucleoside kinase is usually the rate-limiting enzyme in their activation, and the triphosphate usually accounts for more than 90% of the intracellular metabolites.

Clofarabine triphosphate accumulates at high levels in CEM cells [17, 18]: treatment of cells with low concentrations of clofarabine (1–3 μM for 2–4 h) resulted in concentrations of clofarabine triphosphate that were 50–100 μM, which were similar to intracellular dATP concentrations in untreated cells. The accumulation of clofarabine triphosphate was dose dependent up to 10 μM. Similar intracellular concentrations of clofarabine triphosphate were achieved in all phases of the cell cycle (G_1, S, and G_2-M) [18]. Clinical studies have indicated that plasma clofarabine levels of 1.5 μM are achieved at the maximally tolerated dose of clofarabine in patients with acute leukemias after a 1-h infusion, and this treatment resulted in a clofarabine triphosphate concentration of approximately 19 μM in blast cells [20].

When clofarabine was removed from the medium of K562 and CEM cell cultures, clofarabine triphosphate had a half-life in cells of 1–3 h [18, 21]. However, in

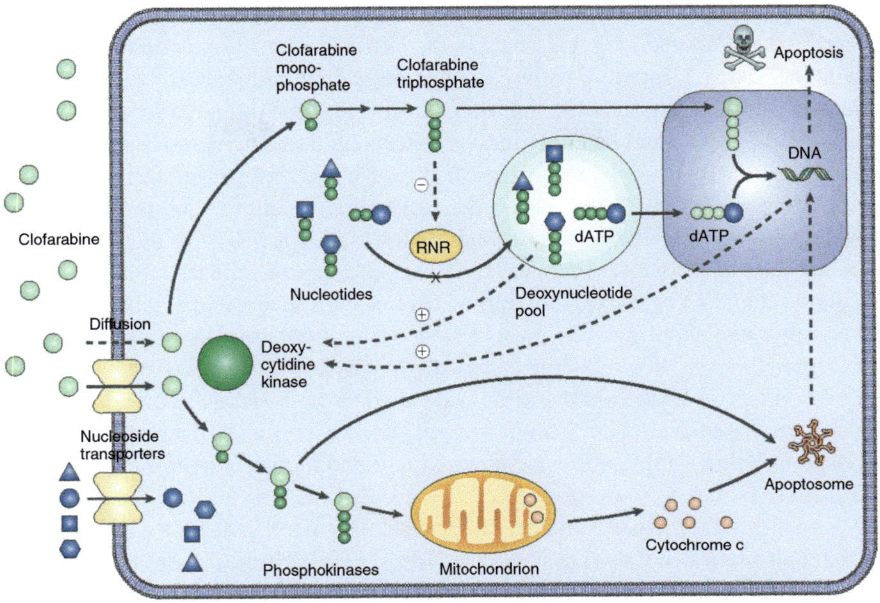

Fig. 16.3 Schematic of clofarabine's mechanism of action. Clofarabine is transported into cells by both diffusion and facilitated diffusion. It is monophosphorylated by deoxycytidine kinase (dCK) and then serially phosphorylated by other kinases to form clofarabine triphosphate, the active moiety. The triphosphate acts to terminate DNA chain elongation and inhibit repair by incorporating it into the DNA chain through competitive inhibition of DNA polymerases. It also inhibits ribonucleotide reductase, with a reduction of dNTP pools, and induces apoptosis through direct and indirect actions on mitochondria by releasing cytochrome *c* and other proapoptotic factors (Obtained with permission from Bonate et al. [73])

circulating leukemic cells, more than 50% of the clofarabine triphosphate was still present 24 h after clofarabine transfusion [20]. The metabolism of clofarabine and cladribine has been compared in ex vivo studies with CLL and AML cells that were obtained from patients [22]. In these studies, the half-life of clofarabine triphosphate was longer than that in CEM cells but similar to that of cladribine triphosphate (7.3 vs. 4.3 h, respectively). The enzymes involved in the degradation of nucleoside triphosphates in cells have not been studied in great detail. Triphosphate metabolites of nucleoside analogs do not readily cross cell membranes and are therefore trapped in the cells in which they were created, whereas nucleosides themselves will freely distribute across the cell membrane. Therefore, the antitumor activity of these agents can be extended well beyond the time that the drug circulates in the plasma because the active metabolite is maintained in tumor cells long after the drug has disappeared from the plasma. The long retention time of clofarabine triphosphate contributes to its lasting antitumor activity, even though the plasma half-life is fairly short [20, 23].

Cytoplasmic 5′-nucleotidase cN-II is one of the seven 5′-nucleotidases found in mammals. This enzyme catalyzes the removal of the 5′-phosphate from purine

5′-monophosphates and is involved in the maintenance of cellular nucleotide pools. Therefore, it can also degrade analogs of purine nucleoside monophosphates and could theoretically interfere with the activation of clofarabine. In cell culture experiments with CEM and RL cells, inhibition of this enzyme did not affect the cytotoxicity of clofarabine and had only modest effects on the induction of apoptosis [24], indicating that it has only a modest effect on the metabolism of clofarabine when clofarabine is constantly present in the cell culture medium. The results of these studies suggest that the monophosphate pool maintained by the dCyd kinase/5′-nucleotidase activity ratio in the presence of excess extracellular clofarabine is sufficient to maintain cytotoxic clofarabine triphosphate levels in the cell. However, it is possible that such inhibitors would have a more dramatic effect on metabolism after the removal of clofarabine from the external environment, which happens in vivo. As clofarabine triphosphate is degraded to the clofarabine monophosphate, inhibition of this enzyme could prevent further degradation, resulting in re-phosphorylation by the monophosphate kinase and an increase in the intracellular half-life of clofarabine triphosphate.

As expected for a dAdo analog, clofarabine was incorporated into DNA, but not RNA, indicating that it is a DNA-directed drug [18]. At low concentrations, clofarabine is mostly incorporated into internal positions in the DNA (>80%), suggesting that DNA synthesis is not inhibited by the incorporation of clofarabine monophosphate into the growing DNA strand. However, at high concentrations (1 or 10 μM), much more clofarabine is found at terminal positions in DNA. At 10 μM, 65% of the clofarabine in DNA is found at terminal positions, which suggests that DNA synthesis is inhibited at the site of incorporation.

The primary enzyme involved in the activation of clofarabine in tumor cells is dCyd kinase [17, 18, 22]. Clofarabine is a very good substrate for this enzyme, with K_m and V_{max} values that are similar to those of dCyd [21] but much better than those of dAdo (the catalytic efficiency of dAdo is only 0.3% that of dCyd). Clofarabine was modestly better substrate for dCyd kinase than was cladribine. Its catalytic efficiency was three to four times that of cladribine, with a V_{max} that was ten times greater. The X-ray crystal structure of dCyd kinase with clofarabine in the active site has been determined [25]. The results of these studies indicate that the conformation of the enzyme/clofarabine complex was similar to structures of the pyrimidine-bound complexes and that the interactions between the 2-Cl group and its surrounding hydrophobic residues contribute to the high catalytic efficiency of dCyd kinase with clofarabine.

Decreased dCyd kinase activity has been shown to result in resistance to clofarabine in various cell culture systems [22, 26–29]. Decreased histone acetylation [28], but not methylation of the dCyd kinase gene [26, 28, 29], was associated with decreased dCyd kinase expression. In HL-60 cells, the decreased activation of clofarabine was associated with decreased expression of dCyd kinase, deoxyguanosine kinase, and hENT1, hENT2, and hCNT3 genes [30]. Studies have shown that there are genetic variations in the expression of dCyd kinase activity in patient populations and suggest that these variations are responsible for the variable rates of activation of clofarabine and other nucleoside analogs [31].

Treatment of cells with clofarabine and other nucleoside analogs can enhance dCyd kinase activity in many, but not all, cell lines [32–34]. Others have shown that inhibition of DNA synthesis can enhance dCyd kinase activity [35, 36] by phosphorylating dCyd kinase at serine 74 [35, 37, 38]. The enhancement of dCyd kinase activity by clofarabine can be exploited to improve antitumor activity by combining clofarabine with other nucleoside analogs that are activated by dCyd kinase [33, 34, 39–41].

Clofarabine is also a good substrate for deoxyguanosine kinase [42], an enzyme that is expressed in mitochondria. The catalytic efficiency of clofarabine with this enzyme is similar to that of both deoxyguanosine and cladribine, although both the K_m and V_{max} values for the two deoxyadenosine analogs are 10–20 times greater than are those for deoxyguanosine. The contribution of deoxyguanosine kinase to the phosphorylation of clofarabine in cells is low due to the much higher expression of dCyd kinase activity in most cell types [43, 44], but it could be important in cells that express low amounts of dCyd kinase. Resistance to clofarabine in CEM cells was correlated with decreased dCyd kinase activity but not with decreased deoxyguanosine kinase [22, 27].

16.5 Mechanisms of Action

The mechanism of action of clofarabine resembles that of other dAdo analogs and is schematically presented in Fig. 16.3. Below, we describe the primary actions of this nucleoside analog.

16.5.1 Inhibition of DNA Synthesis

As with other anticancer nucleoside analogs, the primary activity of clofarabine that is responsible for its antitumor activity is the inhibition of DNA synthesis [17, 18, 21, 45]. RNA and protein synthesis are inhibited by clofarabine only at high concentrations. Clofarabine triphosphate also inhibited yeast poly(A) polymerase activity [46], but it is unclear how much the inhibition of this enzyme contributes to the antitumor activity of clofarabine. DNA synthesis is immediately inhibited in cells treated with clofarabine, and a 3-h incubation with 0.3 μM clofarabine resulted in prolonged inhibition [45], which did not recover to more than 20% of control values 72 h after removal of the drug. The immediate and long-lasting inhibition of DNA synthesis in cells treated with clofarabine strongly suggests that the enzymes that are critical for DNA replication, such as DNA polymerase and ribonucleotide reductase, are the primary targets for clofarabine and that disruption of DNA function as a result of the incorporation of clofarabine into daughter strands is of secondary importance to the activity of clofarabine.

16.5.1.1 Inhibition of Ribonucleotide Reductase

Incubation of cells with clofarabine results in significant decreases in intracellular deoxynucleotide pools [17, 18, 45], suggesting that clofarabine triphosphate is a potent inhibitor of ribonucleotide reductase, a critical enzyme that is involved in the de novo synthesis of deoxynucleotides [47]. This hypothesis was confirmed in experiments in which clofarabine triphosphate potently inhibited ribonucleotide reductase in cell-free extracts [17], and incubation of cells with clofarabine dramatically decreased the conversion of radiolabeled purines and pyrimidines to their respective deoxynucleotide triphosphates [45]. Clofarabine had the most impact on dCTP and dATP pools, a modest impact on dGTP pools, and no effect on dTTP pools [17, 45]. The concentration of clofarabine triphosphate that is required to inhibit ADP reduction from ribonucleotide reductase isolated from K562 cells by 50% is 65 nM, which is similar to that seen with cladribine triphosphate [17].

The activity of ribonucleotide reductase in cells is tightly controlled by the natural nucleotides to ensure that the cell has all of the deoxynucleotides needed for DNA synthesis in the correct concentrations. It is known that dATP is a potent regulator of ribonucleotide reductase activity and inhibits the reduction of ADP, UDP, and CDP [47]. Therefore, the results described above suggest that clofarabine triphosphate interacts with ribonucleotide reductase in the allosteric binding site as an analog of dATP. However, in studies with purified human ribonucleotide reductase, Aye and Stubbe [48] showed that both clofarabine diphosphate and clofarabine triphosphate were potent inhibitors of ribonucleotide reductase activity. They showed that clofarabine triphosphate is a rapid reversible inhibitor, with a K_i of 40 nM, and that clofarabine diphosphate is a slow-binding, reversible inhibitor, with a K_i of 17 nM. Their results indicated that clofarabine triphosphate bound to the allosteric binding site (A site) on the α subunit. The A site controls the rate of the reaction, and when dATP is bound, the enzyme is inactive. Clofarabine diphosphate bound to the substrate-binding site (C site). Although clofarabine diphosphate levels are much lower than clofarabine triphosphate levels in cells [18], the relatively long half-life of the inhibited state means that clofarabine diphosphate could still significantly contribute to the inhibition of ribonucleotide reductase in cells. Finally, inhibition of enzyme activity by either compound was associated with protein oligomerization that was more kinetically stable than were dATP-induced hexamers [48–50].

16.5.1.2 Inhibition of DNA Polymerization

Clearly, inhibition of ribonucleotide reductase is sufficient to result in the inhibition of DNA synthesis; however, clofarabine triphosphate is also a good substrate and inhibitor of DNA polymerases α and ε, two important enzymes that are involved in the replication of chromosomal DNA [17, 45]. Clofarabine triphosphate was found to be a potent inhibitor of the incorporation of dATP by DNA polymerase α, with a K_i value of approximately 1 μM (K_m for dATP was 4 μM), but it was a weak inhibitor of DNA polymerase β (involved in DNA repair) and γ (involved in mitochondrial DNA synthesis). A nucleoside triphosphate analog can interact with a DNA polymerase in one of three ways: it can interfere with DNA synthesis without being used as a substrate; it can be used as a substrate but not interfere with continued

DNA synthesis; or it can be used as a substrate and cause disruption of subsequent DNA chain elongation. The results of studies in intact cells with radiolabeled clofarabine indicate that it is incorporated into DNA in internal and terminal positions [18], but these studies did not indicate whether DNA synthesis was inhibited due to the incorporation. In addition, inhibition of dATP incorporation by isolated polymerases does not indicate that DNA synthesis is actually inhibited because it is possible that clofarabine triphosphate inhibited dATP incorporation by acting as an alternative substrate without interfering with subsequent elongation.

The results of DNA-sequencing studies supported those of the radiolabeled studies, showing that clofarabine triphosphate is used by DNA polymerase α [17], with K_m and V_{max} values that are similar to those of dATP (as well as cladribine triphosphate). These studies also showed that the ability of polymerase α to add new nucleotides after the incorporation of clofarabine triphosphate was significantly less than that after the incorporation of dATP. The K_m of adding dGTP after the incorporation of clofarabine triphosphate was 100-fold greater than that after the incorporation of dAMP. The V_{max} for the incorporation of dGTP was similar, regardless of whether dAMP or clofarabine monophosphate was incorporated previously. Interestingly, the incorporation of cladribine had only a modest effect on the subsequent use of dGTP as a substrate (only a threefold difference to that seen after the incorporation of dAdo). The effect of clofarabine incorporation on subsequent chain elongation was similar to that of fludarabine, an agent known to interfere with DNA synthesis. The effect of clofarabine triphosphate on DNA polymerase ε activity was similar to that seen with DNA polymerase α, except that it more effectively inhibited chain elongation by DNA polymerase ε [45]. This enhanced inhibition of chain elongation resulted in significant inhibition of DNA synthesis by this enzyme at clofarabine triphosphate concentrations that were only 3% those of dATP.

Under conditions in which control reactions extended all of the labeled DNA primer to the end of the template strand, DNA polymerase α was able to extend the DNA chain with clofarabine triphosphate in place of dATP across a single thymidine residue in the template strand, but it was not able to extend past two consecutive thymidine residues [17]. This result was very similar to that seen with fludarabine triphosphate but was different from that seen with cladribine triphosphate. DNA polymerase α was able to extend the DNA chain with cladribine triphosphate across two consecutive thymidine residues in the template strand, but it could not extend beyond three consecutive thymidine residues. These results indicate that clofarabine caused significant chain termination by DNA polymerase α, which is consistent with the immediate and lasting inhibition of DNA synthesis seen in cells treated with clofarabine [18].

These results seem to be in conflict with the results that indicate that at low concentrations, more than 80% of the clofarabine incorporated into DNA is incorporated into internal positions [18], which suggests that elongation of DNA is not inhibited by the incorporation of clofarabine into DNA. The above results indicate that DNA polymerases can easily extend the DNA chain across single thymidine residues with clofarabine triphosphate but that chain extension is dramatically inhibited by the incorporation of two successive clofarabine nucleotides. Since it is likely that single incorporations are more prevalent in DNA than are multiple incorporations, there would be many more internal clofarabine molecules in DNA, even though the inhibition of DNA synthesis due to chain termination is the primary action of clofarabine that is responsible for its antitumor activity. In addition, chain termination caused by two successive clofarabine incorporations would have one internal and one terminal, for a ratio of 50%. These results indicate that DNA replication is severely inhibited, even under circumstances in which most of the incorporated clofarabine is in internal positions in the DNA.

Clofarabine has also been shown to inhibit nucleotide excision DNA repair in chronic lymphocytic leukemia (CLL) lymphocytes isolated from patients that were induced by treatment with 4-hydroperoxycyclophosphamide [51]. Clofarabine was as potent as fludarabine in the inhibition of DNA repair in this model; however, clofarabine triphosphate demonstrated maximal inhibition at one-tenth the concentration of fludarabine triphosphate. Although not directly studied in this paper, the inhibition of nucleotide excision repair could be due to the inhibition of the DNA polymerases involved in the repair or to the inhibition of ribonucleotide reductase activity. In addition, inhibition of DNA repair could explain the activity of clofarabine against resting non-proliferating tumor cells [52].

Collectively, the results presented in the previous paragraphs indicate that DNA synthesis is inhibited in cells treated with clofarabine through two distinct but complementary actions: inhibition of ribonucleotide reductase and DNA polymerase activity. The potent inhibition of ribonucleotide reductase activity by clofarabine nucleotides enhances its inhibition of the replicative DNA polymerases (self-potentiation) by decreasing the intracellular concentration of the natural substrate, dATP, which competes with clofarabine triphosphate for use as a substrate by these enzymes (i.e., in the presence of ribonucleotide reductase inhibition, less clofarabine triphosphate is needed to inhibit DNA polymerase activity). Indeed, clofarabine combines the strong DNA-terminating activity of fludarabine (a weak inhibitor of ribonucleotide reductase) and the strong inhibition of ribonucleotide reductase by cladribine (a weak inhibitor of DNA polymerases) into one molecule that is a strong inhibitor of both DNA elongation and ribonucleotide reductase. The relative importance of clofarabine's actions to the antitumor activity of clofarabine is not known, but it is likely that both targets significantly contribute to its cell-killing action.

16.5.2 Repair of DNA Containing Clofarabine

The removal of clofarabine from the 3′-end of DNA chains by 3′-exonucleases that are associated with the DNA replication complex is an important part of the mechanism of action of this compound that has not yet been evaluated. If clofarabine is quickly removed from the 3′-terminus of the DNA chain, DNA synthesis can continue normally, although the polymerase would still have a chance to incorporate another molecule of clofarabine in the repair site, resulting in a futile incorporation and removal cycle. The incorporation of two or more clofarabine residues sequentially in the DNA may be harder to repair than single incorporations and could represent a greater block to DNA synthesis. Once the DNA polymerase extends beyond the incorporated analog, DNA synthesis can continue normally. It is not known whether clofarabine that is successfully incorporated into the DNA chains (beyond the replication sites) results in DNA that cannot function normally. However, Hentosh and colleagues [53, 54] demonstrated that the random incorporation of cladribine into DNA can disrupt transcriptional regulation by altering DNA binding of TATA-binding protein and can have deleterious effects on cell function. It is likely that the random incorporation of clofarabine would have similar effects. However, if there are negative consequences to the incorporation of clofarabine into DNA chains, these actions are secondary in importance to the cell-killing mechanism of action of clofarabine.

16.5.3 Induction of Apoptosis

The inhibition of replication in cells normally leads to the turning on of replication checkpoint pathways. Stalled replication forks can threaten DNA replication fidelity, and cells respond to replication blocks by triggering checkpoint pathways that monitor replication fork progression [55]. This monitoring of DNA synthesis operates normally during low-intensity replication stress and is required for tumor cells to resume cell cycle progression. However, during chronic or high-intensity replication stress, stalled forks do not restart after removal of the stressor, resulting in irreversible S-phase arrest, possible mitotic catastrophe, and cell death.

The inhibition of DNA synthesis and the DNA damage caused by clofarabine resulted in the induction of apoptosis in CEM and HCT116 cells [56–58]. Replication stress induced by the treatment of CEM cells with 10 μM clofarabine leads to Chk1 phosphorylation, which is accompanied by Chk1 downregulation, concomitant apoptosis, and cell death [5]. Incubation with clofarabine resulted in a dose- and time-dependent downregulation of Bcl-X_L, Mcl-1, and Cdc25A proteins, but it did not affect Cdc25C [57]. Treatment with clofarabine also resulted in the dephosphorylation of Akt and its downstream effectors (Bad and FKHRL1). In addition, there was a marked increase in the population of cells in G1/S and early S phase. Clofarabine led to more apoptotic cell death than did fludarabine, suggesting that DNA damage caused by clofarabine is more easily recognized by the surveillance systems that initiate apoptotic cascades [51].

16.5.4 Activity Against Non-proliferating Cancer Cells

Clofarabine is also active against quiescent human lymphocytes and monocytes [52]. Treatment of these cells with clofarabine induced DNA strand breaks, which were markedly reduced by supplementation of the culture medium with dCyd. Clofarabine also interfered with mitochondrial integrity in primary CLL cells [59], which led to the release of the proapoptotic mitochondrial proteins cytochrome C and apoptosis protein-activating factor (Apaf-1). The activity of clofarabine was similar to that of cladribine, and both agents induced mitochondrial damage more effectively than did fludarabine. The investigators proposed three mechanisms that may be responsible for the mitochondrial damage in non-proliferating CLL cells: (1) incorporation into nuclear DNA, resulting in DNA damage and inducing an apoptotic cascade; (2) binding to Apaf-1, resulting in the induction of apoptosis [60]; and (3) direct interference with mitochondrial function. They felt that mitochondrial damage caused by clofarabine or cladribine resulted from all three effects, whereas mitochondrial damage caused by fludarabine resulted from only nuclear DNA damage and Apaf-1 binding. They suggested that the direct activity against mitochondrial function could be due to the binding of clofarabine and cladribine nucleotides to proteins that are known to regulate mitochondrial functions. Clofarabine triphosphate was able to activate Apaf-1-dependent caspase activity in CLL cell extracts with kinetic parameters that were identical to those of dATP [60].

The caspase cascade is initiated by cytochrome *c* binding to Apaf-1; this induces it to undergo a conformational change in the presence of dATP, leading to the formation of Apaf-1 multimers and the recruitment of procaspase-9, forming a complex known as the apoptosome. The subsequent autocatalysis of procaspase-9 is followed by the proteolytic activation of procaspases 3, 6, and 7. Therefore, clofarabine triphosphate can contribute to the formation and activation of the apoptosome, which results in the activation of the caspase cascade. These studies notwithstanding, the mechanisms responsible for the disruption of mitochondrial integrity have not been fully elucidated, and it is possible that mitochondrial damage is the result of an apoptotic cascade resulting from the inhibition of ribonucleotide reductase or DNA polymerase activity.

Clofarabine has also been shown to inhibit DNA repair in quiescent cells [51]. Although clofarabine triphosphate is a weak inhibitor of DNA polymerase β [17], a polymerase that is involved in base excision repair, it is a potent inhibitor of DNA polymerase ε [45] and likely DNA polymerase δ, two enzymes that are also involved in DNA repair [61]. As noted, clofarabine is a potent inhibitor of ribonucleotide reductase, and the reduction in intracellular deoxynucleotides could inhibit DNA repair due to the lack of substrates. Because DNA is constantly being repaired in quiescent cells due to its spontaneous degradation, inhibition of DNA repair could induce the apoptotic response that has been observed in these cells.

16.5.5 Miscellaneous Activities

Clofarabine and cladribine were both found to bind to the A(2A) receptor, with K_is of 17 and 15 μM, respectively [62]. Clofarabine was the only adenosine analog to bind to the A(3) receptor, with a K_i of 10 μM. None of the adenosine analogs bound to the A(2B) receptor. Clofarabine was an agonist of the A(1) receptor. These results suggest that interaction with the adenosine receptors contributes to the toxicity observed with clofarabine and other deoxyadenosine analogs.

Treatment of breast cancer cell lines with clofarabine has been shown to reactivate silenced tumor suppressor genes such as APC, PTEN, and RARβ2 through hypomethylation and transcriptional upregulation [63, 64]. This action needs to be evaluated in liquid tumor cell lines as well as in primary tumor cells during therapy.

16.6 Cancer Selectivity of Clofarabine

Similar to other nucleoside analogs, clofarabine is not selective to cancer or to a specific cancer histological type. Nonetheless, as described above, most of the cell line studies are directed toward acute myelogenous or lymphoblastic diseases. The activity of the drug in the clinical setting also suggests that it has preferred activity toward ALL and AML. Within AML, cell line data suggest that in cells harboring FLT3 internal tandem duplication, prolonged treatment would be more effective, as there is a failure of the cell cycle checkpoint in FLT3-ITD mutant cells [65]. In addition to leukemias, other hematological malignancies, such as myeloma [41, 66, 67] and lymphoma [68–70], appear to show sensitivity to this analog. Among solid tumors, breast [63, 71], colon [9, 58], and brain tumors [72] have been evaluated.

In the clinical setting, described in detail in the next chapter (Chap. 17), most of clofarabine's activity has been observed in acute leukemias. For these diagnoses, the drug has been approved for pediatric leukemias and is also effective in the treatment of adult leukemias. Solid tumors showed limited activity, perhaps due to myelosuppression as a dose-limiting toxicity. Unlike other drugs, clofarabine was approved first in pediatric leukemias. Clofarabine's development, leading to its approval in acute leukemias, was reviewed in detail by Bonate et al. [73].

16.7 Clinical Pharmacology

To obtain investigational new drug approval and to use clofarabine clinically, MD Anderson conducted animal toxicology and pharmacology studies. On the basis of tolerated doses in mice and dogs, an IC_{10} of 15 mg/m^2/day was selected for humans. Because of clofarabine's similarity to fludarabine, the clinical trial design was based on this dAdo analog (i.e., every cycle consisted of a daily dose for 5 days, and the cycle was repeated every 28 days). The initial phase I investigation of clofarabine was performed in patients with solid tumors and hematological malignancies. As with fludarabine, the dose of clofarabine that was selected as the starting dose was high [74]. Myelosuppression was the dose-limiting toxicity; thus, the maximum tolerated dose in the solid tumor setting was much lower than the starting dose: 2 mg/m^2/day for 5 days. For acute leukemias, where myelosuppression is not a concern, the dose was identified as 40 mg/m^2/day [75].

16.7.1 Plasma Pharmacology

During phase I investigations, a de-escalation of dose in solid tumor patients and an increase in acute leukemia patients resulted in the evaluation of several doses (2, 4,

7.5, 11.25, 15, 22.5, 30, 40, and 55 mg/m^2/day). The number of patients at each dose was low; however, there appeared to be a dose-dependent accumulation of plasma clofarabine (Fig. 16.4). The peak concentration occurred at the end of the 60-min infusion. For adult acute leukemias at the defined MTD, the plasma peak level was 1.5 μM (range, 0.4–3.2 μM) [75]. For pediatric acute leukemias, the doses were tested between 11.25 and 70 mg/m^2/day for 5 days. The MTD was 52 mg/m^2/day, which was slightly higher than what was identified for adult acute leukemia patients. At this MTD, the plasma concentration was a median of 1.1 μM [76]. On the basis of clofarabine's clinical activity, identified specifically in adult acute leukemias during phase I clinical studies, a phase II study was conducted in 62 individuals with acute leukemias [23]. Plasma pharmacological studies in 25 patients elucidated that at the recommended phase II dose in acute leukemias (40 mg/m^2/day × 5 days), the peak plasma concentration of clofarabine was 1 μM (range, 0.26–1.94 μM). Elimination kinetics in five patient samples suggested biphasic kinetics. With this pharmacokinetic profile, there was 0.04 μM clofarabine remaining in plasma at 24 h after infusion. This is when the second dose is administered.

Clofarabine is eliminated renally. In the isolated perfused rat kidney model, clofarabine clearance was nonlinear. However, the concentration of drug was much higher than the physiological level achieved in humans [77]. The findings in a rat in vivo model system suggested that clofarabine is a substrate for the cimetidine-sensitive organic cation transporter (probably OCT2) system in kidneys [77].

Population pharmacokinetic studies, initially in pediatric patients [78] and then in both children and adults, demonstrated [79] that while there were no differences in plasma pharmacology by sex, tumor type, or race, age was a variant. For adults, the volume of distribution and β half-life of clofarabine elimination were much higher, resulting in a higher exposure of the drug. In addition to clofarabine, 6-ketoclofarabine, a metabolite of clofarabine, was also detected in the plasma; however, this was a minor metabolite of no known significance. Since clofarabine is also used in the clinic as an oral drug [68, 80–84], it is important to mention that the bioavailability of oral clofarabine is around 60%, suggesting that this is a viable formulation of this drug [79]. Clofarabine is resistant to purine nucleoside phosphorylase cleavage, which provides a rationale for an oral formulation of clofarabine that is not cleaved by microbial PNP in the gut. Clinically, oral clofarabine was well tolerated and had an MTD of 3 mg/m^2/day for 21 days in relapsed and refractory non-Hodgkin lymphoma [68].

16.7.2 Cellular Pharmacology

As mentioned in the plasma pharmacology section, there were nine different doses used during the phase I clinical trial of clofarabine. The clofarabine triphosphate level analyzed in 40 patients suggested a dose-dependent increase in cellular triphosphate levels. However, there was heterogeneity at each dose level. For adult acute leukemias, at the MTD, the median triphosphate value was 19 μM (range, 3–52 μM) [75], which was similar to that observed in pediatric patients (range, 6

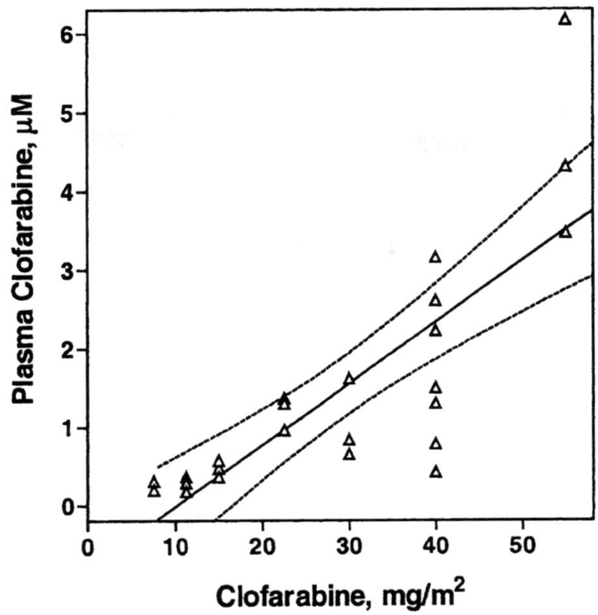

Fig. 16.4 Dose-dependent accumulation of plasma clofarabine. Blood samples were obtained on the first day from each patient at the end of clofarabine infusion. Plasma was separated, and clofarabine concentrations were quantitated as described by Gandhi et al. [20]. The numbers of samples were 2 at 7.5, 3 at 11.5, 3 at 15, 3 at 22.5, 2 at 30, 7 at 40, and 3 at 55 mg/m^2/day. The dashed lines represent 95% confidence intervals (Obtained with permission from Gandhi et al. [20])

and 19 µM). Importantly, this level of cytotoxic triphosphate was sufficient in the complete and sustained inhibition of DNA synthesis [76].

The efficacy of clofarabine in acute leukemia resulted in a phase II investigation in relapsed refractory acute leukemias. At the MTD (40 mg/m^2/day × 5 days), the peak clofarabine triphosphate level was 15 µM (range, 1–44 µM, $n = 29$). The accumulation was similar in different diagnoses, such as AML, ALL, and CML. The elimination profile of clofarabine triphosphate indicated that the triphosphate was retained, with a half-life of 24 h. Interestingly, the 5-day profile of triphosphate accumulation suggested that the levels of triphosphate had an incremental increase in responders, while they remained fairly similar in nonresponders (Fig. 16.5) [23]. A detailed comparison of clofarabine triphosphate pharmacological traits demonstrated that in responders, the peak value at the end of the first infusion was higher (18 µM; range, 5–44 µM; $n = 16$) than that in nonresponders (10 µM; range, 1–23 µM; $n = 11$). Furthermore, because of longer retention of triphosphate in leukemia blasts of responders, the second day end-of-infusion value was 30 µM (1–67 µM, $n = 15$) for responders and 9 µM (1–23 µM, $n = 10$) for nonresponders.

Clofarabine triphosphate competes with the endogenous dATP pool for incorporation into DNA and inhibition of DNA synthesis. The concentration of dATP was a median of 1.8 µM (range, 0.4–22 µM; $n = 9$). These data suggest that the ratio of

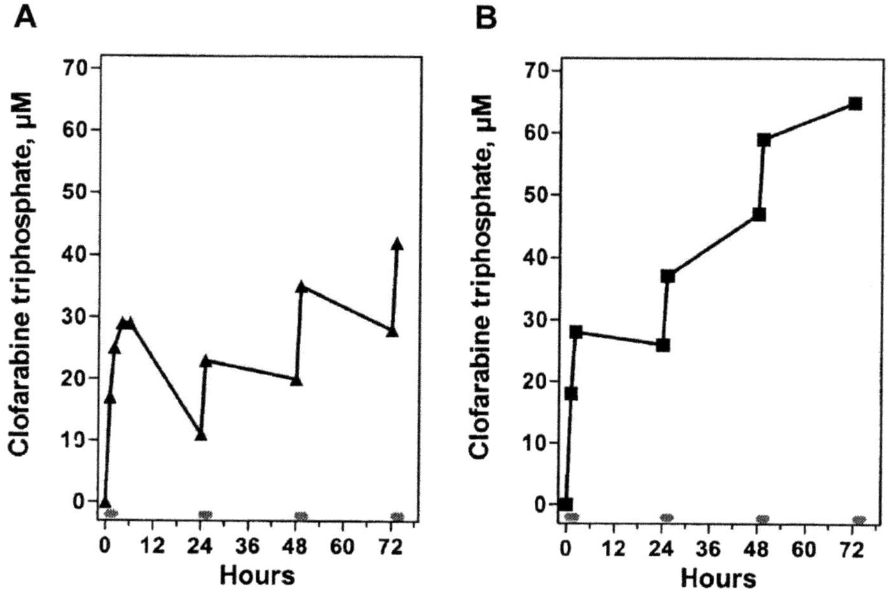

Fig. 16.5 Incremental accumulation of clofarabine triphosphate in two representative patients. Pretreatment and end-of-infusion samples were obtained from two patients after several infusions of clofarabine to quantitate the intracellular levels of triphosphate. Rectangular bars on the abscissa indicate clofarabine infusions. **a** Nonresponder; **b** responder (Obtained with permission from Kantarjian et al. [23])

clofarabine triphosphate to dATP favors incorporation of the analog into DNA. While DNA incorporation was not studied, DNA synthesis inhibition showed a dose-dependent [20] decrease in the DNA synthetic capacity of circulating leukemia cells in patients receiving this therapy. The decline was almost complete and was maintained at higher doses (Fig. 16.6).

16.8 Combination Rationales and Trials

Clinically, the maximum use of clofarabine was in pediatric and adult acute leukemias. The standard of care for AML is high-dose cytarabine (ara-C) or ara-C-containing regimens. Biochemically, it was demonstrated that clofarabine triphosphate modulated the accumulation of ara-C triphosphate (the cytotoxic metabolite of ara-C), resulting in two- to threefold higher levels of ara-C triphosphate in AML cell lines and AML primary blasts [33]. This is similar to the fludarabine- and cladribine-mediated modulation of ara-C triphosphate accumulation in AML [85–87]. The maximum augmentation of ara-C triphosphate accumulation was observed with 1 µM clofarabine, a concentration that is achievable at the MTD (40 mg/m^2/day).

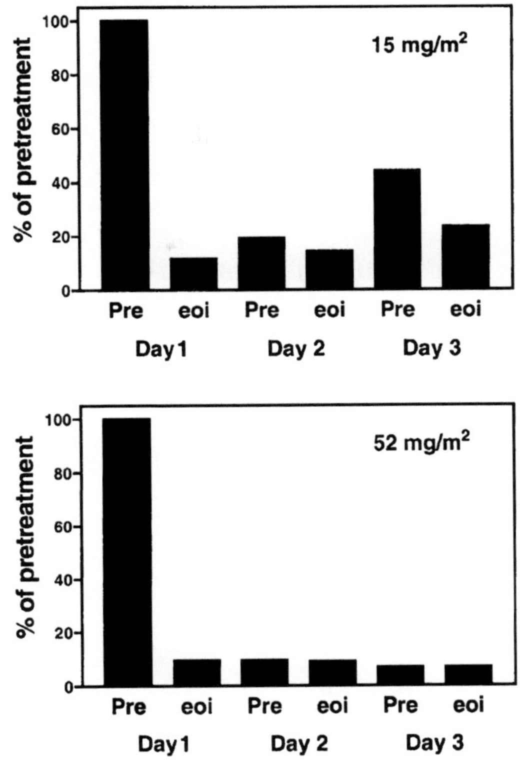

Fig. 16.6 Inhibition of DNA synthesis. Blood samples were obtained from two patients (patients 2 and 23) before and at the end of clofarabine infusion on the indicated days. Leukemia cells were isolated and incubated with thymidine, as described by Jeha et al. [76]. Data are expressed as a percentage of the untreated (control) value. Pre indicates, prior to infusion, and eoi, at the end of infusion (Obtained with permission from Jeha et al. [76])

These observations were the basis of several clinical trials in which clofarabine was combined with ara-C. With these combinations, the plasma pharmacology of clofarabine was not impacted; however, clofarabine infusion prior to ara-C administration resulted in a 1.4-fold median increase in the ara-C triphosphate accumulation in five of eight patients [88]. Because of the phase I nature of this study, the doses of clofarabine varied. Systematic cellular pharmacokinetic studies of ara-C triphosphate are needed to fully evaluate the impact of MTD clofarabine on ara-C triphosphate accumulation in AML blasts. Clinically, a randomized study of ara-C, alone and in combination with clofarabine, demonstrated that the overall response rate was 47% in the combination arm compared to 23% in the single-agent arm. Importantly, the addition of clofarabine doubled the rate of complete remissions from 18% to 35%; however, toxicity was also increased with the combination [89]. A retrospective comparison of the clofarabine and ara-C combination with fludarabine and the ara-C couplet combined with granulocyte colony-stimulating factor suggested that there was an advantage to replacing fludarabine with clofarabine [90].

As described above, clofarabine's actions on DNA replication are also mimicked during DNA repair. Both inhibition of ribonucleotide reductase and incorporation of analog triphosphate in DNA inhibit synthesis of the DNA repair patch [51]. For the initiation of a DNA damage response, alkylating agents such as cyclophosphamide and busulfan have been combined with clofarabine in the preclinical setting [91, 92] and during clinical trials in both adult AML [93] and ALL [94]. During these investigations, it was demonstrated that clofarabine administration, before or after cyclophosphamide, resulted in greater cytotoxicity as well as an increased damage response, measured as phosphorylation of H2AX (γH2AX).

In addition to these above-mentioned combination approaches, sorafenib has been combined with clofarabine and ara-C [95]. Pharmacodynamic endpoints suggested that this combination inhibited the phosphorylation of Akt, S6 ribosomal protein, and 4EBP-1 in leukemia blasts. Although this was a small study, it showed a high response rate. For example, all five patients with FLT3-ITD and four of six patients with wild-type FLT3 showed a response. Such combinations need to be evaluated in a large cohort of patients. Inhibition of the mTOR pathway by temsirolimus was also shown to be effective in combination with clofarabine in AML cell lines [96]. The opposite actions of clofarabine and decitabine on the R2 subunit of ribonucleotide reductase were evaluated and modeled in AML. This modeling study suggested that a synergistic interaction occurs between these two nucleoside analogs [97]. Low-dose decitabine and clofarabine have been combined in the treatment of MDS and AML [98]. In addition, clofarabine has been combined with other therapeutics, such as gemtuzumab ozogamicin [99].

16.9 Summary

Clofarabine's actions, its similarities to and differences from cladribine and fludarabine, and its efficacy in acute leukemias led to its FDA approval. When combined with other chemotherapeutic drugs and targeted agents, it has resulted in clinical improvements in pediatric and adult acute leukemias. New combination strategies are being designed and tested for acute leukemias.

Acknowledgments The authors thank Hima Vangapandu, PhD, for her help with the references. The authors also thank Ms. Ann Sutton for scientific editing.

Conflict of Interest Clofarabine was discovered at Southern Research Institute, which receives licensing fees and royalty payments from its commercial development. Some of this money is distributed to Dr. Parker. Dr. Gandhi has no conflicts of interest to disclose.

References

1. Jordheim LP, Durantel D, Zoulim F, Dumontet C. Advances in the development of nucleoside and nucleotide analogues for cancer and viral diseases. Nat Rev Drug Discov. 2013;12(6):447–64.
2. Parker WB. Enzymology of purine and pyrimidine antimetabolites used in the treatment of cancer. Chem Rev. 2009;109(7):2880–93.
3. Zimmerman TP, Gersten NB, Ross AF, Miech RP. Adenine as substrate for purine nucleoside phosphorylase. Can J Biochem. 1971;49(9):1050–4.
4. Jensen KF, Nygaard P. Purine nucleoside phosphorylase from *Escherichia coli* and Salmonella typhimurium. Purification and some properties. Eur J Biochem/FEBS. 1975;51(1):253–65.

5. Secrist 3rd JA, Thottassery J, Parker WB. Clofarabine: from design to approval. In: Herdewijn P, editor. Modified nucleosides: in biochemistry, biotechnology and medicine. Weinheim: WILEY-VCH Verlag GmbH & Co. KGaA; 2008. p. 631–46.
6. Maguire MH, Sim MK. Studies on adenosine deaminase. 2. Specificity and mechanism of action of bovine placental adenosine deaminase. Eur J Biochem/FEBS. 1971;23(1):22–9.
7. Watanabe KA, Reichman U, Hirota K, Lopez C, Fox JJ. Nucleosides. 110. Synthesis and antiherpes virus activity of some 2′-fluoro-2′-deoxyarabinofuranosylpyrimidine nucleosides. J Med Chem. 1979;22(1):21–4.
8. Montgomery JA, Shortnacy-Fowler AT, Clayton SD, Riordan JM, Secrist 3rd JA. Synthesis and biologic activity of 2′-fluoro-2-halo derivatives of 9-beta-D-arabinofuranosyladenine. J Med Chem. 1992;35(2):397–401.
9. Takahashi T, Kanazawa J, Akinaga S, Tamaoki T, Okabe M. Antitumor activity of 2-chloro-9-(2-deoxy-2-fluoro-beta-D-arabinofuranosyl) adenine, a novel deoxyadenosine analog, against human colon tumor xenografts by oral administration. Cancer Chemother Pharmacol. 1999;43(3):233–40.
10. Waud WR, Schmid SM, Montgomery JA, Secrist 3rd JA. Preclinical antitumor activity of 2-chloro-9-(2-deoxy-2-fluoro-beta-D- arabinofuranosyl)adenine (Cl-F-ara-A). Nucleosides Nucleotides Nucleic Acids. 2000;19(1–2):447–60.
11. Cass CE. Nucleoside transport. In: Georgopapadakou NH, editor. Drug transport in antimicrobial and cancer chemotherapy. New York: Marcel Dekker; 1995. p. 403–51.
12. King KM, Damaraju VL, Vickers MF, Yao SY, Lang T, Tackaberry TE, et al. A comparison of the transportability, and its role in cytotoxicity, of clofarabine, cladribine, and fludarabine by recombinant human nucleoside transporters produced in three model expression systems. Mol Pharmacol. 2006;69(1):346–53.
13. Elwi AN, Damaraju VL, Kuzma ML, Mowles DA, Baldwin SA, Young JD, et al. Transepithelial fluxes of adenosine and 2′-deoxyadenosine across human renal proximal tubule cells: roles of nucleoside transporters hENT1, hENT2, and hCNT3. Am J Physiol Renal Physiol. 2009;296(6):F1439–51.
14. de Wolf C, Jansen R, Yamaguchi H, de Haas M, van de Wetering K, Wijnholds J, et al. Contribution of the drug transporter ABCG2 (breast cancer resistance protein) to resistance against anticancer nucleosides. Mol Cancer Ther. 2008;7(9):3092–102.
15. Nagai S, Takenaka K, Nachagari D, Rose C, Domoney K, Sun D, et al. Deoxycytidine kinase modulates the impact of the ABC transporter ABCG2 on clofarabine cytotoxicity. Cancer Res. 2011;71(5):1781–91.
16. Fukuda Y, Schuetz JD. ABC transporters and their role in nucleoside and nucleotide drug resistance. Biochem Pharmacol. 2012;83(8):1073–83.
17. Parker WB, Shaddix SC, Chang CH, White EL, Rose LM, Brockman RW, et al. Effects of 2-chloro-9-(2-deoxy-2-fluoro-beta-D-arabinofuranosyl)adenine on K562 cellular metabolism and the inhibition of human ribonucleotide reductase and DNA polymerases by its 5′-triphosphate. Cancer Res. 1991;51(9):2386–94.
18. Xie C, Plunkett W. Metabolism and actions of 2-chloro-9-(2-deoxy-2-fluoro-beta-D-arabinofuranosyl)-adenine in human lymphoblastoid cells. Cancer Res. 1995;55(13):2847–52.
19. Avery TL, Rehg JE, Lumm WC, Harwood FC, Santana VM, Blakley RL. Biochemical pharmacology of 2-chlorodeoxyadenosine in malignant human hematopoietic cell lines and therapeutic effects of 2-bromodeoxyadenosine in drug combinations in mice. Cancer Res. 1989;49(18):4972–8.
20. Gandhi V, Kantarjian H, Faderl S, Bonate P, Du M, Ayres M, et al. Pharmacokinetics and pharmacodynamics of plasma clofarabine and cellular clofarabine triphosphate in patients with acute leukemias. Clin Cancer Res. 2003;9(17):6335–42.
21. Parker WB, Shaddix SC, Rose LM, Shewach DS, Hertel LW, Secrist 3rd JA, et al. Comparison of the mechanism of cytotoxicity of 2-chloro-9-(2-deoxy-2- fluoro-beta-D-arabinofuranosyl) adenine, 2-chloro-9-(2-deoxy-2-fluoro- beta-D-ribofuranosyl)adenine, and 2-chloro-9-(2-

deoxy-2,2-difluoro- beta-D-ribofuranosyl)adenine in CEM cells. Mol Pharmacol. 1999;55(3):515–20.
22. Lotfi K, Mansson E, Spasokoukotskaja T, Pettersson B, Liliemark J, Peterson C, et al. Biochemical pharmacology and resistance to 2-chloro-2′-arabino-fluoro-2′-deoxyadenosine, a novel analogue of cladribine in human leukemic cells. Clin Cancer Res. 1999;5(9):2438–44.
23. Kantarjian H, Gandhi V, Cortes J, Verstovsek S, Du M, Garcia-Manero G, et al. Phase 2 clinical and pharmacologic study of clofarabine in patients with refractory or relapsed acute leukemia. Blood. 2003;102(7):2379–86.
24. Jordheim LP, Marton Z, Rhimi M, Cros-Perrial E, Lionne C, Peyrottes S, et al. Identification and characterization of inhibitors of cytoplasmic 5′-nucleotidase cN-II issued from virtual screening. Biochem Pharmacol. 2013;85(4):497–506.
25. Zhang Y, Secrist 3rd JA, Ealick SE. The structure of human deoxycytidine kinase in complex with clofarabine reveals key interactions for prodrug activation. Acta Crystallogr D Biol Crystallogr. 2006;62(Pt 2):133–9.
26. Leegwater PA, De Abreu RA, Albertioni F. Analysis of DNA methylation of the 5′ region of the deoxycytidine kinase gene in CCRF-CEM-sensitive and cladribine (CdA)- and 2-chloro-2′-arabino-fluoro-2′-deoxyadenosine (CAFdA)-resistant cells. Cancer Lett. 1998;130(1–2):169–73.
27. Mansson E, Flordal E, Liliemark J, Spasokoukotskaja T, Elford H, Lagercrantz S, et al. Down-regulation of deoxycytidine kinase in human leukemic cell lines resistant to cladribine and clofarabine and increased ribonucleotide reductase activity contributes to fludarabine resistance. Biochem Pharmacol. 2003;65(2):237–47.
28. Waud WR, Gilbert KS, Parker WB, Secrist JA. Isolation and characterization of a murine P388 leukemia line resistant to clofarabine. Nucleosides Nucleotides Nucleic Acids. 2011;30(11):826–38.
29. Yamauchi T, Uzui K, Nishi R, Shigemi H, Ueda T. Cytarabine-resistant leukemia cells are moderately sensitive to clofarabine in vitro. Anticancer Res. 2014;34(4):1657–62.
30. Shigemi H, Yamauchi T, Tanaka Y, Ueda T. Novel leukemic cell lines resistant to clofarabine by mechanisms of decreased active metabolite and increased antiapoptosis. Cancer Sci. 2013;104(6):732–9.
31. Lamba JK, Crews K, Pounds S, Schuetz EG, Gresham J, Gandhi V, et al. Pharmacogenetics of deoxycytidine kinase: identification and characterization of novel genetic variants. J Pharmacol Exp Ther. 2007;323(3):935–45.
32. Spasokoukotskaja T, Sasvari-Szekely M, Hullan L, Albertioni F, Eriksson S, Staub M. Activation of deoxycytidine kinase by various nucleoside analogues. Adv Exp Med Biol. 1998;431:641–5.
33. Cooper T, Ayres M, Nowak B, Gandhi V. Biochemical modulation of cytarabine triphosphate by clofarabine. Cancer Chemother Pharmacol. 2005;55(4):361–8.
34. Parker WB, Shaddix SC, Gilbert KS, Shepherd RV, Waud WR. Enhancement of the in vivo antitumor activity of clofarabine by 1-beta-D-[4-thio-arabinofuranosyl]-cytosine. Cancer Chemother Pharmacol. 2009;64(2):253–61.
35. Csapo Z, Sasvari-Szekely M, Spasokoukotskaja T, Talianidis I, Eriksson S, Staub M. Activation of deoxycytidine kinase by inhibition of DNA synthesis in human lymphocytes. Biochem Pharmacol. 2001;61(2):191–7.
36. Spasokoukotskaja T, Sasvari-Szekely M, Keszler G, Albertioni F, Eriksson S, Staub M. Treatment of normal and malignant cells with nucleoside analogues and etoposide enhances deoxycytidine kinase activity. Eur J Cancer. 1999;35(13):1862–7.
37. Amsailale R, Van Den Neste E, Arts A, Starczewska E, Bontemps F, Smal C. Phosphorylation of deoxycytidine kinase on Ser-74: impact on kinetic properties and nucleoside analog activation in cancer cells. Biochem Pharmacol. 2012;84(1):43–51.
38. Keszler G, Spasokoukotskaja T, Sasvari-Szekely M, Eriksson S, Staub M. Deoxycytidine kinase is reversibly phosphorylated in normal human lymphocytes. Nucleosides Nucleotides Nucleic Acids. 2006;25(9–11):1147–51.

39. Guo Y, Xu X, Qi W, Xie C, Wang G, Zhang A, et al. Synergistic antitumor interactions between gemcitabine and clofarabine in human pancreatic cancer cell lines. Mol Med Rep. 2012;5(3):734–8.
40. Valdez BC, Li Y, Murray D, Ji J, Liu Y, Popat U, et al. Comparison of the cytotoxicity of cladribine and clofarabine when combined with fludarabine and busulfan in AML cells: enhancement of cytotoxicity with epigenetic modulators. Exp Hematol. 2015;43(6):448–61. e2.
41. Valdez BC, Wang G, Murray D, Nieto Y, Li Y, Shah J, et al. Mechanistic studies on the synergistic cytotoxicity of the nucleoside analogs gemcitabine and clofarabine in multiple myeloma: relevance of p53 and its clinical implications. Exp Hematol. 2013;41(8):719–30.
42. Sjoberg AH, Wang L, Eriksson S. Substrate specificity of human recombinant mitochondrial deoxyguanosine kinase with cytostatic and antiviral purine and pyrimidine analogs. Mol Pharmacol. 1998;53(2):270–3.
43. Arner ES, Eriksson S. Mammalian deoxyribonucleoside kinases. Pharmacol Ther. 1995;67(2):155–86.
44. Lindemalm S, Liliemark J, Gruber A, Eriksson S, Karlsson MO, Wang Y, et al. Comparison of cytotoxicity of 2-chloro- 2′-arabino-fluoro-2′-deoxyadenosine (clofarabine) with cladribine in mononuclear cells from patients with acute myeloid and chronic lymphocytic leukemia. Haematologica. 2003;88(3):324–32.
45. Xie KC, Plunkett W. Deoxynucleotide pool depletion and sustained inhibition of ribonucleotide reductase and DNA synthesis after treatment of human lymphoblastoid cells with 2-chloro-9-(2-deoxy-2-fluoro-beta-D-arabinofuranosyl) adenine. Cancer Res. 1996;56(13):3030–7.
46. Chen LS, Plunkett W, Gandhi V. Polyadenylation inhibition by the triphosphates of deoxyadenosine analogues. Leuk Res. 2008;32:1573–81.
47. Nordlund P, Reichard P. Ribonucleotide reductases. Annu Rev Biochem. 2006;75:681–706.
48. Aye Y, Stubbe J. Clofarabine 5′-di and -triphosphates inhibit human ribonucleotide reductase by altering the quaternary structure of its large subunit. Proc NatAcad Sci. 2011;108(24):9815–20.
49. Aye Y, Brignole EJ, Long MJ, Chittuluru J, Drennan CL, Asturias FJ, et al. Clofarabine targets the large subunit (alpha) of human ribonucleotide reductase in live cells by assembly into persistent hexamers. Chem Biol. 2012;19(7):799–805.
50. Fu Y, Lin HY, Wisitpitthaya S, Blessing WA, Aye Y. A fluorimetric readout reporting the kinetics of nucleotide-induced human ribonucleotide reductase oligomerization. Chem Biochem: Eur J Chem Biol. 2014;15(17):2598–604.
51. Yamauchi T, Nowak BJ, Keating MJ, Plunkett W. DNA repair initiated in chronic lymphocytic leukemia lymphocytes by 4-hydroperoxycyclophosphamide is inhibited by fludarabine and clofarabine. Clin Cancer Res. 2001;7(11):3580–9.
52. Carson DA, Wasson DB, Esparza LM, Carrera CJ, Kipps TJ, Cottam HB. Oral antilymphocyte activity and induction of apoptosis by 2-chloro-2′-arabino-fluoro-2′-deoxyadenosine. Proc Natl Acad Sci. 1992;89(7):2970–4.
53. Hartman WR, Hentosh P. The antileukemia drug 2-chloro-2′-deoxyadenosine: an intrinsic transcriptional antagonist. Mol Pharmacol. 2004;65(1):227–34.
54. Hartman WR, Walters DE, Hentosh P. Presence of the anti-leukemic nucleotide analog, 2-chloro-2′-deoxyadenosine-5′-monophosphate, in a promoter sequence alters DNA binding of TATA-binding protein (TBP). Arch Biochem Biophys. 2007;459(2):223–32.
55. Dimitrova DS, Gilbert DM. Temporally coordinated assembly and disassembly of replication factories in the absence of DNA synthesis. Nat Cell Biol. 2000;2(10):686–94.
56. Lee YJ, Hwang IS, Lee YJ, Lee CH, Kim SH, Nam HS, et al. Knockdown of Bcl-xL enhances growth-inhibiting and apoptosis-inducing effects of resveratrol and clofarabine in malignant mesothelioma H-2452 cells. J Korean Med Sci. 2014;29(11):1464–72.
57. Takahashi T, Shimizu M, Akinaga S. Mechanisms of the apoptotic activity of Cl-F-araA in a human T-ALL cell line. CCRF-CEM Cancer Chemother Pharmacol. 2002;50(3):193–201.

58. Wang X, Albertioni F. Effect of clofarabine on apoptosis and DNA synthesis in human epithelial colon cancer cells. Nucleosides Nucleotides Nucleic Acids. 2010;29(4–6):414–8.
59. Genini D, Adachi S, Chao Q, Rose DW, Carrera CJ, Cottam HB, et al. Deoxyadenosine analogs induce programmed cell death in chronic lymphocytic leukemia cells by damaging the DNA and by directly affecting the mitochondria. Blood. 2000;96(10):3537–43.
60. Genini D, Budihardjo I, Plunkett W, Wang X, Carrera CJ, Cottam HB, et al. Nucleotide requirements for the in vitro activation of the apoptosis protein-activating factor-1-mediated caspase pathway. J Biol Chem. 2000;275(1):29–34.
61. Miura S, Izuta S. DNA polymerases as targets of anticancer nucleosides. Curr Drug Targets. 2004;5(2):191–5.
62. Jensen K, Johnson LA, Jacobson PA, Kachler S, Kirstein MN, Lamba J, et al. Cytotoxic purine nucleoside analogues bind to A1, A2A, and A3 adenosine receptors. Naunyn Schmiedeberg's Arch Pharmacol. 2012;385(5):519–25.
63. Lubecka-Pietruszewska K, Kaufman-Szymczyk A, Stefanska B, Cebula-Obrzut B, Smolewski P, Fabianowska-Majewska K. Clofarabine, a novel adenosine analogue, reactivates DNA methylation-silenced tumour suppressor genes and inhibits cell growth in breast cancer cells. Eur J Pharmacol. 2014;723:276–87.
64. Majda K, Kaufman-Szymczyk A, Lubecka-Pietruszewska K, Bednarek A, Fabianowska-Majewska K. Influence of clofarabine on transcriptional activity of PTEN, APC, RARB2, ZAP70 genes in K562 cells. Anticancer Res. 2010;30(11):4601–6.
65. Seedhouse C, Grundy M, Shang S, Ronan J, Pimblett H, Russell N, et al. Impaired S-phase arrest in acute myeloid leukemia cells with a FLT3 internal tandem duplication treated with clofarabine. Clin Cancer Res. 2009;15(23):7291–8.
66. Krett NL, Ayres M, Nabhan C, Ma C, Nowak B, Nawrocki S, et al. In vitro assessment of nucleoside analogs in multiple myeloma. Cancer Chemother Pharmacol. 2004;54(2):113–21.
67. Uy GL, Tomasson MH, Ruddell A, DiPersio JF, Vij R. The activity and toxicity of low dose clofarabine against relapsed or refractory myeloma. Haematologica. 2006;91(11):1581–2.
68. Abramson JS, Takvorian RW, Fisher DC, Feng Y, Jacobsen ED, Brown JR, et al. Oral clofarabine for relapsed/refractory non-Hodgkin lymphomas: results of a phase 1 study. Leuk Lymphoma. 2013;54(9):1915–20.
69. Blum KA, Hamadani M, Phillips GS, Lozanski G, Johnson AJ, Lucas DM, et al. Prolonged myelosuppression with clofarabine in the treatment of patients with relapsed or refractory, aggressive non-Hodgkin lymphoma. Leuk Lymphoma. 2009;50(3):349–56.
70. Nabhan C, Davis N, Bitran JD, Galvez A, Fried W, Tolzien K, et al. Efficacy and safety of clofarabine in relapsed and/or refractory non-Hodgkin lymphoma, including rituximab-refractory patients. Cancer. 2011;117(7):1490–7.
71. Rahmati-Yamchi M, Zarghami N, Nozad Charoudeh H, Ahmadi Y, Baradaran B, Khalaj-Kondori M, et al. Clofarabine has apoptotic effect on T47D breast cancer cell line via P53R2 gene expression. Adv Pharm Bull. 2015;5(4):471–6.
72. Patel YT, Jacus MO, Boulos N, Dapper JD, Davis AD, Vuppala PK, et al. Preclinical examination of clofarabine in pediatric ependymoma: intratumoral concentrations insufficient to warrant further study. Cancer Chemother Pharmacol. 2015;75(5):897–906.
73. Bonate PL, Arthaud L, Cantrell Jr WR, Stephenson K, Secrist 3rd JA, Weitman S. Discovery and development of clofarabine: a nucleoside analogue for treating cancer. Nat Rev Drug Discov. 2006;5(10):855–63.
74. Collins JM, Grieshaber CK, Chabner BA. Pharmacologically guided phase I clinical trials based upon preclinical drug development. J Natl Cancer Inst. 1990;82(16):1321–6.
75. Kantarjian HM, Gandhi V, Kozuch P, Faderl S, Giles F, Cortes J, et al. Phase I clinical and pharmacology study of clofarabine in patients with solid and hematologic cancers. J Clin Oncol. 2003;21(6):1167–73.
76. Jeha S, Gandhi V, Chan KW, McDonald L, Ramirez I, Madden R, et al. Clofarabine, a novel nucleoside analog, is active in pediatric patients with advanced leukemia. Blood. 2004;103(3):784–9.

77. Ajavon AD, Bonate PL, Taft DR. Renal excretion of clofarabine: assessment of dose-linearity and role of renal transport systems on drug excretion. Eur J Pharm Sci. 2010;40(3):209–16.
78. Bonate PL, Craig A, Gaynon P, Gandhi V, Jeha S, Kadota R, et al. Population pharmacokinetics of clofarabine, a second-generation nucleoside analog, in pediatric patients with acute leukemia. J Clin Pharmacol. 2004;44(11):1309–22.
79. Bonate PL, Cunningham CC, Gaynon P, Jeha S, Kadota R, Lam GN, et al. Population pharmacokinetics of clofarabine and its metabolite 6-ketoclofarabine in adult and pediatric patients with cancer. Cancer Chemother Pharmacol. 2011;67(4):875–90.
80. Rudrapatna VK, Morley K, Boucher KM, Pierson AS, Shull CT, Kushner JP, et al. Phase I trial of low-dose oral Clofarabine in myelodysplastic syndromes patients who have failed frontline therapy. Leuk Res. 2015;39(8):835–9.
81. Jacoby MA, Martin MG, Uy GL, Westervelt P, Dipersio JF, Cashen A, et al. Phase I study of oral clofarabine consolidation in adults aged 60 and older with acute myeloid leukemia. Am J Hematol. 2014;89(5):487–92.
82. Faderl S, Garcia-Manero G, Estrov Z, Ravandi F, Borthakur G, Cortes JE, et al. Oral clofarabine in the treatment of patients with higher-risk myelodysplastic syndrome. J Clin Oncol. 2010;28(16):2755–60.
83. Al Ustwani O, Greene JD, Wetzler M. The use of low-dose protracted oral clofarabine in a patient with myelodysplastic syndrome after failing 5-azacitidine. Leuk Res Rep. 2013;2(1):34–5.
84. Buckley SA, Mawad R, Gooley TA, Becker PS, Sandhu V, Hendrie P, et al. A phase I/II study of oral clofarabine plus low-dose cytarabine in previously treated acute myeloid leukaemia and high-risk myelodysplastic syndrome patients at least 60 years of age. Br J Haematol. 2015;170(3):349–55.
85. Gandhi V, Plunkett W. Modulation of arabinosylnucleoside metabolism by arabinosylnucleotides in human leukemia cells. Cancer Res. 1988;48(2):329–34.
86. Gandhi V, Estey E, Keating MJ, Chucrallah A, Plunkett W. Chlorodeoxyadenosine and arabinosylcytosine in patients with acute myelogenous leukemia: pharmacokinetic, pharmacodynamic, and molecular interactions. Blood. 1996;87(1):256–64.
87. Gandhi V, Estey E, Keating MJ, Plunkett W. Fludarabine potentiates metabolism of cytarabine in patients with acute myelogenous leukemia during therapy. J Clin Oncol. 1993;11(1):116–24.
88. Faderl S, Gandhi V, O'Brien S, Bonate P, Cortes J, Estey E, et al. Results of a phase 1-2 study of clofarabine in combination with cytarabine (ara-C) in relapsed and refractory acute leukemias. Blood. 2005;105(3):940–7.
89. Faderl S, Wetzler M, Rizzieri D, Schiller G, Jagasia M, Stuart R, et al. Clofarabine plus cytarabine compared with cytarabine alone in older patients with relapsed or refractory acute myelogenous leukemia: results from the CLASSIC I Trial. J Clin Oncol. 2012;30(20):2492–9.
90. Becker PS, Kantarjian HM, Appelbaum FR, Petersdorf SH, Storer B, Pierce S, et al. Clofarabine with high dose cytarabine and granulocyte colony-stimulating factor (G-CSF) priming for relapsed and refractory acute myeloid leukaemia. Br J Haematol. 2011;155(2):182–9.
91. Valdez BC, Li Y, Murray D, Champlin RE, Andersson BS. The synergistic cytotoxicity of clofarabine, fludarabine and busulfan in AML cells involves ATM pathway activation and chromatin remodeling. Biochem Pharmacol. 2011;81(2):222–32.
92. Valdez BC, Murray D, Nieto Y, Li Y, Wang G, Champlin RE, et al. Synergistic cytotoxicity of the DNA alkylating agent busulfan, nucleoside analogs and suberoylanilide hydroxamic acid in lymphoma cell lines. Leuk Lymphoma. 2012;53(5):973–81.
93. Karp JE, Ricklis RM, Balakrishnan K, Briel J, Greer J, Gore SD, et al. A phase 1 clinical-laboratory study of clofarabine followed by cyclophosphamide for adults with refractory acute leukemias. Blood. 2007;110(6):1762–9.
94. Faderl S, Balakrishnan K, Thomas DA, Ravandi F, Borthakur G, Burger J, et al. Phase I and extension study of clofarabine plus cyclophosphamide in patients with relapsed/refractory acute lymphoblastic leukemia. Clin Lymph Myelo Leuk. 2014;14(3):231–8.

95. Inaba H, Rubnitz JE, Coustan-Smith E, Li L, Furmanski BD, Mascara GP, et al. Phase I pharmacokinetic and pharmacodynamic study of the multikinase inhibitor sorafenib in combination with clofarabine and cytarabine in pediatric relapsed/refractory leukemia. J Clin Oncol. 2011;29(24):3293–300.
96. Chiarini F, Lonetti A, Teti G, Orsini E, Bressanin D, Cappellini A, et al. A combination of temsirolimus, an allosteric mTOR inhibitor, with clofarabine as a new therapeutic option for patients with acute myeloid leukemia. Oncotarget. 2012;3(12):1615–28.
97. Thudium KE, Ghoshal S, Fetterly GJ, Haese JP, Karpf AR, Wetzler M. Synergism between clofarabine and decitabine through p53R2: a pharmacodynamic drug-drug interaction modeling. Leuk Res. 2012;36(11):1410–6.
98. Faderl S, Ravandi F, Huang X, Wang X, Jabbour E, Garcia-Manero G, et al. Clofarabine plus low-dose cytarabine followed by clofarabine plus low-dose cytarabine alternating with decitabine in acute myeloid leukemia frontline therapy for older patients. Cancer. 2012;118(18):4471–7.
99. Foster MC, Amin C, Voorhees PM, van Deventer HW, Richards KL, Ivanova A, et al. A phase I dose-escalation study of clofarabine in combination with fractionated gemtuzumab ozogamicin in patients with refractory or relapsed acute myeloid leukemia. Leuk Lymphoma. 2012;53(7):1331–7.

Clinical Use of Clofarabine for Adults and Children with Leukemia

17

James McCloskey, Jamie Koprivnikar, Stefan Faderl, Dirk Reinhardt, and Nobuko Hijiya

Abstract

Clofarabine is a second-generation nucleoside analogue designed to be more effective than precursor nucleoside analogues such as fludarabine and cladribine. Early clinical studies of clofarabine demonstrated its activity in hematologic malignancies, and clofarabine was approved by the United States Food and Drug Administration (FDA) for the treatment of relapsed and refractory pediatric acute lymphoblastic leukemia (ALL) in 2004. Clofarabine has significant efficacy in adults and children with hematologic malignancies including ALL, acute myeloid leukemia (AML), and myelodysplastic syndrome (MDS). The unique biochemical modulation properties of clofarabine when used in combination with other established antileukemic drugs also make it an appealing agent for use in combination therapy with purine nucleoside analogues or DNA-damaging agents; these combinations have been tested in a number of studies in patients with ALL or AML. In this chapter, we review the development of clofarabine, the rationale and history of its use in combination regimens, and the potential roles and toxicities of these regimens in the treatment of adult and pediatric leukemias. The use of clofarabine in conditioning regimens prior to stem cell transplantation and for histiocytosis is also discussed.

J. McCloskey • J. Koprivnikar • S. Faderl
Division of Leukemia, John Theurer Cancer Center at Hackensack University Medical Center, Hackensack, NJ, USA

D. Reinhardt
Paediatric Hematology and Oncology, Medical Center, University of Essen, Essen, Germany

N. Hijiya (✉)
Division of Hematology Oncology and Stem Cell Transplant, Ann and Robert H Lurie Children's Hospital of Chicago, Department of Pediatrics, Northwestern University Feinberg School of Medicine, 225E Chicago Avenue, Box #30, Chicago, IL 60611, USA

Department of Pediatrics, Feinberg School of Medicine, Northwestern University, Evanston, IL, USA
e-mail: NHijiya@luriechildrens.org

T. Ueda (ed.), *Chemotherapy for Leukemia*, DOI 10.1007/978-981-10-3332-2_17

Keywords
Clofarabine • Acute myeloid leukemia • Acute lymphoblastic leukemia • Myelodysplastic syndrome • Stem cell transplantation

17.1 Introduction

Clofarabine (Cl-F-ara-A, 2-chloro-2′-fluoro-2′-deoxyarabinosyladenine) is a nucleoside (2′-deoxyadenosine) analogue. Precursor nucleoside drugs include fludarabine and cladribine, which have the disadvantages of being susceptible to bacterial cleavage and causing moderate myelosuppression, profound and prolonged immunosuppression, and neurologic toxicity at high doses [1–3]. While the mechanism of action of clofarabine is similar to that of cladribine, the unique biochemical properties of clofarabine result in a more rapid onset of action with higher efficacy and the potential for increased tolerability. Specifically, compared to cladribine, clofarabine has improved transmembrane transport, causes greater disruption of DNA elongation due to higher substrate specificity for DNA polymerase, and inhibits tumor cell growth at more than tenfold lower concentration [3–5].

Deoxycytidine kinase (dCK) is the key enzyme involved in the activation of nucleoside analogues. Clofarabine is initially phosphorylated into its monophosphate metabolite by dCK. Following additional phosphorylation steps, it is eventually converted to the active triphosphate derivative [3]. Clofarabine is cytotoxic to proliferating cells as well as nondividing cells. The level of cytotoxicity of nucleoside analogues depends on the intracellular accumulation of their triphosphate metabolites. Lymphocytes are especially susceptible because of the high level of dCK and low level of 5′-deoxynucleotidase in these cells [6]. The anticancer activity of clofarabine triphosphate occurs through multiple pathways, which are described in Chap. 16 [3, 6]; here, we focus on the clinical development and evidence of clofarabine efficacy, tolerability, and toxicity in adult and pediatric patients with leukemia.

17.2 Clofarabine for Adult Leukemia

Acute leukemia affects approximately four out of every 100,000 individuals each year, with nearly 20,000 new cases estimated to occur in 2016 [7]. Despite improvements in risk stratification and supportive care, leukemia remains a deadly disease that will claim an estimated 10,430 lives in 2016 [7]. Myelodysplastic syndrome (MDS), which is characterized by dysplastic and ineffective blood cell production and a variable risk of transformation to acute leukemia, is diagnosed in more than 20,000 people annually [8]. Acute myeloid leukemia (AML) and MDS predominantly affect patients ≥60 years of age in which myelosuppression, immunosuppression, and neurologic toxicities are often amplified by comorbid conditions. Even in the era of targeted therapy and immunotherapy, there remains a significant unmet need among patients with these diseases. Standard treatment remains suboptimal, with low response rates of brief duration.

Clofarabine has demonstrated antitumor activity in various in vitro [9, 10] and in vivo [9–12] models of both solid [13] and hematological tumors [14]. Initially, there was little interest in clofarabine as an anticancer agent, and it was not studied in humans until more than a decade after these preclinical studies. Kantarjian and colleagues conducted the first phase 1 study of clofarabine in 51 patients with hematologic and solid malignancies [15]. Patients with solid tumors experienced dose-limiting myelosuppression at 2 mg/m^2 intravenously (IV) daily for 5 days. However, those with acute leukemia were able to tolerate higher doses, up to 55 mg/m^2 IV daily for 5 days. Dose-limiting, but reversible, hepatotoxicity was observed at this higher dose. Subsequent studies using 40 mg/m^2 IV daily for 5 days in patients with acute leukemia demonstrated a tolerable safety profile, and this dosing schedule was subsequently used in phase 2 studies. In these studies, clofarabine also showed promising activity in patients with leukemia and MDS. Patients with AML, acute lymphoblastic leukemia (ALL), chronic myeloid leukemia-blast phase (CML-BP), and high-risk MDS receiving clofarabine had an overall response rate (ORR) of 48% ($n = 62$) [16]. These trials laid the groundwork for further investigations into the efficacy of clofarabine in subsequent clinical studies.

17.2.1 Acute Myeloid Leukemia (AML)

Cure for AML is achieved in up to 40% of patients under the age of 60 years, with the best available therapy including chemotherapy and allogenic stem cell transplant (alloSCT). For older individuals, however, cure rates drop to less than 10% [7, 17]. While our understanding of AML has increased in recent years, this has not translated to substantial advances in therapies delivered or outcomes achieved. For more than 40 years, standard induction therapy has consisted of 7 days of cytarabine and 3 days of an anthracycline (i.e., 7 + 3); however, 7 + 3 is a challenging regimen to tolerate. It is associated with 10–30% mortality at 30 days post-induction in patients >60 years of age and has a 8- to 12-month median survival for unselected older individuals [18]. Patients with AML have a high rate of relapse after initial response, with treatment of relapsed individuals posing additional challenges, including low response rates and the presence of cumulative toxicities.

17.2.1.1 Clofarabine Monotherapy in Adults with AML

The CLASSIC II trial was a phase 2 study that looked at clofarabine efficacy as an outpatient-based induction monotherapy in 112 untreated patients with AML who were ≥60 years of age. Subjects enrolled in the trial were a median age of 71 [19]. The ORR was 46%, of which 38% achieved complete response (CR) and 8% achieved CR with incomplete platelet recovery (CRp). Of the study population with unfavorable prognostic factors, the ORR was 39% for patients ≥70 years, 32% with

Table 17.1 Studies of first-line clofarabine in adults with AML

Reference	Regimen	Patients (no.)	Median age (years)	ORR (%)	CR (%)	OS
Kantarjian et al. [19]	Clofarabine monotherapy	112	71	46	38	41 weeks
Faderl et al. [26][a]	Clofarabine + cytarabine	70	71	31–63	31–63	5.8–11.4 months
Burnett et al. [20]	Clofarabine monotherapy	406	74	38	22	12%[b]
Kadia et al. [25][c]	Clofarabine + cytarabine	118	74	68	60	11.1 and 18.5 months
Foran et al. [21]	Clofarabine monotherapy	727	68	42.8	42.8	1.41[d]

CR complete response, *ORR* overall response rate, *OS* overall survival
[a]Study evaluated clofarabine + idarubicin and clofarabine monotherapy; ranges represent (clofarabine + idarubicin) – clofarabine monotherapy
[b]2-year OS was 12% for clofarabine monotherapy compared to 13% for LDAC; demonstrated no OS benefit
[c]Median OS was 11.1 months for all patients and 18.5 months for responders
[d]Represents the weighted hazard ratio of clofarabine/7 + 3 instead of OS

Eastern Cooperative Oncology Group (ECOG) performance status of 2. 42% with unfavorable cytogenetics, and 51% with antecedent hematologic disease. The median overall survival (OS) was 41 weeks with a 30-day all-cause mortality of 9.8% (Table 17.1).

A large randomized ECOG trial established that clofarabine does not increase survival for older patients with de novo or secondary AML [20]. Burnett et al. compared clofarabine and low-dose cytarabine (LDAC), a common treatment for induction in elderly patients unable to tolerate 7 + 3, in 406 patients (median age of 74 years) with newly diagnosed de novo AML, secondary AML, or high-risk MDS. The ORR was 38% in the clofarabine arm compared to 19% in the LDAC arm, and 2-year survival was 13% for clofarabine compared to 12% for LDAC. While there was no difference in OS, relapse-free survival was 20% for the clofarabine arm compared to 8% for the LDAC arm.

Clofarabine monotherapy was unable to improve survival compared to 7 + 3 in a recent trial sponsored by ECOG. A total of 727 patients ≥60 years of age and newly diagnosed with AML were randomized to clofarabine monotherapy or 7 + 3 with the option of decitabine maintenance following induction. Preliminary results presented at the American Society of Hematology Annual Meeting in 2015 revealed no significant difference in OS, with a hazard ratio (HR) of 1.41 [21]. Furthermore, CR rates were nearly identical: 42.8% for the clofarabine arm and 43.8% in the 7 + 3 arm.

Table 17.2 Clofarabine studies in adults with relapsed AML

Reference	Regimen	Patients (no.)	Median age (years)	ORR (%)	CR (%)	OS (months)
Faderl et al. [28][a]	Clofarabine + cytarabine	25	59	42	25	7.9
Faderl et al. [26][b]	Clofarabine + idarubicin + cytarabine	44	56–58	48	48	Not reported
Becker et al. [22]	Clofarabine + cytarabine	46	53	61	46	Not reported
Faderl et al. [23]	Clofarabine + cytarabine	320	67	46.9	35.2	6.6

ALL acute lymphoblastic leukemia, *AML* acute myeloid leukemia, *CML-BP* chronic myeloid leukemia-blast phase, *CR* complete response, *MDS* myelodysplastic syndrome, *ORR* overall response rate, *OS* overall survival

[a]Median age of entire study population which included ALL, MDS, and CML-BP, ORR/CR includes AML and MDS patients; OS of the entire study population

[b]ORR was not a primary end point

17.2.1.2 Clofarabine/Cytarabine Combination Therapy in Adults with AML

The promising responses observed with clofarabine monotherapy in hematologic malignancies led to the studies of clofarabine in combination with other cytotoxic agents in patients with AML. FLAG [i.e., fludarabine and cytarabine with granulocyte-colony stimulating factor (G-CSF) priming] is a common regimen used for patients with relapsed AML and has been in use since the 1990s. Becker et al. substituted clofarabine for fludarabine, based on their structural similarity and the higher response rates achieved with clofarabine [22]. The study evaluated 46 patients with refractory/relapsed AML and a median age of 53 years and demonstrated an ORR of 61% with CR rate of 46%. The authors suggested that this combination therapy could be a viable option for this patient population given the lack of dose-limiting toxicity (DLT; Table 17.2).

In 2012, the CLASSIC I trial was conducted as a follow-up to the phase 1/2 study that had established the activity of clofarabine in relapsed AML [23]. This phase 3 trial was a double-blind, placebo-controlled study that compared clofarabine combined with cytarabine to cytarabine and placebo in patients ≥55 years of age with relapsed or refractory AML. A total of 320 patients with a median age of 67 were evaluated. Patients in the clofarabine + cytarabine arm had a better ORR than cytarabine + placebo (46.9% vs. 22.9%). Clofarabine also had a 37.7% 4-month event-free survival (EFS) compared to 16.6% with placebo; however, there was no significant difference in the median OS between clofarabine and placebo (6.6 vs. 6.3 months, $P = 1.00$).

Similar results were seen when 5 days of clofarabine monotherapy at 30 mg/m^2 was compared to clofarabine + LDAC dosed subcutaneously for 14 days at 20 mg/m^2 [24]. In this study, 70 patients ≥60 years of age with AML or high-risk MDS were randomized. The median age of the patients was 71 years. Clofarabine combined with LDAC had a CR rate of 63% with an induction mortality of 19%, whereas clofarabine monotherapy had a CR rate of 31% with an induction mortality of 31%. OS was equivalent between clofarabine combined with LDAC and clofarabine monotherapy (11.4 vs. 5.8 months; $P = 0.10$). In another study, Kadia et al. evaluated 118 patients with a median age of 74 and newly diagnosed AML and treated with clofarabine and LDAC followed by alternating cycles of decitabine maintenance/consolidation [25]. Though there was no comparator arm, the ORR was 68% with a 60% CR rate, which was higher than any rates seen in any prior induction AML clofarabine trials.

17.2.1.3 Clofarabine/Anthracycline Combination Therapy in Adults with AML

A phase 1 study investigated the efficacy of clofarabine in 44 patients ≥18 years of age in the first relapse or with primary refractory AML [26]. Patients were randomized to either clofarabine and idarubicin or clofarabine, idarubicin, and cytarabine (CIA). The maximum tolerated dose (MTD) in the clofarabine/idarubicin arm was clofarabine 22.5 mg/m^2 IV daily for 5 days and idarubicin 10 mg/m^2 IV daily for 3 days. The MTD for CIA was the same, with the addition of cytarabine 0.75/m^2 IV for 5 days. DLTs were hyperbilirubinemia, hepatic transaminitis, mucositis, and diarrhea. Though it was not a primary end point of the study, a response rate of 48% was seen.

This study was followed by a phase 2 study of CIA in patients with newly diagnosed AML 60 years of age or younger [27]. Induction therapy consisted of clofarabine given at a dose of 20 mg/m^2 for 5 days, idarubicin given at a dose of 10 mg/m^2 on days 1–3, and cytarabine given at a dose of 1 g/m^2 on days 1–5. Patients in remission were consolidated with up to six cycles of CIA given on an attenuated dosing schedule. Of the 57 patients evaluable, an ORR of 79% was attained, with the median OS not yet reached after a median follow-up of 10.9 months. Median EFS was 13.5 months. Therapy was well tolerated with 4-week mortality rate of 2%. OS and EFS of patients treated with CIA compared favorably to historical controls treated with 7 + 3, even after multivariate analysis.

17.2.2 Myelodysplastic Syndrome (MDS)

In addition to activity in AML, the previously discussed study by Faderl et al. also demonstrated clofarabine activity in patients with MDS [28]. In a small patient population, a CR rate of 25% was achieved in high-risk MDS patients. Subsequent studies looked at oral dosing of clofarabine and higher-risk MDS (Table 17.3). Thirty-two patients with intermediate- and high-risk disease based on the International Prognostic Scoring System were evaluated [29]. Nearly all of the patients had secondary MDS or were refractory to hypomethylating agents (HMA). Despite the population having a median age of 70 years, an ORR of 43% was seen, with 25% achieving complete remission. Toxicity increased at higher doses. Of

Table 17.3 Clofarabine studies in adults with higher-risk MDS

Study	Regimen	Patients (no.)	Median age (years)	ORR (%)	CR (%)	OS (months)
Faderl et al. [28][a]	Clofarabine + cytarabine	25	59	42	25	7.9
Faderl et al. [29][b]	Oral clofarabine	32	70	43	25	9.2 and 13.8
Faderl et al. [30][c]	Clofarabine	58	68	36	26	7.4, 13.4, and 21.7
Ghanem et al. [31][d]	Clofarabine	109	67	Not evaluated	Not evaluated	4.3

ALL acute lymphoblastic leukemia, *AML* acute myeloid leukemia, *CML-BP* chronic myeloid leukemia-blast phase, *CMML* chronic myelomonocytic leukemia, *CR* complete response, *MDS* myelodysplastic syndrome, *ORR* overall response rate, *OS* overall survival

[a]Median age of entire study population, which included ALL, MDS, and CML-BP, ORR/CR includes AML and MDS patients; OS of the entire study population

[b]OS, entire study population, 9.2 months; responders, 13.8 months

[c]OS, entire study population, 7.4 months; responders, 13.4 months; complete responders, 21.7 months

[d]MDS and CMML patients, post-clofarabine failure

note, 16% of patients experienced acute renal failure. Hepatic and gastrointestinal adverse events (AEs) were seen at all doses. The toxicity profile was studied further in a phase 2 trial; the results of which were reported in 2012. Fifty-eight patients with a median age of 68 years and higher-risk MDS were adaptively randomized to lower- and higher-dose treatment arms [30]. The side effect profile was similar for both arms and consistent with prior reports but more severe at the higher-dose level. The ORR was 36% with a CR rate of 26%. Despite the response rate seen in these trials, the majority of high-risk MDS patients will fail all available therapy or relapse quickly after response [31]. One hundred and nine patients with MDS or chronic myelomonocytic leukemia (CMML) and a median age of 67 years were evaluated. Of the patients evaluated, 38 had received clofarabine as first-line therapy, 59 received it after failing an HMA, and 22 had failed 2 or more MDS-directed therapies. Following failure, the OS in this patient population was 4.3 months, which correlates closely with OS post-HMA failure [31, 32]. Given that survival for high-risk MDS patients is between 11 and 13 months after clofarabine therapy, there remains significant opportunity to research and improve the outcomes of these patients [30, 31].

17.2.3 Acute Lymphoblastic Leukemia (ALL)

Two Southwest Oncology Group (SWOG) studies, led by Advani and colleagues, explored the use of clofarabine in adult ALL. In the first study, 37 patients were treated with clofarabine 40 mg/m^2/day and cytarabine 1 g/m^2/day on days 1–5 [33]. The median age was 41 years; 44% of patients were in a second or subsequent relapse or had refractory disease and 59% of patients had high-risk cytogenetics. Six out of thirty-six patients (17%) achieved a complete remission with or without complete count recovery. Median OS was 3 months. In the second study, SWOG study S0910, epratuzumab, a humanized monoclonal antibody against CD22, was combined with clofarabine and cytarabine in adults with relapsed/refractory pre-B ALL [34]. The complete remission rate with or without complete count recovery with the addition of epratuzumab was 52%.

Faderl and colleagues treated 50 patients with a median age of 30 years with clofarabine 40 mg/m^2 daily for 3 days and cyclophosphamide 200 mg/m^2 every 12 h for 3 days [35]. The response rate of the whole study group was 14%, including 10% of patients who achieved CR or CR without hematologic recovery. Three responses occurred in patients with primary refractory disease. The early mortality rate (<30 days) was 6%. The median duration of response was 69 days, and the median OS was 3 months. Another retrospective study of 55 patients treated with clofarabine combination therapy showed a 50% remission rate in relapsed/refractory patients, with 17–35% of patients proceeding to alloSCT [36].

17.3 Clofarabine for Pediatric Leukemia

Since the first phase 1 study of clofarabine was initiated in 1993 in adult patients with hematologic and solid malignancies [37], several clinical trials have demonstrated the clinical activity of clofarabine monotherapy for hematological malignancies. Moreover, combination regimens have been tested that leverage the pharmacological properties of clofarabine by combining it with traditional antileukemic drugs, revealing promising results [38–40]. Development of new therapeutic agents for children has historically lagged behind their introduction in adults. Most published studies of clofarabine have been conducted in adult patients with AML or MDS. However, unlike its predecessors, clofarabine was approved by the FDA in 2004 specifically for use in pediatric patients with relapsed or refractory ALL who have failed treatment with at least two prior regimens.

17.3.1 Clofarabine in Pediatric Acute Lymphoblastic Leukemia (ALL)

With contemporary first-line chemotherapy regimens, the vast majority of newly diagnosed pediatric patients with ALL will achieve remission, and the OS rate is approaching 90% [41]. Despite our overall success in treating newly diagnosed ALL, long-term cure rates for children who relapse remain poor, and relapsed ALL is still the leading cause of death among pediatric oncology patients [41]. The FDA approval of clofarabine was based on phase 1 and 2 studies in pediatric patients with refractory or relapsed ALL in which clofarabine monotherapy had demonstrated activity [42]. Based on the promising monotherapy data, several combinations of

Table 17.4 Published studies of clofarabine in children with ALL

	Phase	Combination	References
	Phase 1	CLO	[47]
CLO212	Phase 2	CLO	[42]
A report from UK	–	CLO (n = 5) CLO, CTX, VP (n = 18)	[83]
CLO21800205	Phase 1/2	CLO, CTX, VP	[43, 44]
Italian multicenter study	Phase 2	CLO, CTX, VP	[46]
Italian study	–	CLO, CTX, VP (n = 24)	[58]
COG AALL1131	Phase 3	CLO, CTX, VP, PEG, VCR	[57]
COG AAML0523	Phase 1/2	CLO, ara-C	[45]
POE07–01	Phase 1	CLO, CTX	[52]
VANDEVOL Study	Phase 1	CLO, Mito, VP, Asp, Dex	[53]
TVTC protocol	Phase 2	CLO, Thio, Topo, Vinorel, Dex	[59]
CoALL trial 08–09	Phase 2	CLO, PEG	[84]

ALL acute lymphoblastic leukemia, *ara-C* cytarabine, *Asp* L-asparaginase, *CLO* clofarabine, *CoALL* the German Co-operative Study Group for treatment of ALL, *CTX* cyclophosphamide, *Dex* dexamethasone, *Mito* mitoxantrone, *PEG* PEG-asparaginase, *Thio* thiotepa, *Topo* topotecan, *VCR* vincristine, Vinorel, vinorelbine, *VP* etoposide

clofarabine with other agents were subsequently evaluated in pediatric patients with relapsed ALL [43–46].

17.3.1.1 Clofarabine Monotherapy in Pediatric ALL

The initial phase 1 study of clofarabine monotherapy for children with ALL was done at MD Anderson Cancer Center in conjunction with a study in adults [15, 47] (Table 17.4). Twenty-five children with ALL (n = 8) or AML (n = 17) received six dose levels between 11.25 and 70 mg/m^2 IV over 1 h for 5 consecutive days. Five patients (one AML and four ALL) achieved CR, and three patients (two AML and one ALL) achieved a partial response (PR), yielding an ORR of 32%. Four out of 17 children (24%) with ALL and one of eight patients with AML (13%) attained CR. The DLTs were reversible hepatotoxicity and skin rash, which were seen at 70 mg/m^2/day for 5 days, and the MTD was 52 mg/m^2/day for 5 days.

A phase 2 study of clofarabine monotherapy was conducted in several institutions across the US [42]. Sixty-one children with ALL had received a median number of three prior regimens (range 2–6), including prior hematopoietic stem cell transplantation (HSCT) in 30% of the patients, and 35 patients (57%) were refractory to the last salvage regimen received before clofarabine. Patients received clofarabine at the MTD of 52 mg/m^2/day for 5 days every 2–6 weeks [42] (Table 17.4). Of the 61 children in the study, seven (12%) attained CR and five (8%) CR without platelet recovery (CRp) for an ORR of 20%; 10% had PR. The remission was durable, and patients were able to proceed to HSCT after receiving clofarabine. Remissions were sustained in patients who did not undergo an HSCT for a median of 6 weeks. Four patients remained in CR or CRp for 8+, 12, 37+, and 48 weeks after receiving only clofarabine. Febrile neutropenia, anorexia, hypotension, and nausea were the most common side effects.

Another phase 2 study of clofarabine monotherapy was conducted in Europe [48]. In this study, 65 pediatric patients with relapsed/refractory ALL were enrolled, and data from the first 53 patients have been presented. In this study, patients received clofarabine also at the MTD of 52 mg/m^2 for 5 days. Fourteen of fifty-three (26%) patients who received at least one course of clofarabine had a response: six achieved CR, seven CRp, and one PR. Four patients proceeded to HSCT after receiving clofarabine, and one patient had durable remission for 20+ months. Three patients developed liver toxicity (hyperbilirubinemia, transaminitis).

17.3.1.2 Clofarabine Combination Therapy

There are a few clofarabine combinations that have been studied based on the mechanism of action of clofarabine. As an inhibitor of ribonucleotide reductase (RnR), clofarabine accumulates cytarabine triphosphate in leukemic cells, thereby increasing the antileukemic activity of cytarabine [40, 49]. Clofarabine also causes depletion of dNTPs, resulting in the inhibition of deoxycytidine kinase through a feedback mechanism. Thus, a combination of clofarabine and cytarabine increases retention of ara-CTP. This combination has been widely investigated in various studies in adult AML [28], pediatric ALL [50], and pediatric AML [51].

Clofarabine inhibits DNA synthesis as well as repair [43]; therefore, combinations of clofarabine and different DNA-damaging agents such as cyclophosphamide [38, 44, 52], epipodophyllotoxins [44, 53], anthracyclines [26], and anthracenedione [53, 54] have also been explored. An in vitro study showed that the cross-links were rapidly repaired in chronic lymphocytic lymphoma (CLL) lymphocytes after exposure to activated cyclophosphamide or 4-hydroperoxycyclophosphamide (4-HC), but DNA repair was impaired when the cells were pretreated with clofarabine [55]. A combination treatment with 4-HC and clofarabine had a synergistic effect on apoptotic cell death, greater than the sum of the effect of each agent [55]. In a phase 1 study of clofarabine and cyclophosphamide in adult patients with leukemia [38], 18 patients received cyclophosphamide (200 mg/m^2) alone on day 0 and clofarabine (20 mg/m^2 and 10 mg/m^2 as dose level 1 [n = 6] and 0 [n = 12], respectively) plus cyclophosphamide on day 1. Prolonged bone marrow suppression was seen as the DLT at dose level 1. Increased DNA damage measured as H2AX phosphorylation was observed in 12 of 13 patients with clofarabine and cyclophosphamide compared with cyclophosphamide alone.

17.3.1.3 Clofarabine Combination Therapy Studies in Pediatric ALL

Clofarabine in Combination with Cyclophosphamide and Etoposide

A combination of clofarabine with cyclophosphamide and etoposide was designed based on evidence of the synergistic effect of clofarabine and DNA-damaging agents [38, 55], as well as previous experience with a regimen of cyclophosphamide and etoposide [56] (Table 17.4). A phase 1/2 study [43, 44] of this combination was conducted. In the phase 1 portion, the primary objectives were to determine the DLT, MTD, and recommended doses for the phase 2 portion of the study [44]. All three drugs were given IV for 5 consecutive days in induction and for 4 consecutive days in consolidation, for a maximum of eight cycles. G-CSF was given to 25 patients (20 with ALL and five with AML) enrolled in 5 cohorts starting 1 day after the last dose of study treatment and continuing until an absolute neutrophil count of 0.75×10^9/L was reached. No DLT was seen in cohorts 1–3. A patient in cohort 4 (clofarabine 30 mg/m^2/day, cyclophosphamide 440 mg/m^2/day, and etoposide 100 mg/m^2/day) had a DLT of grade 3 lipase elevation, grade 3 abdominal pain, and hepatomegaly. Symptoms for which veno-occlusive disease (VOD) could not be excluded occurred in this patient but resolved without any sequelae. Pancreatitis (grade 2) and lipase elevation (grade 3) were observed in another patient in this cohort, but neither met the DLT criteria. This cohort was expanded to ten patients, and no further DLTs occurred. In cohort 5 (clofarabine 40 mg/m^2/day, cyclophosphamide 440 mg/m^2/day, and etoposide 100 mg/m^2/day), a DLT of prolonged bone marrow aplasia beyond day 42 was observed in one patient. Five additional patients were enrolled in cohort 5, and no further DLTs occurred; therefore, MTD was not reached, and the recommended phase 2 doses were determined to be clofarabine 40 mg/m^2/day, cyclophosphamide 440 mg/m^2/day, and etoposide 100 mg/m^2/day for 5 consecutive days. In the phase 1 study, CR was attained in nine patients and CRp in two patients among the 20 patients with ALL. All five patients with AML attained CR ($n = 1$) or CRp ($n = 4$). Nine out of sixteen responders proceeded to HSCT.

In the phase 2 portion of the study [43], patients aged 1–21 years with refractory/relapsed ALL were enrolled and received treatment at the recommended dose determined in the phase 1 study (Table 17.4). The primary end point of this study was an overall remission rate (ORR = CR + CRp). Minimal residual disease (MRD) by flow cytometry was evaluated as an exploratory end point. Among the 25 patients enrolled in this study, 14 had two prior induction regimens, seven had three prior induction regimens, and four had one prior induction regimen. Notably, 15 patients (60%) had disease refractory to the immediately preceding regimen and four patients had received a prior HSCT. The ORR was 44%, which comprised seven patients who achieved CR (28%) and four who achieved CRp (16%). In addition, three patients (12%) achieved PR. MRD was evaluable in eight patients. Five of the eight patients were MRD negative (defined as <0.01%), and three were MRD positive. A total of 10 patients, which included 7 of 11 responders, proceeded to HSCT. The median number of cycles patients received was one (range: 1–3). Ten of eleven responders achieved the best response after one cycle. Treatment-related AEs that occurred in ≥25% of patients were as follows: vomiting (88%); nausea (72%); febrile neutropenia and thrombocytopenia (60% each); anemia (56%); neutropenia and pyrexia (52% each); decreased appetite (44%); ALT increased, AST increased, hypokalemia, and hypotension (36% each); diarrhea (28%); and hyperbilirubinemia (28%). Treatment was discontinued for one patient because of fungal sinusitis, which occurred 17 days after the last dose of study drug. Eighty-eight percent of patients had serious AEs, regardless of relationship to study drug. It should be noted that six patients (24%) died within 30 days of the last dose of study treatment; these deaths were attributed to hepatic VOD (two patients), septic shock (two patients), pulmonary edema (one patient), and infection (one patient). Four of the initial eight patients developed severe hepatotoxicity, and two of the patients with VOD had prior HSCT within 12 months. Therefore, the protocol was amended to exclude patients with prior HSCT, viral hepatitis and/or cirrhosis, or elevated conjugated bilirubin levels at study entry; there were no further events of severe liver toxicity in the remaining 17 patients. Nevertheless, among all 25 patients enrolled, the incidence of severe infections (grade 3 or greater) was high (72%). The study concluded that the combination treatment of clofarabine, etoposide, and cyclophosphamide in pediatric patients with refractory or relapsed ALL was effective in heavily treated patients but also suggested a need for optimization of the regimen with careful patient selection, dosing, and better supportive care to minimize toxicity.

The Children's Oncology Group (COG) included this regimen in the post-induction consolidation phase for newly diagnosed, very high-risk patients with pre-B ALL [57]. The patients were randomized to a control arm (cyclophosphamide, fractionated cytarabine, mercaptopurine), experimental arm 1 (cyclophosphamide and etoposide), or experimental arm 2 (clofarabine 30 mg/m^2 for 5 days, cyclophosphamide, and etoposide). All arms included vincristine and PEG-asparaginase, which were identical. More grade 4–5 infections and pancreatitis were seen in experimental arm 2 compared to the control arm or experimental arm 1. The dose of clofarabine was then reduced to 20 mg/m^2 for 5 days and myeloid growth factor was required. However, 3 of 39 patients in experimental arm 2 with clofarabine developed grade 4 infections, compared to none in the control arm (n = 20) or experimental arm (n = 47). In addition, one of the patients who had a grade 4 infection developed grade 5 renal toxicity. Based on these results, experimental arm 2 was permanently closed.

Other studies using the same drug combination (clofarabine, cyclophosphamide, etoposide) [46, 58] had more favorable toxicity profiles but a similar efficacy. A study by Miano et al. investigated the same doses of the drugs used in the study described above (clofarabine 40 mg/m^2/day, cyclophosphamide 440 mg/m^2/day, and etoposide 100 mg/m^2/day for 5 days). A total of 40 children with refractory or relapsed acute leukemia (24 ALL and 16 AML) were treated. Twenty of forty patients (50%) had prior HSCT. Seventeen patients (43%) had an overall response after the first cycle, which included nine CR (22%), eight CRp (15%), and two PR (5%). Seven of sixteen AML patients (44%) and ten of twenty-four ALL patients (42%) were responders. Twenty-six patients (65%) had at least one grade 3–4 toxicity, of which the most common toxicity was infection. Two patients who received the study treatment after HSCT died due to infection following prolonged bone marrow suppression after the first cycle. However, no death from liver toxicity was reported in this study. Locatelli et al. [46] used a slightly different dosing schedule: clofarabine 40 mg/m^2/day, cyclophosphamide 400 mg/m^2/day, and etoposide 150 mg/m^2/day for 5 days (Table 17.4). Twenty-five children with refractory or multiple-relapsed ALL were enrolled in this study. Among them, eight patients were in a second (n = 6) or third (n = 2) relapse, and 17 patients were resistant to the last course of chemotherapy. Thirteen patients (52%) achieved CR and one (4%) achieved CRp; therefore, the ORR was 56%. Seven of the 13 patients (54%) who achieved a response proceeded to HSCT. The regimen was reported to be well tolerated. Febrile neutropenia, mucositis, and reversible liver toxicity were the most common AEs, but there were no cases of VOD, and most notably, no patients died of treatment-related complications. It should be noted that all patients received prophylactic antibiotics. Vigilant supportive care and dose modification may help to improve toxicity profiles with this regimen.

Clofarabine in Combination with Cytarabine

The COG conducted a phase 1/2 study of the combination of clofarabine and cytarabine in pediatric patients with ALL in second or subsequent relapse and AML in first relapse [50, 51] (Table 17.4). In the phase 1 portion of the study, cytarabine 1 g/m^2 was given on days 1–5, and clofarabine in varying doses was given on days 2–6. Ten patients were enrolled in each dose cohort. The first cohort of patients received clofarabine at 40 mg/m^2/day. Among the ten patients enrolled on the first cohort, eight patients had ALL and two had AML. Fever and neutropenia, infection, and transaminitis were the most common grade 3 or greater toxicities. DLT was observed in two ALL patients with prior HSCT: grade 4 fungal infection and pneumonitis in one patient and grade 4 fungal infection in the other. The MTD was not reached, and ten patients (three patients with ALL in second relapse and seven with AML) were enrolled in the second cohort with clofarabine 52 mg/m^2, which is the pediatric single-agent MTD. Ten patients completed cycle 1, and seven of them also received cycle 2. Diarrhea, nausea, febrile neutropenia, and infection were the most common grade 3 or greater toxicities in both cycles. In this cohort, one patient with AML experienced DLT of prolonged bone marrow aplasia, grade 4 hypokalemia, grade 3 nausea, and grade 3 dehydration.

Other Combinations of Clofarabine

Other combinations of clofarabine investigated in pediatric clinical trials are summarized in Table 17.4. Time sequential combination of clofarabine followed by cyclophosphamide was tested in a phase 1 study by POETIC (Pediatric Oncology Experimental Therapeutics Investigator's Consortium) [52]. Another objective of that study was to determine the MTD of this combination in children with relapsed/refractory leukemia as well as test whether clofarabine would augment cyclophosphamide-mediated toxicity by inhibiting repair of cyclophosphamide-induced DNA strand breaks.

The VANDEVOL study of the French SFCE Acute Leukemia Committee was a phase 1 study of escalating doses of clofarabine (20–40 mg/m^2) with fixed doses of mitoxantrone, etoposide, asparaginase, and dexamethasone [53]. Twenty patients with very early, second, or posttransplant relapse of ALL were enrolled and 19 of them were evaluable. DLT (liver) occurred at the clofarabine dose of 32 mg/m^2 in one of six patients. Four patients treated at the dose level of clofarabine 40 mg/m^2 had DLT (two fungal infections and two liver). MTD was determined to be 32 mg/m^2. Eleven of nineteen patients (57.9%) achieved CR. There were no deaths related to the treatment in this study.

The TVTC regimen (clofarabine with topotecan, vinorelbine, and thiotepa) was tested in a phase 1/2 study. In the phase 2 portion of the study, 17 patients with relapsed or refractory ALL, AML, or biphenotypic leukemia were treated [59]. The

ORR was 69%, which included ten patients who achieved CR and one who achieved CRp. Of note, 8 of 12 (67%) patients with relapsed/refractory AML achieved CR or CRp. The most common grade 3 or greater toxicities were febrile neutropenia (82%) and transaminitis (47%).

17.3.2 Clofarabine for Pediatric AML

The OS rate in pediatric acute myeloid leukemia has improved significantly in recent decades, from less than 40% to more than 70% [60, 61]. This has been achieved by treatment intensification, improved supportive care, and progress in alloSCT. The most important and effective anticancer agents used in AML are anthracyclines and cytarabine, including their analogues, and the combination of cytarabine, daunorubicin, and etoposide has been established as standard in both children and adults with AML. Variations in scheduling of formulation (i.e., liposomal daunorubicin) aimed to increase intensity or to reduce toxicities. Despite all these efforts, approximately 30% of children with AML relapse and succumb to the disease. In AML relapse, a combination of fludarabine and cytarabine is one of the most commonly used treatment regimens. It is typically used with G-CSF, which is considered to have priming effect (FLAG). The recent International AML Relapse 2001/01 trial showed an OS rate of 38% in children with first relapse or primary refractory disease [62, 63]. The re-induction utilized the synergism of cytarabine and fludarabine. The randomized addition of liposomal daunorubicin demonstrated benefit mostly in relapsed core-binding leukemia (t (8; 21); inv. (16)). The OS rate in this study was approximately 60% [63]. Nevertheless, further improvement of outcomes of both de novo and relapsed pediatric AML is urgently needed. Although it would be preferable to develop compounds that have precise targets or use immunotherapies, only conventional cytotoxic chemotherapeutic drugs with or without alloSCT have been proven to cure children with AML.

As described above, clofarabine, as a structural hybrid of fludarabine and cladribine, inhibits both DNA polymerase and RnR and results in induction of apoptosis [64] and enhanced accumulation of cytarabine in lymphocytes [65]. In vitro studies showed a particular sensitivity of AML blasts to the combination and synergy of clofarabine with cytarabine, but epigenetic drugs such as decitabine have also been shown to have synergy with clofarabine in vitro [25, 40, 66].

The initial phase 1 trial of clofarabine monotherapy in pediatric ALL described above included children with AML ($n = 8$) who were heavily pretreated. Only one of the eight patients achieved CR [47]. The phase 2 trial in relapsed/refractory pediatric AML enrolled 42 children, and only 11 responded. The ORR was just 26% (1 CRp and 10 PR). Following alloSCT, three children remained in remission for more than a year [67]. Usually, children with AML in a second relapse or refractory to relapse treatment receive a significant amount of purine analogues including similar compounds such as cytarabine, fludarabine, and cladribine. This might explain the limited efficacy in these heavily pretreated patient groups.

In adults with AML, several clinical trials at different stages of disease and ages have been performed. In most trials, superior response rates in comparison to placebo or other chemotherapy-based regimens have been reported [19, 20, 23, 27, 68]. Regarding OS, the results are conflicting. In trials enrolling elderly patients with AML (median age >70 years), not unexpectedly, higher morbidity and mortality, mostly due to infections, have been observed that counterbalance the higher response rates [20]. By contrast, in younger adults with AML, some trials demonstrated a better EFS, disease-free survival (DFS), or OS in patients treated with combinations including clofarabine. In a randomized trial of clofarabine/cytarabine versus idarubicin/cytarabine, Nazha et al. showed an improved EFS, DFS, and OS in AML patients younger than 60 years of age [27]. The detailed analysis confirmed that this result was mainly due to improvements in patients younger than 40 years and in those in an unfavorable genetic risk group.

Supported by these data, several pediatric study groups evaluated clofarabine in pediatric AML. The CLOUD trial applied an intermediate dosage of clofarabine (30 mg/m^2) in combination with liposomal daunorubicin (60 mg/m^2) in children with relapse within 12 months of initial AML diagnosis, refractory to induction therapy, or in a second or subsequent relapse [69]. Out of nine children, three achieved CR and proceeded to alloSCT (personal communication). The St. Jude Group demonstrated the feasibility of combining clofarabine, cytarabine, and the multikinase inhibitor sorafenib in refractory and relapsed pediatric AML [70]. The COG AAML0523 study (cytarabine 1 g/m^2 with clofarabine 52 mg/m^2) almost exclusively focused on children at first relapse [51]. The study resulted in an ORR of 48% in 48 evaluable patients, and 21 of 23 responders underwent alloSCT. The OS rate at 3 years was 46% ± 27% for responders, which included mostly patients with low-risk characteristics, compared to a 3-year OS rate of 16% for nonresponders.

A recently completed phase 1/2 trial with 34 heavily pretreated children with refractory or relapsed AML (early first relapse, n = 15; refractory first relapse, n = 11; second or subsequent relapse, n = 8) combined clofarabine, liposomal daunorubicin, and cytarabine (CLARA-L-DNR). The response rate, including CR and CR with incomplete hematological recovery, was 59%. The treatment schedule was based on an adapted Faderl regimen developed in adult AML [23, 71, 72]. The final recommended schedule was clofarabine 40 mg/m^2 for 5 days, liposomal daunorubicin 60 mg/m^2 for 3 days, and cytarabine 2 g/m^2 for 5 days. Subsequent stem cell transplantation (SCT) was left at the discretion of the treating physician. No particular toxicities were noted during the SCT procedure, and pretreatment with this chemotherapy combination did not preclude a successful SCT procedure. The 1-year projected overall survival (pOS) was 53 ± 9%. This was even higher in responding patients (n = 21) with a 1-year pOS of 75.9% (SE 9.4%) and a 1-year projected event-free survival (pEFS) of 56.1% (SE 11%) [73]. In general, the combination of clofarabine, liposomal daunorubicin, and high-dose cytarabine was well tolerated, after excluding patients with subclinical fungal infections. Most observed AEs were expected (febrile neutropenia and infections, gastrointestinal symptoms, dermatological manifestations, and pain).

Based on the promising data in adults with AML and subsequent pediatric trials, the AML-BFM study group investigated clofarabine as a first-line treatment. The prospective randomized AML-BFM 2012 trial compared standard ADxE (cytarabine, liposomal daunorubicin, etoposide) and a combination of clofarabine, cytarabine, and liposomal daunorubicin (CDxA). In this ongoing trial, the toxicity rates were closely monitored because intensification and the occurrence of unusual side effects should be documented. Since clofarabine is clearly an effective cytostatic drug, myelosuppression and all associated complications are expected. Specifically, a greater incidence of clofarabine-associated skin toxicities and capillary leak syndrome is anticipated. On the other hand, better efficacy in acute monoblastic leukemia, and possibly in cytogenetically high-risk patients, may also be possible.

17.4 Other Aspects of Clofarabine

17.4.1 Clofarabine as a Conditioning Regimen for Allogeneic Stem Cell Transplant (alloSCT)

Conditioning regimens for alloSCT are used for immunosuppression to prevent graft rejection and for eradiating residual tumor cells. Fludarabine is a potent immunosuppressant but does not have great anticancer activity against leukemia or MDS [74]. Given the antileukemic activity of clofarabine and its similar mechanism of action to fludarabine, a number of studies have substituted clofarabine in place of fludarabine in conditioning regimens. Some utilized a clofarabine combination to reduce the intensity or toxicity of the conditioning regimens. Table 17.5 summarizes pediatric and adult studies of the use of clofarabine as a conditioning regimen for alloSCT.

Several studies have evaluated the use clofarabine-based conditioning regimens for patients with active disease at the time of transplantation [75, 76]. Chevallier reported a retrospective study of 90 patients with acute leukemia receiving a clofarabine-containing reduced-intensity conditioning regimen. In this series, 73% of patients had active disease at the time of transplantation, and 38 patients had received prior SCT. The 2-year OS rate of patients with AML was 35%, compared to 0% in ALL. To better evaluate the utility of clofarabine, Chevallier designed a prospective, multicenter phase 2 trial testing the use of clofarabine as part of the conditioning regimen in combination with IV busulfan and antithymocyte globulin [77]. Thirty patients with high-risk myelodysplastic syndromes (MDS) or acute leukemia in remission at the time of transplantation were treated. Engraftment occurred in 100% of patients. The 1-year OS rate was 63%. Patients with MDS and AML had better outcomes in terms of survival and relapse than patients with ALL or biphenotypic leukemia [77]. Conditioning regimens using clofarabine in combination with melphalan with and without alemtuzumab have also been studied [74, 78]. These studies show a similarly favorable engraftment rate and toxicity profile.

Table 17.5 Clofarabine as part of a conditioning regimen before hematopoietic stem cell transplant for leukemia in adults and children

	Patient population			
Combination	Diagnosis	Median age (range) (years)	Note	References
Bu, CLO	AML, ALL, MDS	63.5 (25–74)	Phase 2, reduced intensity	[85]
Flu, CLO, Thio, Mel	ALL, MDS/JMML, relapsed solid tumors, nonmalignant diseases	9 (2–18)	αβ T- and B-cell–depleted allografts from haploidentical family donors	[86]
CLO, Bu	AML ALL, MDS biphenotypic leukemia	59 (20.6–64.5)	Reduced toxicity	[77]
Bu, CLO	ALL	36 (20–64)		[87]
CLO, Mel	AML, MDS, NHL, other hem malignancy	54 (21–73)	Phase 1 and 2	[78]
CLO, Mel	AML, ALL, or MDS	62.8 (30.5–65.7)	Reduced intensity	[74]
Bu, CLO	AML, CML, ALL, CLL, NHL, MDS, MM	53 (1–68)	Phase 1 and 2	[88]
CLO, ara-C, ATG	AML, MDS	54 (24–68)	Reduced intensity	[76]
CLO, Bu, ATG	AML, MDS, ALL, biphenotypic leukemia	59 (20.6–64.5)	Phase 2, reduced toxicity	[77]

ALL acute lymphoblastic leukemia, *AML* acute myeloid leukemia, *ara-C* cytarabine, *ATG* antithymocyte globulin, *Bu* busulfan, *CLO* clofarabine, *CLL* chronic lymphocytic leukemia, *CML* chronic myeloid leukemia, *Flu* fludarabine, *JMML* juvenile myelomonocytic leukemia, *MDS* myelodysplastic syndrome, *Mel* melphalan, *MM* multiple myeloma, *NHL* non-Hodgkin's lymphoma, *Thio* thiotepa

17.4.2 Clofarabine for Refractory Histiocytosis

In the last several years, clofarabine has emerged as a promising agent for refractory histiocytosis. Prednisone and vinblastine have been considered to be a standard treatment for patients with refractory Langerhans cell histiocytosis (LCH) who require systemic therapy, but agents used for AML, including clofarabine, cladribine, and cytarabine, have shown efficacy in refractory patients [79]. This efficacy of purine analogues is thought to be attributed to an effect on immature myeloid precursors identified at the origin of LCH pathogenesis [79]. Clofarabine has shown activity in patients with LCH who were refractory to cytarabine or cladribine [80–82], as well as in children with other histiocytic disorders such as juvenile xanthogranuloma and Rosai-Dorfman disease [80]. In one of the case series [80], 18 children (11 LCH, 4 juvenile xanthogranuloma, and 3 Rosai-Dorfman disease) received clofarabine monotherapy after a median of 3 prior regimens. Most patients received clofarabine 25 mg/m^2/day for 5 days, which was repeated every 28 days for a median of six cycles (range 2–8 cycles). Seventeen patients were alive and showed disease improvement after two to four cycles of clofarabine. Eleven of seventeen patients achieved CR and 4 achieved PR. All patients developed neutropenia [80].

17.5 Conclusion

Clofarabine is a cytotoxic, second-generation purine nucleoside analogue with significant activity against leukemia as a single agent. Several clofarabine combination regimens have been explored and have shown promising results. For adult leukemia, clofarabine is generally well tolerated; however, its efficacy as monotherapy is disappointing, particularly in AML, where it has been most extensively studied. Preliminary efficacy data in MDS and ALL has not been impressive enough to move the drug forward into routine use. Clofarabine does have a role in the treatment of AML when combined with other agents. In pediatric ALL and AML, several clofarabine combination regimens have been explored. Despite encouraging efficacy results, there is concern regarding significant toxicities with some combinations. Dose modifications or supportive care may be helpful. Clofarabine has also shown promise as a conditioning regimen for SCT and in the treatment of refractory histiocytosis.

References

1. Hijiya N, Barry E, Arceci RJ. Clofarabine in pediatric acute leukemia: current findings and issues. Pediatr Blood Cancer. 2012;59(3):417–22. doi:10.1002/pbc.24112.
2. Parker WB, Shaddix SC, Chang CH, White EL, Rose LM, Brockman RW, et al. Effects of 2-chloro-9-(2-deoxy-2-fluoro-beta-D-arabinofuranosyl)adenine on K562 cellular metabolism and the inhibition of human ribonucleotide reductase and DNA polymerases by its 5′-triphosphate. Cancer Res. 1991;51(9):2386–94.
3. Lotfi K, Mansson E, Spasokoukotskaja T, Pettersson B, Liliemark J, Peterson C, et al. Biochemical pharmacology and resistance to 2-chloro-2′-arabino-fluoro-2′-deoxyadenosine, a novel analogue of cladribine in human leukemic cells. Clin Cancer Res. 1999;5(9):2438–44.
4. Parker WB, Allan PW, Hassan AE, Secrist 3rd JA, Sorscher EJ, Waud WR. Antitumor activity of 2-fluoro-2′-deoxyadenosine against tumors that express *Escherichia coli* purine nucleoside phosphorylase. Cancer Gene Ther. 2003;10(1):23–9. doi:10.1038/sj.cgt.7700520.
5. Xie C, Plunkett W. Metabolism and actions of 2-chloro-9-(2-deoxy-2-fluoro-beta-D-arabinofuranosyl)-adenine in human lymphoblastoid cells. Cancer Res. 1995;55(13):2847–52.
6. Genini D, Adachi S, Chao Q, Rose DW, Carrera CJ, Cottam HB, et al. Deoxyadenosine analogs induce programmed cell death in chronic lymphocytic leukemia cells by damaging the DNA and by directly affecting the mitochondria. Blood. 2000;96(10):3537–43.
7. American Cancer Society. Cancer facts and figures 2016. http://www.cancer.org/acs/groups/content/@research/documents/document/acspc-047079.pdf. Accessed 20 June 2016.
8. Howlader N, Noone A, Krapcho M, Miller D, Bishop K, Altekruse S, et al., editors. SEER cancer statistics review, 1975–2013. Bethesda: National Cancer Institute; 2014.
9. Waud WR, Schmid SM, Montgomery JA, Secrist 3rd JA. Preclinical antitumor activity of 2-chloro-9-(2-deoxy-2-fluoro-beta-D- arabinofuranosyl)adenine (Cl-F-ara-A). Nucleosides Nucleotides Nucleic Acids. 2000;19(1–2):447–60. doi:10.1080/15257770008033020.
10. Montgomery JA, Shortnacy-Fowler AT, Clayton SD, Riordan JM, Secrist III JA. Synthesis and biologic activity of 2′-fluoro-2-halo derivatives of 9-beta-D-arabinofuranosyladenine. J Med Chem. 1992;35(2):397–401.
11. Takahashi T, Kanazawa J, Akinaga S, Tamaoki T, Okabe M. Antitumor activity of 2-chloro-9-(2-deoxy-2-fluoro-beta-D-arabinofuranosyl) adenine, a novel deoxyadenosine analog, against

human colon tumor xenografts by oral administration. Cancer Chemother Pharmacol. 1999;43(3):233–40.
12. Carson DA, Wasson DB, Esparza LM, Carrera CJ, Kipps TJ, Cottam HB. Oral antilymphocyte activity and induction of apoptosis by 2-chloro-2′-arabino-fluoro-2′-deoxyadenosine. Proc Natl Acad Sci U S A. 1992;89(7):2970–4.
13. Dykes D. Response of subcutaneous HT-29 colon tumor to combination treatment with oxaliplatin and clofarabine. Birmingham: Southern Research Institute; 2003.
14. Dykes D. Response of subcutaneous CCRF-CEM leukemia to combination treatment with Ara C and clofarabine. Birmingham: Southern Research Institute; 2002.
15. Kantarjian HM, Gandhi V, Kozuch P, Faderl S, Giles F, Cortes J, et al. Phase I clinical and pharmacology study of clofarabine in patients with solid and hematologic cancers. J Clin Oncol. 2003;21(6):1167–73.
16. Kantarjian H, Gandhi V, Cortes J, Verstovsek S, Du M, Garcia-Manero G, et al. Phase 2 clinical and pharmacologic study of clofarabine in patients with refractory or relapsed acute leukemia. Blood. 2003;102(7):2379–86. doi:10.1182/blood-2003-03-0925.
17. Dohner H, Weisdorf DJ, Bloomfield CD. Acute myeloid leukemia. N Engl J Med. 2015;373(12):1136–52. doi:10.1056/NEJMra1406184.
18. Estey E. Acute myeloid leukemia and myelodysplastic syndromes in older patients. J Clin Oncol. 2007;25(14):1908–15. doi:10.1200/JCO.2006.10.2731.
19. Kantarjian HM, Erba HP, Claxton D, Arellano M, Lyons RM, Kovascovics T, et al. Phase II study of clofarabine monotherapy in previously untreated older adults with acute myeloid leukemia and unfavorable prognostic factors. J Clin Oncol. 2010;28(4):549–55. doi:10.1200/JCO.2009.23.3130.
20. Burnett AK, Russell NH, Hunter AE, Milligan D, Knapper S, Wheatley K, et al. Clofarabine doubles the response rate in older patients with acute myeloid leukemia but does not improve survival. Blood. 2013;122(8):1384–94. doi:10.1182/blood-2013-04-496596.
21. Foran J, Sun Z, Claxton D, et al. North American Leukemia, Intergroup phase III randomized trial of single-agent clofarabine as induction and post-remission therapy, and decitabine as maintenance therapy in newly-diagnosed acute myeloid leukemia in older adults (age > 60 years): a trial of the ECOG-ACRIN Cancer Research Group. Paper presented at the American Society of Hematology Annual Meeting, December 3; 2015.
22. Becker PS, Kantarjian HM, Appelbaum FR, Petersdorf SH, Storer B, Pierce S, et al. Clofarabine with high dose cytarabine and granulocyte colony-stimulating factor (G-CSF) priming for relapsed and refractory acute myeloid leukaemia. Br J Haematol. 2011;155(2):182–9. doi:10.1111/j.1365-2141.2011.08831.x.
23. Faderl S, Wetzler M, Rizzieri D, Schiller G, Jagasia M, Stuart R, et al. Clofarabine plus cytarabine compared with cytarabine alone in older patients with relapsed or refractory acute myelogenous leukemia: results from the CLASSIC I trial. J Clin Oncol. 2012;30(20):2492–9. doi:10.1200/JCO.2011.37.9743.
24. Faderl S, Ravandi F, Huang X, Garcia-Manero G, Ferrajoli A, Estrov Z, et al. A randomized study of clofarabine versus clofarabine plus low-dose cytarabine as front-line therapy for patients aged 60 years and older with acute myeloid leukemia and high-risk myelodysplastic syndrome. Blood. 2008;112(5):1638–45. doi:10.1182/blood-2007-11-124602.
25. Kadia TM, Faderl S, Ravandi F, Jabbour E, Garcia-Manero G, Borthakur G, et al. Final results of a phase 2 trial of clofarabine and low-dose cytarabine alternating with decitabine in older patients with newly diagnosed acute myeloid leukemia. Cancer. 2015;121(14):2375–82. doi:10.1002/cncr.29367.
26. Faderl S, Ferrajoli A, Wierda W, Huang X, Verstovsek S, Ravandi F, et al. Clofarabine combinations as acute myeloid leukemia salvage therapy. Cancer. 2008;113(8):2090–6. doi:10.1002/cncr.23816.
27. Nazha A, Kantarjian H, Ravandi F, Huang X, Choi S, Garcia-Manero G, et al. Clofarabine, idarubicin, and cytarabine (CIA) as frontline therapy for patients </=60 years with newly diagnosed acute myeloid leukemia. Am J Hematol. 2013;88(11):961–6. doi:10.1002/ajh.23544.

28. Faderl S, Gandhi V, O'Brien S, Bonate P, Cortes J, Estey E, et al. Results of a phase 1-2 study of clofarabine in combination with cytarabine (ara-C) in relapsed and refractory acute leukemias. Blood. 2005;105(3):940–7. doi:10.1182/blood-2004-05-1933.
29. Faderl S, Garcia-Manero G, Estrov Z, Ravandi F, Borthakur G, Cortes JE, et al. Oral clofarabine in the treatment of patients with higher-risk myelodysplastic syndrome. J Clin Oncol. 2010;28(16):2755–60. doi:10.1200/JCO.2009.26.3509.
30. Faderl S, Garcia-Manero G, Jabbour E, Ravandi F, Borthakur G, Estrov Z, et al. A randomized study of 2 dose levels of intravenous clofarabine in the treatment of patients with higher-risk myelodysplastic syndrome. Cancer. 2012;118(3):722–8. doi:10.1002/cncr.26327.
31. Ghanem H, Garcia-Manero G, Faderl S, Ravandi F, Cortes J, Katragadda L, et al. Outcomes of patients with myelodysplatic syndrome and chronic myelomonocytic leukemia post clofarabine failure. Ther Adv Hematol. 2014;5(2):29–34. doi:10.1177/2040620713519742.
32. Jabbour E, Garcia-Manero G, Batty N, Shan J, O'Brien S, Cortes J, et al. Outcome of patients with myelodysplastic syndrome after failure of decitabine therapy. Cancer. 2010;116(16):3830–4. doi:10.1002/cncr.25247.
33. Advani AS, Gundacker HM, Sala-Torra O, Radich JP, Lai R, Slovak ML, et al. Southwest Oncology Group Study S0530: a phase 2 trial of clofarabine and cytarabine for relapsed or refractory acute lymphocytic leukaemia. Br J Haematol. 2010;151(5):430–4.
34. Advani AS, McDonough S, Coutre S, Wood B, Radich J, Mims M, et al. SWOG S0910: a phase 2 trial of clofarabine/cytarabine/epratuzumab for relapsed/refractory acute lymphocytic leukaemia. Br J Haematol. 2014;165(4):504–9. doi:10.1111/bjh.12778.
35. Faderl S, Balakrishnan K, Thomas DA, Ravandi F, Borthakur G, Burger J, et al. Phase I and extension study of clofarabine plus cyclophosphamide in patients with relapsed/refractory acute lymphoblastic leukemia. Clin Lymphoma Myeloma Leuk. 2014;14(3):231–8. doi:10.1016/j.clml.2013.12.001.
36. Huguet F, Leguay T, Raffoux E, Rousselot P, Vey N, Pigneux A, et al. Clofarabine for the treatment of adult acute lymphoid leukemia: the Group for Research on Adult Acute Lymphoblastic Leukemia intergroup. Leuk Lymphoma. 2015;56(4):847–57. doi:10.3109/10428194.2014.887708.
37. Faderl S, Gandhi V, Keating MJ, Jeha S, Plunkett W, Kantarjian HM. The role of clofarabine in hematologic and solid malignancies – development of a next-generation nucleoside analog. Cancer. 2005;103(10):1985–95. doi:10.1002/cncr.21005.
38. Karp JE, Ricklis RM, Balakrishnan K, Briel J, Greer J, Gore SD, et al. A phase 1 clinical-laboratory study of clofarabine followed by cyclophosphamide for adults with refractory acute leukemias. Blood. 2007;110(6):1762–9. doi:10.1182/blood-2007-03-081364.
39. Faderl S, Verstovsek S, Cortes J, Ravandi F, Beran M, Garcia-Manero G, et al. Clofarabine and cytarabine combination as induction therapy for acute myeloid leukemia (AML) in patients 50 years of age or older. Blood. 2006;108(1):45–51.
40. Ghanem H, Jabbour E, Faderl S, Ghandhi V, Plunkett W, Kantarjian H. Clofarabine in leukemia. Expert Rev Hematol. 2010;3(1):15–22. doi:10.1586/ehm.09.70.
41. Smith MA, Seibel NL, Altekruse SF, Ries LA, Melbert DL, O'Leary M, et al. Outcomes for children and adolescents with cancer: challenges for the twenty-first century. J Clin Oncol. 28(15):2625–34.
42. Jeha S, Gaynon PS, Razzouk BI, Franklin J, Kadota R, Shen V, et al. Phase II study of clofarabine in pediatric patients with refractory or relapsed acute lymphoblastic leukemia. J Clin Oncol. 2006;24(12):1917–23.
43. Hijiya N, Thomson B, Isakoff MS, Silverman LB, Steinherz PG, Borowitz MJ, et al. Phase 2 trial of clofarabine in combination with etoposide and cyclophosphamide in pediatric patients with refractory or relapsed acute lymphoblastic leukemia. Blood. 2011;118(23):6043–9. doi:10.1182/blood-2011-08-374710.
44. Hijiya N, Gaynon P, Barry E, Silverman L, Thomson B, Chu R, et al. A multi-center phase I study of clofarabine, etoposide and cyclophosphamide in combination in pediatric patients with refractory or relapsed acute leukemia. Leukemia. 2009;23(12):2259–64.

45. Cooper T, Alonzo, TA, Gerbing, RB, Perentesis, J, Whitlock, JA, Raetz, E, Carroll, WL, Gamis, AS, Razzouk, BI. A report from the Children's Oncology Group On the Safety of Clofarabine in combination with cytarabine in pediatric patients with relapsed acute leukemia. The American Society of Hematology 53rd annual meeting. 2010;(3076)
46. Locatelli F, Testi AM, Bernardo ME, Rizzari C, Bertaina A, Merli P, et al. Clofarabine, cyclophosphamide and etoposide as single-course re-induction therapy for children with refractory/ multiple relapsed acute lymphoblastic leukaemia. Br J Haematol. 2009;147(3):371–8.
47. Jeha S, Gandhi V, Chan KW, McDonald L, Ramirez I, Madden R, et al. Clofarabine, a novel nucleoside analog, is active in pediatric patients with advanced leukemia. Blood. 2004;103(3):784–9.
48. Kearns P, Michel G, Nelken B, et al. BIOV-111a European phase II trial of clofarabine (Evoltra) in refractory and relapsed childhood acute lymphoblastic leukemia. Blood. 2006;108(527a):Abstract #1859
49. Bonate PL, Arthaud L, Cantrell Jr WR, Stephenson K, Secrist III JA, Weitman S. Discovery and development of clofarabine: a nucleoside analogue for treating cancer. Nat Rev Drug Discov. 2006;5(10):855–63.
50. Cooper TM, Razzouk BI, Gerbing R, Alonzo TA, Adlard K, Raetz E, et al. Phase I/II trial of clofarabine and cytarabine in children with relapsed/refractory acute lymphoblastic leukemia (AAML0523): a report from the Children's Oncology Group. Pediatr Blood Cancer. 2013;60(7):1141–7. doi:10.1002/pbc.24398.
51. Cooper TM, Alonzo TA, Gerbing RB, Perentesis JP, Whitlock JA, Taub JW, et al. AAML0523: a report from the Children's Oncology Group on the efficacy of clofarabine in combination with cytarabine in pediatric patients with recurrent acute myeloid leukemia. Cancer. 2014;120(16):2482–9. doi:10.1002/cncr.28674.
52. Abd Elmoneim A, Gore L, Ricklis RM, Boklan J, Cooper T, Narendran A, et al. Phase I dose-escalation trial of clofarabine followed by escalating doses of fractionated cyclophosphamide in children with relapsed or refractory acute leukemias. Pediatr Blood Cancer. 2012;59(7):1252–8. doi:10.1002/pbc.24264.
53. Nelken B, Cave H, Leverger G, Galambrun C, Plat G, Schmitt C, et al. A phase I study of clofarabine with multiagent chemotherapy in childhood high risk relapse of acute lymphoblastic leukemia (VANDEVOL Study of the French SFCE Acute Leukemia Committee). Pediatr Blood Cancer. 2016;63(2):270–5. doi:10.1002/pbc.25751.
54. Abbi KK, Rybka W, Ehmann WC, Claxton DF. Phase I/II study of clofarabine, etoposide, and mitoxantrone in patients with refractory or relapsed acute leukemia. Clin Lymphoma Myeloma Leuk. 2015;15(1):41–6. doi:10.1016/j.clml.2014.06.005.
55. Yamauchi T, Nowak BJ, Keating MJ, Plunkett W. DNA repair initiated in chronic lymphocytic leukemia lymphocytes by 4-hydroperoxycyclophosphamide is inhibited by fludarabine and clofarabine. Clin Cancer Res. 2001;7(11):3580–9.
56. Raetz EA, Borowitz MJ, Devidas M, Linda SB, Hunger SP, Winick NJ, et al. Reinduction platform for children with first marrow relapse of acute lymphoblastic leukemia: a Children's Oncology Group Study [corrected]. J Clin Oncol. 2008;26(24):3971–8.
57. Burke M, Devidas M, Chen S, Gore L, Larsen E, Hilden JM, et al. Feasibility of intensive post-Induction therapy incorporating clofarabine (CLOF) in the very high risk (VHR) stratum of patients with newly diagnosed high risk B-lymphoblastic leukemia (HR B-ALL): Children's Oncology Group AALL1131. J Clin Oncol. 2015;33(15 Suppl, May 20 Supplement):Abstract 10007.
58. Miano M, Pistorio A, Putti MC, Dufour C, Messina C, Barisone E, et al. Clofarabine, cyclophosphamide and etoposide for the treatment of relapsed or resistant acute leukemia in pediatric patients. Leuk Lymphoma. 2012;53(9):1693–8. doi:10.3109/10428194.2012.663915.
59. Shukla N, Kobos R, Renaud T, Steinherz LJ, Steinherz PG. Phase II trial of clofarabine with topotecan, vinorelbine, and thiotepa in pediatric patients with relapsed or refractory acute leukemia. Pediatr Blood Cancer. 2014;61(3):431–5. doi:10.1002/pbc.24789.
60. Creutzig U, Zimmermann M, Bourquin JP, Dworzak MN, Fleischhack G, Graf N, et al. Randomized trial comparing liposomal daunorubicin with idarubicin as induction for pediatric

acute myeloid leukemia: results from Study AML-BFM 2004. Blood. 2013;122(1):37–43. doi:10.1182/blood-2013-02-484097.
61. Zwaan CM, Kolb EA, Reinhardt D, Abrahamsson J, Adachi S, Aplenc R, et al. Collaborative efforts driving progress in pediatric acute myeloid leukemia. J Clin Oncol. 2015;33(27):2949–62. doi:10.1200/JCO.2015.62.8289.
62. Creutzig U, Zimmermann M, Dworzak MN, Gibson B, Tamminga R, Abrahamsson J, et al. The prognostic significance of early treatment response in pediatric relapsed acute myeloid leukemia: results of the international study relapsed AML 2001/01. Haematologica. 2014;99(9):1472–8. doi:10.3324/haematol.2014.104182.
63. Kaspers GJ, Zimmermann M, Reinhardt D, Gibson BE, Tamminga RY, Aleinikova O, et al. Improved outcome in pediatric relapsed acute myeloid leukemia: results of a randomized trial on liposomal daunorubicin by the International BFM Study Group. J Clin Oncol. 2013;31(5):599–607. doi:10.1200/JCO.2012.43.7384.
64. Lech-Maranda E, Korycka A, Robak T. Clofarabine as a novel nucleoside analogue approved to treat patients with haematological malignancies: mechanism of action and clinical activity. Mini-Rev Med Chem. 2009;9(7):805–12.
65. Nagai S, Takenaka K, Nachagari D, Rose C, Domoney K, Sun D, et al. Deoxycytidine kinase modulates the impact of the ABC transporter ABCG2 on clofarabine cytotoxicity. Cancer Res. 2011;71(5):1781–91. doi:10.1158/0008-5472.CAN-10-1919.
66. Thudium KE, Ghoshal S, Fetterly GJ, Haese JP, Karpf AR, Wetzler M. Synergism between clofarabine and decitabine through p53R2: a pharmacodynamic drug-drug interaction modeling. Leuk Res. 2012;36(11):1410–6. doi:10.1016/j.leukres.2012.07.015.
67. Jeha S, Razzouk B, Rytting M, Rheingold S, Albano E, Kadota R, et al. Phase II study of clofarabine in pediatric patients with refractory or relapsed acute myeloid leukemia. J Clin Oncol. 2009;27(26):4392–7. doi:10.1200/JCO.2008.18.8706.
68. Buckley SA, Mawad R, Gooley TA, Becker PS, Sandhu V, Hendrie P, et al. A phase I/II study of oral clofarabine plus low-dose cytarabine in previously treated acute myeloid leukaemia and high-risk myelodysplastic syndrome patients at least 60 years of age. Br J Haematol. 2015;170(3):349–55. doi:10.1111/bjh.13437.
69. Graham NJ, Johnson PJ, Cummins M, et al. A phase I study of clofarabine and liposomal daunorubicin in childhood and adolescent acute myeloid leukemia. J Clin Oncol. 2012;28:TPS327.
70. Inaba H, Rubnitz JE, Coustan-Smith E, Li L, Furmanski BD, Mascara GP, et al. Phase I pharmacokinetic and pharmacodynamic study of the multikinase inhibitor sorafenib in combination with clofarabine and cytarabine in pediatric relapsed/refractory leukemia. J Clin Oncol. 2011;29(24):3293–300. doi:10.1200/JCO.2011.34.7427.
71. Agura E, Cooper B, Holmes H, Vance E, Berryman RB, Maisel C, et al. Report of a phase II study of clofarabine and cytarabine in de novo and relapsed and refractory AML patients and in selected elderly patients at high risk for anthracycline toxicity. Oncologist. 2011;16(2):197–206. doi:10.1634/theoncologist.2010-0220.
72. Faderl S, Ravandi F, Huang X, Wang X, Jabbour E, Garcia-Manero G, et al. Clofarabine plus low-dose cytarabine followed by clofarabine plus low-dose cytarabine alternating with decitabine in acute myeloid leukemia frontline therapy for older patients. Cancer. 2012;118(18):4471–7. doi:10.1002/cncr.27429.
73. Zwaan CM, Dworzak M, Klingebiel T, et al. Clofarabine in combination with high-dose cytarabine and liposomal daunorubicin in pediatric AML: results of a Phase 1B combination study by the ITCC Consortium. Blood. 2014;124:989.
74. Kirschbaum MH, Stein AS, Popplewell L, Delioukina M, Chen R, Nakamura R, et al. A phase I study in adults of clofarabine combined with high-dose melphalan as reduced-intensity conditioning for allogeneic transplantation. Biol Blood Marrow Transplant. 2012;18(3):432–40. doi:10.1016/j.bbmt.2011.07.017.
75. Chevallier P, Labopin M, Buchholz S, Ganser A, Ciceri F, Lioure B, et al. Clofarabine-containing conditioning regimen for allo-SCT in AML/ALL patients: a survey from the Acute

Leukemia Working Party of EBMT. Eur J Haematol. 2012;89(3):214–9. doi:10.1111/j.1600-0609.2012.01822.x.
76. Martin MG, Uy GL, Procknow E, Stockerl-Goldstein K, Cashen A, Westervelt P, et al. Allo-SCT conditioning for myelodysplastic syndrome and acute myeloid leukemia with clofarabine, cytarabine and ATG. Bone Marrow Transplant. 2009;44(1):13–7. doi:10.1038/bmt.2008.423.
77. Chevallier P, Labopin M, Socie G, Tabrizi R, Furst S, Lioure B, et al. Results from a clofarabine-busulfan-containing, reduced-toxicity conditioning regimen prior to allogeneic stem cell transplantation: the phase 2 prospective CLORIC trial. Haematologica. 2014;99(9):1486–91. doi:10.3324/haematol.2014.108563.
78. van Besien K, Stock W, Rich E, Odenike O, Godley LA, O'Donnell PH, et al. Phase I-II study of clofarabine-melphalan-alemtuzumab conditioning for allogeneic hematopoietic cell transplantation. Biol Blood Marrow Transplant. 2012;18(6):913–21. doi:10.1016/j.bbmt.2011.10.041.
79. Allen CE, Ladisch S, McClain KL. How I treat Langerhans cell histiocytosis. Blood. 2015;126(1):26–35. doi:10.1182/blood-2014-12-569301.
80. Simko SJ, Tran HD, Jones J, Bilgi M, Beaupin LK, Coulter D, et al. Clofarabine salvage therapy in refractory multifocal histiocytic disorders, including Langerhans cell histiocytosis, juvenile xanthogranuloma and Rosai-Dorfman disease. Pediatr Blood Cancer. 2014;61(3):479–87. doi:10.1002/pbc.24772.
81. Abraham A, Alsultan A, Jeng M, Rodriguez-Galindo C, Campbell PK. Clofarabine salvage therapy for refractory high-risk langerhans cell histiocytosis. Pediatr Blood Cancer. 2013;60(6):E19–22. doi:10.1002/pbc.24436.
82. Rodriguez-Galindo C, Jeng M, Khuu P, McCarville MB, Jeha S. Clofarabine in refractory Langerhans cell histiocytosis. Pediatr Blood Cancer. 2008;51(5):703–6. doi:10.1002/pbc.21668.
83. O'Connor D, Sibson K, Caswell M, Connor P, Cummins M, Mitchell C, et al. Early UK experience in the use of clofarabine in the treatment of relapsed and refractory paediatric acute lymphoblastic leukaemia. Br J Haematol. 2011;154(4):482–5. doi:10.1111/j.1365-2141.2011.08752.x.
84. Escherich G, Zur Stadt U, Zimmermann M, Horstmann MA. Co ALLsg. Clofarabine in combination with pegylated asparaginase in the frontline treatment of childhood acute lymphoblastic leukaemia: a feasibility report from the CoALL 08-09 trial. Br J Haematol. 2013;163(2):240–7. doi:10.1111/bjh.12520.
85. El-Jawahri A, Li S, Ballen KK, Cutler C, Dey BR, Driscoll J, et al. Phase II trial of reduced-intensity Busulfan/Clofarabine conditioning with allogeneic hematopoietic stem cell transplantation for patients with acute myeloid leukemia, myelodysplastic syndromes, and acute lymphoid leukemia. Biol Blood Marrow Transplant. 2016;22(1):80–5. doi:10.1016/j.bbmt.2015.08.001.
86. Lang P, Feuchtinger T, Teltschik HM, Schwinger W, Schlegel P, Pfeiffer M, et al. Improved immune recovery after transplantation of TCRalphabeta/CD19-depleted allografts from haploidentical donors in pediatric patients. Bone Marrow Transplant. 2015;50(Suppl 2):S6–10. doi:10.1038/bmt.2015.87.
87. Kebriaei P, Basset R, Ledesma C, Ciurea S, Parmar S, Shpall EJ, et al. Clofarabine combined with busulfan provides excellent disease control in adult patients with acute lymphoblastic leukemia undergoing allogeneic hematopoietic stem cell transplantation. Biol Blood Marrow Transplant. 2012;18(12):1819–26. doi:10.1016/j.bbmt.2012.06.010.
88. Magenau J, Tobai H, Pawarode A, Braun T, Peres E, Reddy P, et al. Clofarabine and busulfan conditioning facilitates engraftment and provides significant antitumor activity in nonremission hematologic malignancies. Blood. 2011;118(15):4258–64. doi:10.1182/blood-2011-06-358010.

Re-emerging Antimetabolites with Novel Mechanism of Action with Respect to Epigenetic Regulation: Basic Aspects

18

Dzjemma Sarkisjan, Renske D.M. Steenbergen, Jacqueline Cloos, and Godefridus J. Peters

Abstract

Azacitidine (AzaC) and decitabine (DAC) are epigenetic modulators, which are used for treatment of several hematological malignancies. The epigenetic mode of action of these compounds comprises reduction of DNA methylation by inhibition of DNA methyltransferases (DNMTs), which include the maintenance DNA methyltransferase 1 and de novo methyltransferase DNMT3A and DNMT3B. This property leads to a decrease in CpG island methylation and a reactivation of tumor suppressor genes that are silenced by promoter hypermethylation, thereby contributing to the anti-tumor effect. Insight in the mechanisms of action of these drugs is essential for our understanding how synthetic epigenetic modulators can affect cellular processes. In this review the intracellular metabolism of these cytidine analogs and some novel cytidine analogs are summarized. In addition, the mechanism of DNMT downregulation is discussed, which besides the incorporation of modified nucleotides into the DNA, more recently was also shown to involve proteasomal degradation.

Keywords

Cancer • DNA methyltransferase • Azacitidine • Decitabine

D. Sarkisjan • G.J. Peters (✉)
Department of Medical Oncology, VU University Medical Center,
De Boelelaan 1117, 1081HV Amsterdam, The Netherlands
e-mail: gj.peters@vumc.nl

R.D.M. Steenbergen
Department of Pathology, VU University Medical Center, Amsterdam, The Netherlands

J. Cloos
Department of Pediatric Oncology/Hematology and Hematology, VU University Medical Center, Amsterdam, The Netherlands

T. Ueda (ed.), *Chemotherapy for Leukemia*, DOI 10.1007/978-981-10-3332-2_18

18.1 Introduction

Alterations in the DNA sequence, such as mutations, can give rise to various malignancies, when accumulated. Modifications in the DNA architecture can also contribute to tumorigenesis and disease progression [1]. Changes in DNA architecture are called epigenetic modifications. DNA methylation is an example of an epigenetic modification that is gene suppressive. Gene promoter methylation is deregulated in cancers [2]. Synthetic formulations have been designed to interfere with this aberrant DNA methylation [3].

The cytidine analogs 5-azacytidine (AzaC, Vidaza) and 5-aza-2′-deoxycytidine (DAC, decitabine, Dacogen) are antimetabolites [4]. The chemical structures of cytidine and the cytidine analogs AzaC and DAC are shown in Fig. 18.1. The base of AzaC and DAC is modified on the C5 position. The carbon is replaced by a nitrogen molecule. The difference between AzaC and DAC is that AzaC has a ribose molecule attached to the base, while DAC consists of deoxyribose.

Naturally, deoxycytidine is incorporated into the DNA chain during replication and forms a bridge with the corresponding guanine base. Sequences in the DNA with deoxycytidine–deoxyguanosine (CpG) dinucleotides occur at a high frequency, i.e., an observed-to-expected CpG ratio that is greater than 60%, are referred to as CpG islands [5]. These CpG islands are predominantly located in the promoter region of genes. Gene promoters of human genome consist 72% of high CpG content [6]. Deoxycytidine within CpG dinucleotides can be methylated to form 5-methyldeoxycytidine. By DNA methylation of a gene promoter, a gene can be silenced. In eukaryotes DNA methylation is essential for development, genomic

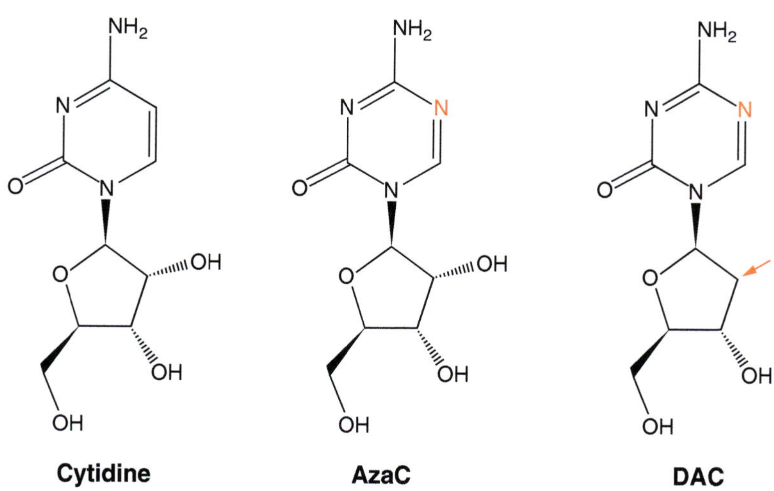

Fig. 18.1 Chemical structures of cytidine and the cytidine analogs azaC (azacytidine) and DAC (aza-2′-deoxycytidine). The modifications of nitrogen in the base are depicted with *red* color. The *red arrow* highlights the deficiency of the deoxy group on the ribose molecule of DAC compared to cytidine and AzaC

imprinting, and X chromosome inactivation. DNA methylation is also implicated in cancer development and progression by silencing of tumor suppressor genes upon promoter methylation. DNA methylation is a reversible process that can be exploited for cancer treatment. Since AzaC and DAC interfere with the process of methylation, these drugs function as epigenetic modulators [3] and can reverse the cancer phenotype. Genes silenced by promoter CpG island hypermethylation in cancers, that are reported to be reactivated after treatment with AzaC or DAC, are summarized elsewhere [7].

Methylation of deoxycytidines, also called cytosine methylation, is carried out by DNA methyltransferases. The methylation pattern is read and copied to a newly synthesized DNA strand by the maintenance methyltransferase DNMT1, which has affinity for hemi-methylated DNA strands [8]. A novel (not earlier present on the DNA) methyl group can be added by DNMT3A or DNMT3B, which are de novo DNA methyltransferases with prevalence for unmethylated DNA [9, 10].

DNMTs use S-adenosyl methionine as the methyl donor (AdoMet). The catalytic mechanism of DNA methyltransferase involves a covalent bond formation between a cysteine residue in the active site of the enzyme and carbon 6 of cytosine in DNA. Thereby, an increase in the flow of electrons to carbon 5 is initiated generating an attack on AdoMet. Extraction of a proton from carbon 5 subsequently follows β-elimination, and a double bond between carbon 5 and carbon 6 is formed. As a result the enzyme and S-adenosyl-homocysteine (AdoHcy) are released, leaving methylated cytosine in the DNA. Cytosine is suitable as methyl-binding moiety because the cytosine is a flexible base, which flips out of the DNA prior to receiving the methyl group. This phenomenon has been described as base-flipping mechanism in various studies [11–13].

The effectivity of epigenetic modifiers as anti-cancer agents is depending on several cellular processes such as uptake and metabolism of the drugs and cell proliferation. Moreover, several effects can be anticipated both on DNA and RNA. To optimize the epigenetic treatment for different cell types, currently several novel (antimetabolite) drugs have been developed, which are described in detail in this review.

18.2 Uptake and Metabolism of AzaC and DAC

In order for nucleoside analogs, such as AzaC and DAC, to function, they need to be internalized into the cells. The nucleoside transporter family SLC29A gene codes for the equilibrative nucleoside transporter (ENTs) proteins and the SLC28A gene for concentrative nucleoside transporters proteins (CNTs). These transporters are responsible for intracellular transport and have been related to nucleoside analog sensitivity in leukemia [14–17]. AzaC is a substrate for hCNT1 and hCNT3. Transport of AzaC into the cell is therefore mediated by these cell membrane transporters (Fig. 18.2) [18, 19]. Moreover, the human ENT is also involved in the transport of AzaC and DAC [20]. Transporter deficiency can lead to resistance to these drugs.

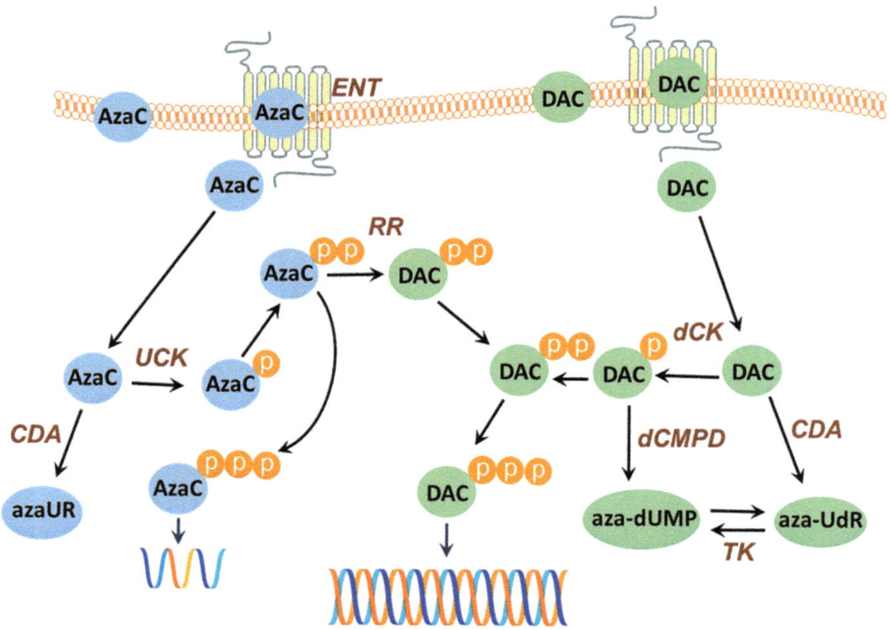

Fig. 18.2 Uptake and metabolism of AzaC and DAC. Compounds enter the cell by diffusion or membrane transporter-mediated influx (human equilibrative nucleoside transporter, hENT). Human concentrative nucleoside transporters (hCNTs) can also play a role in the uptake. The drugs can be inactivated by deamination, catalyzed by cytidine deaminase (CDA). In the cell the metabolic inactive AzaC and DAC are activated by means of phosphorylation, azaC by uridine–cytidine kinase (UCK), and DAC by deoxycytidine kinase (dCK). DAC-MP can also be inactivated by dCMP-deaminase (dCMPD) to aza-dUMP. The deaminated DAC, aza-UdR, is a substrate for thymidine kinase (TK), which catalyzes the transfer of aza-UdR to aza-dUMP. AzaC-DP is reduced by ribonucleotide reductase (RR) to its deoxy-form, aza-2′-deoxycytidine diphosphate (DAC-DP). AzaC-TP is incorporated into RNA; DAC-TP is incorporated into DNA. Incorporation of DAC-TP into DNA leads to hypo-methylation since this will inhibit DNA methyltransferase

After the translocation of the nucleosides into the cells, the prodrugs have to be activated in order to exert their antimetabolite activity [21]. The activation is carried out by phosphorylation. The phosphorylation cycle of AzaC generates AzaC-MP, AzaC-DP, and AzaC-TP (Fig. 18.2). When AzaC is phosphorylated to the AzaC-TP form, it can be incorporated into the RNA. For incorporation into the DNA, the ribose of AzaC-DP needs to be reduced to deoxyribose, which relies on ribonucleotide reductase (RR) [22]. The activating enzyme for AzaC is the uridine–cytidine kinase (UCK) [23], while for DAC deoxycytidine kinase is responsible for activation/phosphorylation of the drug [24]. A known mechanism of deactivation of cytidine analogs is deamination. Both AzaC and DAC are substrates for cytidine deaminase and can be deaminated within the cells, while aza-dCMP can also be deaminated by deoxycytidylate deaminase (Fig. 18.2) [22, 25, 26].

The epigenetic modifying drugs interfere with the activity of DNA-methylating enzymes (DNA methyltransferases), which are often deregulated in cancer.

18.3 The Maintenance DNA Methyltransferase 1 Protein

The maintenance DNA methyltransferase DNMT1 is ubiquitously expressed and has several interacting proteins that are listed elsewhere [27]. DNMT1 is composed of different domains that can be given a functional importance. The N-terminal site of DNMT1 is a regulatory region and consists of proliferating cell nuclear antigen (PCNA) binding domain, (PBD), a heterochromatin targeting sequence (TS), a CXXC-type zinc finger domain, and two bromo-adjacent homology domains (BAH1 and BAH2). The C terminus has the catalytic activity. PCNA targets DNMT1 to the DNA replication site and DNA repair sites in order to restore the DNA methylation pattern [28–31]. It is important to note that methylation is enhanced when the replication machinery is involved, but the assembly of replication fork is not necessary to maintain DNA methylation [32, 33]. The heterochromatin targeting domain was shown to recruit DNMT1 to heterochromatin independent of DNA replication [30]. The CXXC-type zinc finger domain interacts with DNA and ensures that the enzyme is in an auto-inhibitory state in the presence of unmethylated DNA [34]. The N terminus and C terminus of the protein are connected by lysyl–glysyl dipeptide repeats linker ($(KG)_7$) [35]. The function of the C terminus is the catalytic activity of the enzyme, which uses AdoMet as a donor. Several post-transcriptional modifications have been reported to be important for stability and activity of DNMT1. The decay of the protein is proteasome mediated whereby the protein is tagged by ubiquitination [36]. The E3 ligase activity containing protein UHRF1 can ubiquitinate DNMT1 [37]. Phosphorylation and methylation of DNMT1 are reported to increase the stability of the protein [38–41]. In addition, SUMOylation increases in DNMT1 activity [42]. A critical role for DNMT1 in development was demonstrated in animal models; DNMT1 null mice die after gastrulation [43]. DNMT1 overexpression and/or hyperactivity has been reported in various tumors [44–46].

18.4 De Novo Methyltransferases in Health and Disease

In comparison to DNMT1, de novo DNA methyltransferases are tissue-specific [44] smaller proteins. DNMT3A is comprised of 912 amino acids, while DNMT3B is even smaller and is comprised of 853 amino acids. DNMT3A persists in three isoforms. The canonical isoform is 912 amino acids long and the others 723 and 166 amino acids, respectively [10]. The isoform variants are generated by means of alternative splicing. In non-diseased conditions a cell uses alternative splicing to ensure proteomic diversity [47]. Functionally different proteins are then formed from one gene [48]. Alternative splicing is deregulated during cancer development and progression and can cause drug resistance [49, 50]. Interestingly, an alternative spliced variant of DNMT3B was found in tumors, which has an altered functionality [51]. DNMT3A acts in complex with DNMT3L [52, 53], which is inactive on its own [54]. DNMT3L is a stimulatory cofactor of the DNMT3A and DNMT3B enzymes [55]. The DNMT3A gene is frequently mutated in acute myeloid leukemia (AML)

[56, 57] and chronic myelomonocytic leukemia (CMML) [58], and recently a condition named Tatton–Brown syndrome was reported with mutations in DNMT3A gene [59]. On the other hand, mutations in DNMT3B gene cause immunodeficiency–centromeric instability–facial anomalies syndrome 1 (ICF1) [60–64]. For this gene eight different isoforms have been reported. DNMT3A and DNMT3B enzymes are thought to have preference for target sites [65, 66].

18.5 The Mechanism of DNMT1 Downregulation Upon AzaC and DAC Treatment and Beyond

18.5.1 Replication-Based DNMT1 Downregulation

AzaC and DAC have an effect on the DNA methylation pattern. Therefore, these compounds are known as epigenetic modulators. The mechanism of epigenetic modulation involves downregulation of DNA methyltransferases (DNMTs). DAC is able to downregulate DNMT1, DNMT3A, and DNMT3B. Because of the implication of DNMT1 in tumor suppressor gene promoter hypermethylation, interest in DNMT1 downregulating agents has been increasing. Early studies indicated downregulation of DNMT1 by a trapping mechanism. Thereby aza-dCTP is incorporated into the DNA, and a covalent binding is formed between the false cytosine and DNMT1 (Fig. 18.3). Subsequently, the methyltransferase is degraded [67–69]. Mass spectrometry analysis of DNA isolated from DAC-treated cells also revealed

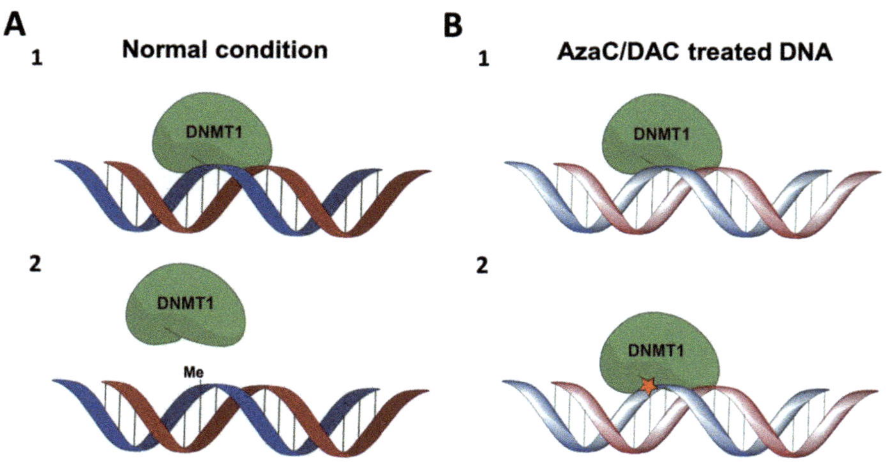

Fig. 18.3 Simplified overview of DNMT1 trapping by AzaC and DAC. **a** Normal condition of DNA methylation by DNMT1. *1* DNMT1 recognizes hemi-methylated DNA and interacts with it, in order to methylate the cytosine base. *2* The cytosine methylation has occurred; DNMT1 release takes place. **b** DNA methylation by DNMT1 after treatment with AzaC and DAC. *1* DNMT1 recognizes hemi-methylated DNA and interacts with it. *2* Because of incorporated DAC, DNMT1 forms covalent binding with DNA; the enzyme is not released instantly

an open-ringed aza-cytosine lacking its carbon 6. It was proposed that the enzyme can still be bound to the base in the open-ring format [70].

18.5.2 Ubiquitination of DNMT1 Upon DAC Exposure

Ubiquitination plays a role in DAC-induced DNMT1 downregulation [71]. Cellular protein degradation is mediated but not limited by ubiquitination, which tags protein for proteasomal degradation. Ubiquitin itself is a polypeptide of 76 amino acids. The cascade of polyubiquitination starts by the ubiquitin-activating enzyme E1 [72]. E1 catalyzes in an ATP-dependent manner the covalent binding of ubiquitin to the cysteine residue of the E1 active site. Then the activated ubiquitin is transferred to ubiquitin-conjugating enzymes, E2. E2 transfers ubiquitin to the third enzyme, ubiquitin protein ligase, E3. Glycine (ubiquitin)–lysine (protein residue) bound is thereby formed. It is generally believed that lysine 48 polyubiquitin chain is a signal for proteasomal degradation [73–76]. Therefore, lysine 48 is a known tag for proteins to degrade. Evidence for ubiquitin-associated degradation of DNMT1 upon DAC exposure was demonstrated, in that upon inhibition of proteasomal activity using the compound MG 132, no DNMT1 downregulation was seen in DAC-treated cells [71, 77].

18.5.3 The Effect of AzaC on RNA

One of the additional characteristics of AzaC is the ability to be incorporated into the RNA. Next to affecting RNA synthesis, incorporation of AzaC into the tRNA was shown to inhibit tRNA methyltransferases, which results in interference with tRNA methylation and processing leading to defective acceptor function of tRNA [78–80]. In addition, incorporation of AzaC into the nucleolar RNA was shown; ribosomal precursor RNA containing AzaC was suggested to have an altered structure [81]. Since methylation is of great importance for ribosomal RNA processing, incorporation of AzaC into RNA will affect protein synthesis as well [82–85]. Interestingly, the deamination products of AzaC and DAC, azauridine (when sequentially phosphorylated to aza-UMP and aza-UDP, which will be reduced to aza-dUDP and dephosphorylated to aza-dUMP) and azadeoxyuridine (when phosphorylated directly to aza-dUMP) interfere with de novo thymidylate synthesis, since aza-dUMP is a poor inhibitor of thymidylate synthase, which may enhance cytotoxic effect of both compounds [86]. Aza-dUMP can also be formed by deamination of aza-dCMP.

18.6 Novel DNMT Inhibitors

Because of the chemical instability of both azacytidine and DAC, prodrugs and novel analogs of both compounds have been designed. Moreover, several compounds were also designed to offer the possibility for oral administration. Zebularine [87–89], SGI-110 (oligonucleotide consisting of DAC linked through a phosphodiester bond to the endogenous nucleoside deoxyguanosine) [90, 91], TAC (2′,3′,5′-triacetyl-5-azacytidine) [92], CP-4200 (elaidic acid ester derivative of AzaC) [93], T-dCyd (4′-thio-2′-deoxycytidine) [94], and Aza-T-dCyd (5-aza-4′-thio-2′-deoxycytidine) [94] are examples of second-generation cytidine nucleoside analogs. The structure and update on clinical trials of these compounds are listed in Table 18.1.

The uptake of the cytidine analog zebularine into the cell is mediated by hCNT1, hCNT3, and hENT2 [95]. When phosphorylated the compound has a potent inhibitory effect on DNMT1 protein, and to a lesser extent, it inhibits also DNMT3A and DNMT3B [96]. Zebularine exerts its action by trapping DNMT1 and preventing its turnover [97]. In addition to downregulation of DNMTs, zebularine was shown to inhibit CDA by an adduct formation with the active site of CDA [98]. Zebularine has no clinical trial records registered yet. On the other hand, the dinucleoside SGI-110 is designed to take care of deamination and instability of DAC [99] and showed potent activity in malignant xenograft models [91]. Currently, there are 13 clinical trials in phases 1, 2, and 3, evaluating this compound alone or in combination with other compounds commonly used in cancer treatment. The compound is being tested in various malignancies.

The compound TAC ,which is a prodrug of AzaC, performed better in terms of oral bioavailability, stability, and solubility as it was initially aimed for clinical studies [92]. However, to the best of our knowledge, the drug did not enter a clinical trial yet. Interestingly, T-dCyd is activated by dCK and incorporated into the DNA without DNA synthesis inhibition and downregulation of DNMT1. The modification in this compound enabled poor deamination, and it can be administered orally. The compound recently entered phase 1 clinical trials and is being studied in advanced solid tumors [100]. Both, T-dCyd and Aza-T-dCyd had in vivo efficacy and are thought to have limited ability to inhibit thymidylate synthase. However, both compounds remain an experimental drug [94].

Cellular uptake of cytidine analogs and clinical efficacy, however, rely often on membrane transporters. AzaC uptake is transporter mediated and was shown to have limited drug uptake. To overcome this limitation, CP-4200 was designed. CP-4200 uptake into the cytosol was independent of nucleoside transporters. In the cell the elaidic acid chain is cleaved off, and azaC is released. Therefore, the mechanism of action is similar to AzaC by DNMT downregulation by trapping of the enzyme [93]. CP-4200 is an interesting experimental drug for its potential to overcome transporter-mediated resistance to AzaC [101].

A chemically different but functionally similar DNMT downregulator is the cytidine analog fluorocyclopentenylcytosine (RX-3117) [106–109]. Initial studies on its mechanism of action and metabolism have been published recently. Uptake of RX-3117 is mediated by hENT1 and its phosphorylation by UCK2 [107]. UCK2 is overexpressed in tumors, which makes RX-3117 specific for cancer cells and possibly will

Table 18.1 Overview of the next generation DNMTs downregulators

Chemical structure/compound name	Type of cancer	Status/ administration	References
Prodrugs			
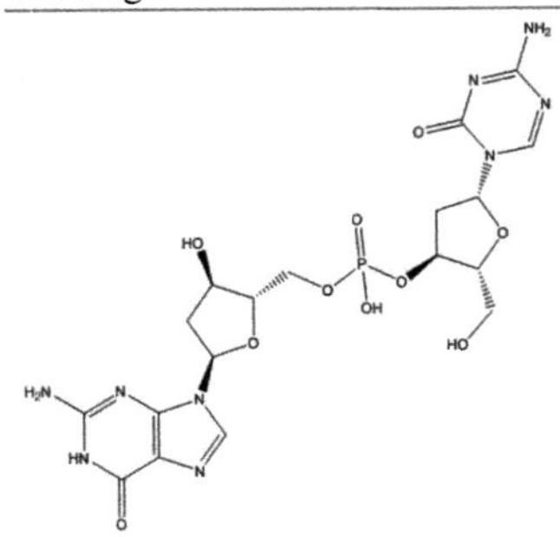 SGI-110	AML	Clinical studies	[102]
	MDS	Phase 1, 2, and 3	[90]
	CMML	s.c. injection	
	Advanced HCC		
	Metastatic melanoma		
	Metastatic colorectal cancer		
	Ovarian cancer		
	Germ cell tumor		
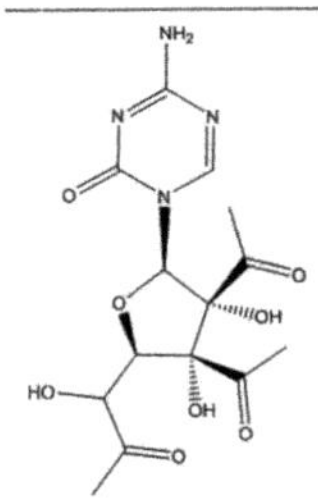 TAC	In vivo model:	Preclinical studies	[92]
	Antileukemic activity in L1210 BDF1 female mice	Oral administration	
		i.p. injection	
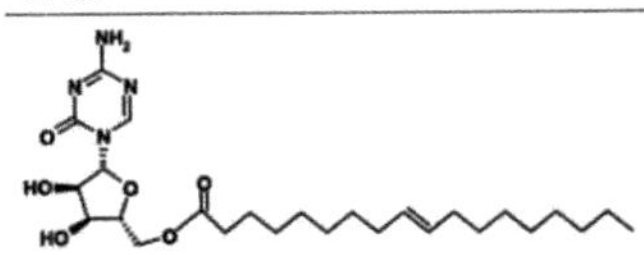 CP-4200	In vivo model:	Preclinical studies i.p/i.v. injection	[93]
	ALL SCID6 diabedic/ severe immunodeficient female mice		
Analogs			
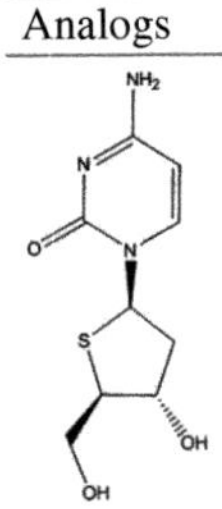 T-dCyd	Advanced solid tumors	Clinical studies Phase 1	[94]
		Oral administration	
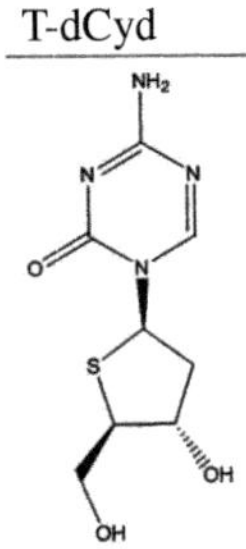 Aza-T-dCyd	In vivo model:	Preclinical studies	[94]
	Antitumor effect in NCI-H23 lung tumor implanted nude mice	i.p. injection	

(continued)

Table 18.1 (continued)

Chemical structure/compound name	Type of cancer	Status/ administration	References
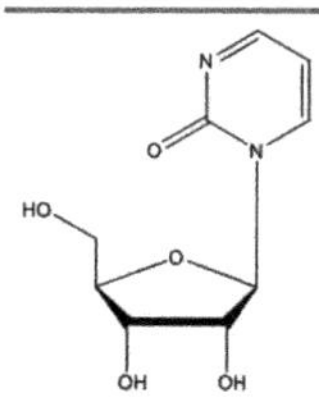 Zebularine	In vivo models:	Preclinical studies	[103]
	Effective in genetically engineerd MMTV-PyMT mammary tumor mice	Oral administration	[104]
	Inhibition of adenoma formation in C57/BL6 female Apc $^{Min/+}$ mice		
	Activity in Panc-89 injected NMRI mice	i.p. injection	[105]
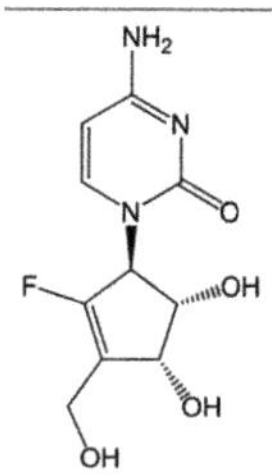 RX-3117	Advanced solid tumors	Clinical studies	[106]
		Phase 1 and 2	
		Oral administration	

The chemical structures, (clinical) trial status, drug administration, and the type of the tumors in which the drugs are being evaluated for are grouped in the table

have a low systemic toxicity [107]. Furthermore, it was shown that RX-3117, contrary to AzaC and DAC, is not deaminated by cytidine deaminase (CDA) and that RX-3117 causes both inhibition of DNA and RNA synthesis, although the inhibition of the former is more pronounced. By doing so, RX-3117 induces DNA double-strand break damage [110]. Interestingly, RX-3117 also targets DNA methyltransferase (DNMT). In two studies a decrease in DNMT1 expression was found in cell lines treated with RX-3117, while this was not the case for DNMT3A [106]. RX-3117 is able to reactivate functional proteins, such as the proton-coupled folate transporter, and repair enzymes, such as O-6-methylguanine DNA methyltransferase and tumor suppressor genes [109]. The mechanism of DNMT1 downregulation by RX-3117, however, is unknown yet. Together these data indicate that RX-3117 might be an effective demethylating agent, comparable to decitabine (Aza-CdR) and azacytidine (Aza-CR) [21].

Since the nucleoside cytidine analogs showed dose-limiting toxicity, non-nucleoside DNMT1 inhibitors have also been developed. The design of such inhibitors is based on computer modeling of catalytic domain of the protein. The non-nucleoside DNMT1 downregulator, N-phthalyl-L-tryptophan (RG108) [111], has shown a potent demethylation effect in vitro [112–114]. Naturally occurring non-nucleoside analogs also exist: tea polyphenol, epigallocatechin- 3gallate (EGCG), genistein, nanomycin A, psammaplin A, and the laccaic acid A. The mechanism of DNMT downregulation of these non-nucleoside compounds is not described yet. These compounds also differ considerably in chemical structure [111].

18.7 Conclusions

Major efforts have been put into the development of novel DNA-demethylating agents. Increasing knowledge from existing drugs permits us to learn about their mechanism of action and enables to develop superior derivatives. A compound can be modified to overcome very well-known existing resistance mechanism or to increase its efficacy. The availability of improved techniques for structural studies on target proteins will likely result in the development of more specific drugs in the future. Application of cancer biology led to the development of a unique novel DNMT1 downregulator, RX-3117. This drug combines a cancer-specific key enzyme necessary for the activation of metabolic inactive drug, with DNMT1 as the ultimate target, which makes this drug a promising anticancer treatment.

References

1. Calcagno DQ, de Arruda Cardoso Smith M, Burbano RR. Cancer type-specific epigenetic changes: gastric cancer. Methods Mol Biol. 2015;1238:79–101.
2. Rodriguez-Paredes M, Esteller M. Cancer epigenetics reaches mainstream oncology. Nat Med. 2011;17(3):330–9.
3. Creusot F, Acs G, Christman JK. Inhibition of DNA methyltransferase and induction of friend erythroleukemia cell differentiation by 5-azacytidine and 5-aza-2′-deoxycytidine. J Biol Chem. 1982;257(4):2041–8.
4. Sorm F, Piskala A, Cihak A, Vesely J. 5-Azacytidine, a new, highly effective cancerostatic. Experientia. 1964;20(4):202–3.
5. Gardiner-Garden M, Frommer M. CpG islands in vertebrate genomes. J Mol Biol. 1987;196(2):261–82.
6. Saxonov S, Berg P, Brutlag DL. A genome-wide analysis of CpG dinucleotides in the human genome distinguishes two distinct classes of promoters. Proc Natl Acad Sci U S A. 2006;103(5):1412–7.
7. Christman JK. 5-Azacytidine and 5-aza-2′-deoxycytidine as inhibitors of DNA methylation: mechanistic studies and their implications for cancer therapy. Oncogene. 2002;21(35):5483–95.
8. Bestor TH, Ingram VM. Two DNA methyltransferases from murine erythroleukemia cells: purification, sequence specificity, and mode of interaction with DNA. Proc Natl Acad Sci U S A. 1983;80(18):5559–63.
9. Okano M, Xie S, Li E. Cloning and characterization of a family of novel mammalian DNA (cytosine-5) methyltransferases. Nat Genet. 1998;19(3):219–20.
10. Xie S, Wang Z, Okano M, Nogami M, Li Y, He WW, et al. Cloning, expression and chromosome locations of the human DNMT3 gene family. Gene. 1999;236(1):87–95.
11. Klimasauskas S, Kumar S, Roberts RJ, Cheng X. HhaI methyltransferase flips its target base out of the DNA helix. Cell. 1994;76(2):357–69.
12. Bianchi C, Zangi R. Base-flipping propensities of unmethylated, hemimethylated, and fully methylated CpG sites. J Phys Chem B. 2013;117(8):2348–58.
13. Bianchi C, Zangi R. Dual base-flipping of cytosines in a CpG dinucleotide sequence. Biophys Chem. 2014;187–188:14–22.
14. Molina-Arcas M, Bellosillo B, Casado FJ, Montserrat E, Gil J, Colomer D, et al. Fludarabine uptake mechanisms in B-cell chronic lymphocytic leukemia. Blood. 2003;101(6):2328–34.
15. Pastor-Anglada M, Molina-Arcas M, Casado FJ, Bellosillo B, Colomer D, Gil J. Nucleoside transporters in chronic lymphocytic leukaemia. Leukemia. 2004;18(3):385–93.

16. Hubeek I, Stam RW, Peters GJ, Broekhuizen R, Meijerink JP, van Wering ER, et al. The human equilibrative nucleoside transporter 1 mediates in vitro cytarabine sensitivity in childhood acute myeloid leukaemia. Br J Cancer. 2005;93(12):1388–94.
17. Marce S, Molina-Arcas M, Villamor N, Casado FJ, Campo E, Pastor-Anglada M, et al. Expression of human equilibrative nucleoside transporter 1 (hENT1) and its correlation with gemcitabine uptake and cytotoxicity in mantle cell lymphoma. Haematologica. 2006;91(7):895–902.
18. Rius M, Stresemann C, Keller D, Brom M, Schirrmacher E, Keppler D, et al. Human concentrative nucleoside transporter 1-mediated uptake of 5-azacytidine enhances DNA demethylation. Mol Cancer Ther. 2009;8(1):225–31.
19. Rius M, Keller D, Brom M, Hummel-Eisenbeiss J, Lyko F, Keppler D. Vectorial transport of nucleoside analogs from the apical to the basolateral membrane in double-transfected cells expressing the human concentrative nucleoside transporter hCNT3 and the export pump ABCC4. Drug Metab Dispos. 2010;38(7):1054–63.
20. Huang Y, Anderle P, Bussey KJ, Barbacioru C, Shankavaram U, Dai Z, et al. Membrane transporters and channels: role of the transportome in cancer chemosensitivity and chemoresistance. Cancer Res. 2004;64(12):4294–301.
21. Peters GJ. Novel developments in the use of antimetabolites. Nucleosides Nucleotides Nucleic Acids. 2014;33(4–6):358–74.
22. Li LH, Olin EJ, Buskirk HH, Reineke LM. Cytotoxicity and mode of action of 5-azacytidine on L1210 leukemia. Cancer Res. 1970;30(11):2760–9.
23. Van Rompay AR, Norda A, Linden K, Johansson M, Karlsson A. Phosphorylation of uridine and cytidine nucleoside analogs by two human uridine-cytidine kinases. Mol Pharmacol. 2001;59(5):1181–6.
24. Momparler RL, Derse D. Kinetics of phosphorylation of 5-aza-2′-deoxyycytidine by deoxycytidine kinase. Biochem Pharmacol. 1979;28(8):1443–4.
25. Chabner BA, Drake JC, Johns DG. Deamination of 5-azacytidine by a human leukemia cell cytidine deaminase. Biochem Pharmacol. 1973;22(21):2763–5.
26. Laliberte J, Marquez VE, Momparler RL. Potent inhibitors for the deamination of cytosine arabinoside and 5-aza-2′-deoxycytidine by human cytidine deaminase. Cancer Chemother Pharmacol. 1992;30(1):7–11.
27. Qin W, Leonhardt H, Pichler G. Regulation of DNA methyltransferase 1 by interactions and modifications. Nucleus. 2011;2(5):392–402.
28. Leonhardt H, Page AW, Weier HU, Bestor TH. A targeting sequence directs DNA methyltransferase to sites of DNA replication in mammalian nuclei. Cell. 1992;71(5):865–73.
29. Chuang LS, Ian HI, Koh TW, Ng HH, Xu G, Li BF. Human DNA-(cytosine-5) methyltransferase-PCNA complex as a target for p21WAF1. Science. 1997;277(5334):1996–2000.
30. Easwaran HP, Schermelleh L, Leonhardt H, Cardoso MC. Replication-independent chromatin loading of Dnmt1 during G2 and M phases. EMBO Rep. 2004;5(12):1181–6.
31. Mortusewicz O, Schermelleh L, Walter J, Cardoso MC, Leonhardt H. Recruitment of DNA methyltransferase I to DNA repair sites. Proc Natl Acad Sci U S A. 2005;102(25):8905–9.
32. Schermelleh L, Haemmer A, Spada F, Rosing N, Meilinger D, Rothbauer U, et al. Dynamics of Dnmt1 interaction with the replication machinery and its role in postreplicative maintenance of DNA methylation. Nucleic Acids Res. 2007;35(13):4301–12.
33. Spada F, Haemmer A, Kuch D, Rothbauer U, Schermelleh L, Kremmer E, et al. DNMT1 but not its interaction with the replication machinery is required for maintenance of DNA methylation in human cells. J Cell Biol. 2007;176(5):565–71.
34. Song J, Rechkoblit O, Bestor TH, Patel DJ. Structure of DNMT1-DNA complex reveals a role for autoinhibition in maintenance DNA methylation. Science. 2011;331(6020):1036–40.
35. Margot JB, Aguirre-Arteta AM, Di Giacco BV, Pradhan S, Roberts RJ, Cardoso MC, et al. Structure and function of the mouse DNA methyltransferase gene: Dnmt1 shows a tripartite structure. J Mol Biol. 2000;297(2):293–300.

36. Agoston AT, Argani P, Yegnasubramanian S, De Marzo AM, Ansari-Lari MA, Hicks JL, et al. Increased protein stability causes DNA methyltransferase 1 dysregulation in breast cancer. J Biol Chem. 2005;280(18):18302–10.
37. Qin W, Leonhardt H, Spada F. Usp7 and Uhrf1 control ubiquitination and stability of the maintenance DNA methyltransferase Dnmt1. J Cell Biochem. 2011;112(2):439–44.
38. Sun L, Zhao H, Xu Z, Liu Q, Liang Y, Wang L, et al. Phosphatidylinositol 3-kinase/protein kinase B pathway stabilizes DNA methyltransferase I protein and maintains DNA methylation. Cell Signal. 2007;19(11):2255–63.
39. Esteve PO, Chin HG, Benner J, Feehery GR, Samaranayake M, Horwitz GA, et al. Regulation of DNMT1 stability through SET7-mediated lysine methylation in mammalian cells. Proc Natl Acad Sci U S A. 2009;106(13):5076–81.
40. Wang J, Hevi S, Kurash JK, Lei H, Gay F, Bajko J, et al. The lysine demethylase LSD1 (KDM1) is required for maintenance of global DNA methylation. Nat Genet. 2009;41(1):125–9.
41. Lavoie G, St-Pierre Y. Phosphorylation of human DNMT1: implication of cyclin-dependent kinases. Biochem Biophys Res Commun. 2011;409(2):187–92.
42. Lee B, Muller MT. SUMOylation enhances DNA methyltransferase 1 activity. Biochem J. 2009;421(3):449–61.
43. Li E, Bestor TH, Jaenisch R. Targeted mutation of the DNA methyltransferase gene results in embryonic lethality. Cell. 1992;69(6):915–26.
44. Robertson KD, Uzvolgyi E, Liang G, Talmadge C, Sumegi J, Gonzales FA, et al. The human DNA methyltransferases (DNMTs) 1, 3a and 3b: coordinate mRNA expression in normal tissues and overexpression in tumors. Nucleic Acids Res. 1999;27(11):2291–8.
45. Rahman WF, Rahman KS, Nafi SN, Fauzi MH, Jaafar H. Overexpression of DNA methyltransferase 1 (DNMT1) protein in astrocytic tumour and its correlation with O6-methylguanine-DNA methyltransferase (MGMT) expression. Int J Clin Exp Pathol. 2015;8(6):6095–106.
46. Furst AL, Barton JK. DNA electrochemistry shows DNMT1 methyltransferase hyperactivity in colorectal tumors. Chem Biol. 2015;22(7):938–45.
47. Wang ET, Sandberg R, Luo S, Khrebtukova I, Zhang L, Mayr C, et al. Alternative isoform regulation in human tissue transcriptomes. Nature. 2008;456(7221):470–6.
48. Kelemen O, Convertini P, Zhang Z, Wen Y, Shen M, Falaleeva M, et al. Function of alternative splicing. Gene. 2013;514(1):1–30.
49. Dehm SM. mRNA splicing variants: exploiting modularity to outwit cancer therapy. Cancer Res. 2013;73(17):5309–14.
50. Stark M, Wichman C, Avivi I, Assaraf YG. Aberrant splicing of folylpolyglutamate synthetase as a novel mechanism of antifolate resistance in leukemia. Blood. 2009;113(18):4362–9.
51. Gopalakrishnan S, Van Emburgh BO, Shan J, Su Z, Fields CR, Vieweg J, et al. A novel DNMT3B splice variant expressed in tumor and pluripotent cells modulates genomic DNA methylation patterns and displays altered DNA binding. Mol Cancer Res. 2009;7(10):1622–34.
52. Aapola U, Kawasaki K, Scott HS, Ollila J, Vihinen M, Heino M, et al. Isolation and initial characterization of a novel zinc finger gene, DNMT3L, on 21q22.3, related to the cytosine-5-methyltransferase 3 gene family. Genomics. 2000;65(3):293–8.
53. Jia D, Jurkowska RZ, Zhang X, Jeltsch A, Cheng X. Structure of Dnmt3a bound to Dnmt3L suggests a model for de novo DNA methylation. Nature. 2007;449(7159):248–51.
54. Hata K, Okano M, Lei H, Li E. Dnmt3L cooperates with the Dnmt3 family of de novo DNA methyltransferases to establish maternal imprints in mice. Development. 2002;129(8):1983–93.
55. Suetake I, Shinozaki F, Miyagawa J, Takeshima H, Tajima S. DNMT3L stimulates the DNA methylation activity of Dnmt3a and Dnmt3b through a direct interaction. J Biol Chem. 2004;279(26):27816–23.
56. Ley TJ, Ding L, Walter MJ, McLellan MD, Lamprecht T, Larson DE, et al. DNMT3A mutations in acute myeloid leukemia. N Engl J Med. 2010;363(25):2424–33.
57. Yan XJ, Xu J, Gu ZH, Pan CM, Lu G, Shen Y, et al. Exome sequencing identifies somatic mutations of DNA methyltransferase gene DNMT3A in acute monocytic leukemia. Nat Genet. 2011;43(4):309–15.

58. Jankowska AM, Makishima H, Tiu RV, Szpurka H, Huang Y, Traina F, et al. Mutational spectrum analysis of chronic myelomonocytic leukemia includes genes associated with epigenetic regulation: UTX, EZH2, and DNMT3A. Blood. 2011;118(14):3932–41.
59. Tatton-Brown K, Seal S, Ruark E, Harmer J, Ramsay E, Del Vecchio Duarte S, et al. Mutations in the DNA methyltransferase gene DNMT3A cause an overgrowth syndrome with intellectual disability. Nat Genet. 2014;46(4):385–8.
60. Hansen RS, Wijmenga C, Luo P, Stanek AM, Canfield TK, Weemaes CM, et al. The DNMT3B DNA methyltransferase gene is mutated in the ICF immunodeficiency syndrome. Proc Natl Acad Sci U S A. 1999;96(25):14412–7.
61. Jiang YL, Rigolet M, Bourc'his D, Nigon F, Bokesoy I, Fryns JP, et al. DNMT3B mutations and DNA methylation defect define two types of ICF syndrome. Hum Mutat. 2005;25(1):56–63.
62. Okano M, Bell DW, Haber DA, Li E. DNA methyltransferases Dnmt3a and Dnmt3b are essential for de novo methylation and mammalian development. Cell. 1999;99(3):247–57.
63. Wijmenga C, Hansen RS, Gimelli G, Bjorck EJ, Davies EG, Valentine D, et al. Genetic variation in ICF syndrome: evidence for genetic heterogeneity. Hum Mutat. 2000;16(6):509–17.
64. Xu GL, Bestor TH, Bourc'his D, Hsieh CL, Tommerup N, Bugge M, et al. Chromosome instability and immunodeficiency syndrome caused by mutations in a DNA methyltransferase gene. Nature. 1999;402(6758):187–91.
65. Hsieh CL. In vivo activity of murine de novo methyltransferases, Dnmt3a and Dnmt3b. Mol Cell Biol. 1999;19(12):8211–8.
66. Handa V, Jeltsch A. Profound flanking sequence preference of Dnmt3a and Dnmt3b mammalian DNA methyltransferases shape the human epigenome. J Mol Biol. 2005;348(5):1103–12.
67. Schermelleh L, Spada F, Easwaran HP, Zolghadr K, Margot JB, Cardoso MC, et al. Trapped in action: direct visualization of DNA methyltransferase activity in living cells. Nat Methods. 2005;2(10):751–6.
68. Taylor SM, Jones PA. Mechanism of action of eukaryotic DNA methyltransferase. Use of 5-azacytosine-containing DNA. J Mol Biol. 1982;162(3):679–92.
69. Wu JC, Santi DV. Kinetic and catalytic mechanism of HhaI methyltransferase. J Biol Chem. 1987;262(10):4778–86.
70. Guimil Garcia R, Brank AS, Christman JK, Marquez VE, Eritja R. Synthesis of oligonucleotide inhibitors of DNA (Cytosine-C5) methyltransferase containing 5-azacytosine residues at specific sites. Antisense Nucleic Acid Drug Dev. 2001;11(6):369–78.
71. Ghoshal K, Datta J, Majumder S, Bai S, Kutay H, Motiwala T, et al. 5-Aza-deoxycytidine induces selective degradation of DNA methyltransferase 1 by a proteasomal pathway that requires the KEN box, bromo-adjacent homology domain, and nuclear localization signal. Mol Cell Biol. 2005;25(11):4727–41.
72. Snoek BC, de Wilt LH, Jansen G, Peters GJ. Role of E3 ubiquitin ligases in lung cancer. World J Clin Oncol. 2013;4(3):58–69.
73. Ciechanover A. N-terminal ubiquitination. Methods Mol Biol. 2005;301:255–70.
74. Groettrup M, Pelzer C, Schmidtke G, Hofmann K. Activating the ubiquitin family: UBA6 challenges the field. Trends Biochem Sci. 2008;33(5):230–7.
75. Hershko A. The ubiquitin system for protein degradation and some of its roles in the control of the cell-division cycle (Nobel lecture). Angew Chem Int Ed Eng. 2005;44(37):5932–43.
76. Rodrigo-Brenni MC, Morgan DO. Sequential E2s drive polyubiquitin chain assembly on APC targets. Cell. 2007;130(1):127–39.
77. Patel K, Dickson J, Din S, Macleod K, Jodrell D, Ramsahoye B. Targeting of 5-aza-2′-deoxycytidine residues by chromatin-associated DNMT1 induces proteasomal degradation of the free enzyme. Nucleic Acids Res. 2010;38(13):4313–24.
78. Lu LJ, Randerath K. Mechanism of 5-azacytidine-induced transfer RNA cytosine-5-methyltransferase deficiency. Cancer Res. 1980;40(8 Pt 1):2701–5.
79. Lee TT, Karon MR. Inhibition of protein synthesis in 5-azacytidine-treated HeLa cells. Biochem Pharmacol. 1976;25(15):1737–42.

80. Schaefer M, Hagemann S, Hanna K, Lyko F. Azacytidine inhibits RNA methylation at DNMT2 target sites in human cancer cell lines. Cancer Res. 2009;69(20):8127–32.
81. Weiss JW, Pitot HC. Effects of 5-azacytidine on nucleolar RNA and the preribosomal particles in Novikoff hepatoma cells. Biochemistry. 1975;14(2):316–26.
82. Weiss JW, Pitot HC. Alteration of ribosomal precursor RNA in Novikoff hepatoma cells by 5-azacytidine. Studies on methylation of 45S and 32S RNA. Arch Biochem Biophys. 1974;165(2):588–96.
83. Weiss JW, Pitot HC. Inhibition of ribosomal RNA maturation in Novikoff hepatoma cells by toyocamycin, tubercidin, and 6-thioguanosine. Cancer Res. 1974;34(3):581–7.
84. Weiss JW, Pitot HC. Inhibition of ribosomal ribonucleic acid maturation by 5-azacytidine and 8-azaguanine in Novikoff hepatoma cells. Arch Biochem Biophys. 1974;160(1):119–29.
85. Glazer RI, Peale AL, Beisler JA, Abbasi MM. The effect of 5-azacytidine and dihydro-5-azacytidine on nuclear ribosomal RNA and poly(A) RNA synthesis in L1210 cells in vitro. Mol Pharmacol. 1980;17(1):111–7.
86. Vesely J, Gostof R, Cihak A, Sorm F. Radioprotective effect of 5-azacytidine in AKR mice. Z Naturforsch B. 1969;24(3):318–20.
87. Cheng JC, Weisenberger DJ, Gonzales FA, Liang G, Xu GL, Hu YG, et al. Continuous zebularine treatment effectively sustains demethylation in human bladder cancer cells. Mol Cell Biol. 2004;24(3):1270–8.
88. Cheng JC, Yoo CB, Weisenberger DJ, Chuang J, Wozniak C, Liang G, et al. Preferential response of cancer cells to zebularine. Cancer Cell. 2004;6(2):151–8.
89. Cheng JC, Matsen CB, Gonzales FA, Ye W, Greer S, Marquez VE, et al. Inhibition of DNA methylation and reactivation of silenced genes by zebularine. J Natl Cancer Inst. 2003;95(5):399–409.
90. Griffiths EA, Choy G, Redkar S, Taverna P, Azab M, Karpf AR. SGI-110: DNA methyltransferase inhibitor oncolytic. Drugs Future. 2013;38(8):535–43.
91. Chuang JC, Warner SL, Vollmer D, Vankayalapati H, Redkar S, Bearss DJ, et al. S110, a 5-Aza-2′-deoxycytidine-containing dinucleotide, is an effective DNA methylation inhibitor in vivo and can reduce tumor growth. Mol Cancer Ther. 2010;9(5):1443–50.
92. Ziemba A, Hayes E, Freeman 3rd BB, Ye T, Pizzorno G. Development of an oral form of azacytidine: 2′3′5′triacetyl-5-azacytidine. Chemother Res Pract. 2011;2011:965826.
93. Brueckner B, Rius M, Markelova MR, Fichtner I, Hals PA, Sandvold ML, et al. Delivery of 5-azacytidine to human cancer cells by elaidic acid esterification increases therapeutic drug efficacy. Mol Cancer Ther. 2010;9(5):1256–64.
94. Thottassery JV, Sambandam V, Allan PW, Maddry JA, Maxuitenko YY, Tiwari K, et al. Novel DNA methyltransferase-1 (DNMT1) depleting anticancer nucleosides, 4′-thio-2′-deoxycytidine and 5-aza-4′-thio-2′-deoxycytidine. Cancer Chemother Pharmacol. 2014;74(2):291–302.
95. Arimany-Nardi C, Errasti-Murugarren E, Minuesa G, Martinez-Picado J, Gorboulev V, Koepsell H, et al. Nucleoside transporters and human organic cation transporter 1 determine the cellular handling of DNA-methyltransferase inhibitors. Br J Pharmacol. 2014;171(16):3868–80.
96. Le Gac G, Esteve PO, Ferec C, Pradhan S. DNA damage-induced down-regulation of human Cdc25C and Cdc2 is mediated by cooperation between p53 and maintenance DNA (cytosine-5) methyltransferase 1. J Biol Chem. 2006;281(34):24161–70.
97. Champion C, Guianvarc'h D, Senamaud-Beaufort C, Jurkowska RZ, Jeltsch A, Ponger L, et al. Mechanistic insights on the inhibition of c5 DNA methyltransferases by zebularine. PLoS ONE. 2010;5(8):e12388.
98. McCormack JJ, Marquez VE, Liu PS, Vistica DT, Driscoll JS. Inhibition of cytidine deaminase by 2-oxopyrimidine riboside and related compounds. Biochem Pharmacol. 1980;29(5):830–2.
99. Yoo CB, Jeong S, Egger G, Liang G, Phiasivongsa P, Tang C, et al. Delivery of 5-aza-2′-deoxycytidine to cells using oligodeoxynucleotides. Cancer Res. 2007;67(13):6400–8.

100. Parker WB, Shaddix SC, Rose LM, Waud WR, Shewach DS, Tiwari KN, et al. Metabolism of 4′-thio-beta-D-arabinofuranosylcytosine in CEM cells. Biochem Pharmacol. 2000;60(12):1925–32.
101. Hummel-Eisenbeiss J, Hascher A, Hals PA, Sandvold ML, Muller-Tidow C, Lyko F, et al. The role of human equilibrative nucleoside transporter 1 on the cellular transport of the DNA methyltransferase inhibitors 5-azacytidine and CP-4200 in human leukemia cells. Mol Pharmacol. 2013;84(3):438–50.
102. Issa JP, Roboz G, Rizzieri D, Jabbour E, Stock W, O'Connell C, et al. Safety and tolerability of guadecitabine (SGI-110) in patients with myelodysplastic syndrome and acute myeloid leukaemia: a multicentre, randomised, dose-escalation phase 1 study. Lancet Oncol. 2015;16(9):1099–110.
103. Chen M, Shabashvili D, Nawab A, Yang SX, Dyer LM, Brown KD, et al. DNA methyltransferase inhibitor, zebularine, delays tumor growth and induces apoptosis in a genetically engineered mouse model of breast cancer. Mol Cancer Ther. 2012;11(2):370–82.
104. Yoo CB, Chuang JC, Byun HM, Egger G, Yang AS, Dubeau L, et al. Long-term epigenetic therapy with oral zebularine has minimal side effects and prevents intestinal tumors in mice. Cancer Prev Res (Phila). 2008;1(4):233–40.
105. Neureiter D, Zopf S, Leu T, Dietze O, Hauser-Kronberger C, Hahn EG, et al. Apoptosis, proliferation and differentiation patterns are influenced by Zebularine and SAHA in pancreatic cancer models. Scand J Gastroenterol. 2007;42(1):103–16.
106. Choi WJ, Chung HJ, Chandra G, Alexander V, Zhao LX, Lee HW, et al. Fluorocyclopentenylcytosine with broad spectrum and potent antitumor activity. J Med Chem. 2012;55(9):4521–5.
107. Sarkisjan D, Julsing JR, Smid K, de Klerk D, van Kuilenburg AB, Meinsma R, et al. The cytidine analog fluorocyclopentenylcytosine (RX-3117) is activated by uridine-cytidine kinase 2. PLoS ONE. 2016;11(9):e0162901.
108. Peters GJ, Smid K, Vecchi L, Kathmann I, Sarkisjan D, Honeywell RJ, et al. Metabolism, mechanism of action and sensitivity profile of fluorocyclopentenylcytosine (RX-3117; TV-1360). Investig New Drugs. 2013;31(6):1444–57.
109. Peters GJ, Sarkisjan D, Julsing JR, Hassan A, Smid K, Kathmann I, Lee Y, Kim DJ. Inhibition of DNA methyltransferase by RX-3117 (fluorocyclopentenylcytosine) leads to upregulation of hypomethylated targets. Proc AACR 107th annual meeting 2016. Abstract #4725.
110. Sarkisjan D, Van den Berg J, Smit E, Lee YB, Kim DJ, Peters GJ. The radiosensitizing effect of fluorocyclopentenyl-cytosine (RX-3117) in lung cancer cell lines. Nucleosides Nucleotides Nucleic Acids. 2016;35:619–30.
111. Asgatay S, Champion C, Marloie G, Drujon T, Senamaud-Beaufort C, Ceccaldi A, et al. Synthesis and evaluation of analogues of N-phthaloyl-l-tryptophan (RG108) as inhibitors of DNA methyltransferase 1. J Med Chem. 2014;57(2):421–34.
112. Brueckner B, Garcia Boy R, Siedlecki P, Musch T, Kliem HC, Zielenkiewicz P, et al. Epigenetic reactivation of tumor suppressor genes by a novel small-molecule inhibitor of human DNA methyltransferases. Cancer Res. 2005;65(14):6305–11.
113. Schirrmacher E, Beck C, Brueckner B, Schmitges F, Siedlecki P, Bartenstein P, et al. Synthesis and in vitro evaluation of biotinylated RG108: a high affinity compound for studying binding interactions with human DNA methyltransferases. Bioconjug Chem. 2006;17(2):261–6.
114. Stresemann C, Brueckner B, Musch T, Stopper H, Lyko F. Functional diversity of DNA methyltransferase inhibitors in human cancer cell lines. Cancer Res. 2006;66(5):2794–800.

Epigenetic Regulator, Re-emerging Antimetabolites with Novel Mechanism of Action (Azacitidine and Decitabine): Clinical Pharmacology and Therapeutic Results

19

Shinya Sato and Yasushi Miyazaki

Abstract

Hypomethylating agents, such as azacitidine (AZA) and decitabine (DAC), are antimetabolites with a very unique mechanism of action as epigenetic regulator. After being incorporated into the DNA, these inhibit the enzyme, DNA methyltransferase, resulting in the hypomethylation of DNA, and change the expression of many genes. AZA is also incorporated into RNA, which will also disturb protein synthesis. AZA and DAC are now used to treat some hematological neoplasms, especially for the treatment of myelodysplastic syndromes (MDS). After several clinical trials, AZA became the first agent shown to prolong overall survival for higher-risk MDS. Treatment with AZA or DAC is also showed to improve cytopenia in MDS and to provide longer leukemia-free survival than other treatment. Although the precise mechanism is not revealed yet, AZA is widely used to treat MDS and, recently, acute leukemia of the elderly. Oral AZA is also under clinical development.

Keywords

Myelodysplastic syndrome (MDS) • Epigenetics • Azacitidine (AZA) • Decitabine (DAC)

19.1 Introduction

It has been shown that the suppression of gene expression by DNA methylation is associated with the development and the progression of various malignancies [1]. The modification of the cytosine base of the CpG region (CpG islands), repeating

S. Sato • Y. Miyazaki (✉)
Department of Hematology, Atomic Bomb Disease Institute, Nagasaki University, 1-12-4 Sakamoto, Nagasaki 852-8523, Japan
e-mail: y-miyaza@nagasaki-u.ac.jp

T. Ueda (ed.), *Chemotherapy for Leukemia*, DOI 10.1007/978-981-10-3332-2_19

cytosine and guanine bases, by DNA metyltransferase (DNMT) leads to the DNA methylation which is one of the epigenetic alterations of the genome [2]. The DNA methylation in the promotor region of the genes generally results in the suppression of transcription, leading to the low expression of the particular protein; however, the mechanism to cause aberrant DNA methylation is not completely understood. The recent discovery of mutations involving some of the genes encoding the methylation regulators, such as the ten-eleven translocation (TET) family of proteins, the DNA methyltransferase (DNMT), and isocitrate dehydrogenase 1 and 2 (IDH1 and IDH2), may help to show some of these mechanisms [3–5]. The mutations of methylation regulators in the myelodysplastic syndromes (MDS) and acute myeloid leukemia (AML) are hoped to become novel therapeutic targets to develop new drugs. Azacitidine (AZA) and decitabine (DAC), which act as DNMT inhibitors, were relatively old drugs, which originally developed for AML, and now they are used in the treatment of MDS and AML. AZA was proven to improve the survival of high-risk MDS compared with conventional care regimes in a randomized clinical trial. AZA is the first drug proven and still the only one agent to provide survival benefit for high-risk MDS patients. Clinical pharmacology and therapeutic results of azacitidine and decitabine are described in this chapter.

19.2 Mechanism of Action of the Methylation Inhibitor

Azacitidine and decitabine are the cytosine analogs and were originally developed in 1964 as derivatives of cytarabine, aiming for better clinical efficacy. The clinical trial with high-dose azacitidine was conducted for AML, in which AZA was used like cytarabine in the treatment, but the clinical development was discontinued because of limited response and frequent adverse events in both the groups treated with AZA or DAC compared with cytarabine. In the initial trials for patients with AML, AZA was administered as a bolus infusion at a dose of 150–200 mg/m^2 [6, 7]. The treatment schedule was a 5-day regime repeated every 14 days. Although some responses were observed for AML, severe toxicities for gastrointestinal tract, such as nausea and vomiting, led to discontinue this injection method, and a continuous intravenous infusion was used in subsequent studies [8]. Significant gastrointestinal toxicity was still observed with continuous infusion, and the subcutaneous administration method was tried [9, 10]. However, there was no clear clinical superiority over cytarabine. Since the importance of DNA methylation pathway was revealed in the differentiation and the control of gene expression in normal and abnormal cells, the mode of action of AZA and DAC obtained the attention as DNA methylation inhibitors with low-dose AZA and DAC. For example, AZA was tried to treat sickle cell anemia and thalassemia patients expecting to induce differentiation of erythroblasts to improve anemia of these conditions. In these trials, low-dose AZA treatment was reported to increase the gamma/beta hemoglobin ratio and the expression of fetal hemoglobin, which suggested the differentiation-inducing activity on human hematopoietic cells [11]. The pharmacokinetics (PK) of azacitidine was performed in six patients following a single 75 mg/m^2 subcutaneous administration (s.c.) dose and a single 75 mg/m^2 intravenous injection (i.v.) dose. The mean maximum observed plasma concentration (Cmax) of azacitidine was 750+403 ng/ml, reaching within 0.5 h. The plasma half-life was 22 min for i.v. and 41 min for s.c. The bioavailability of s.c. azacitidine relative to i.v. azacitidine was approximately 89% [34].

After DAC is taken into cells, it is serially triphosphorylated to become DAC triphosphate (DAC-P3) by nucleotide kinase, and DAC-P3 is incorporated into DNA-like cytidine triphosphate (CTP). Once DAC-P3 is incorporated into DNA, when bound to the enzyme, DNMT, a covalent bond, is generated between DAC-P3 and DNMT, holding DNMT at the DAC-P3 site. This results in low methylation of other CTPs in DNA, which is the low-methylation level of the whole DNA. With regard to AZA, it has been shown that AZA is serially phosphorylated by uridine/cytidine kinase to finally become AZA-triphosphate (AZA-P3), which is incorporated into RNA-like uridine triphosphate (UTP). About 80–90% of the azacitidine is taken into RNA after phosphorylation. Other 10–20% of AZA is reduced by ribonucleotide reductase into deoxyazacitidine diphosphate, DAC-P2, and then DAC-P3 by phosphorylation. Thus, 10–20% of AZA take the same role as DAC, but most of AZA is in RNA [12]. The functional consequences of AZA-P3 incorporation into RNA include alteration of the processing of tRNA and rRNAs, leading to inhibition of protein synthesis [13–17]. Then, AZA will have two functions, inhibition of protein synthesis and inhibition of DNA methylation, both of which are thought to be important for the clinical efficacy of AZA [18]. The study of PK analysis of decitabine was performed, administered decitabine as a 3 h intravenous infusion of 15 mg/m^2 every 8 h for 3 days. The Cmax, the time to the maximum concentration (Tmax) and the terminal phase elimination half-life ($T_{1/2}$) of decitabine were 64.8–77.0 ng/ml and 2.29–2.53 h, and 0.62–0.78 h, respectively [35].

19.2.1 Clinical Studies of Azacitidine in MDS

After AZA is recognized as a differentiation inducer in some clinical trials mentioned above, clinical investigators started to use AZA for anemia of other diseases, including MDS. The Cancer and Leukemia Group B (CALGB) conducted a phase II clinical trial of low-dose azacitidine as a single agent for patients with MDS (CALGB 8421). Primary endpoint was response rate, which meant the improvement of cytopenia and bone marrow failure. This trial enrolled 43 patients with advanced (high-risk) MDS (refractory anemia of excess blasts [RAEB] and RAEB in transformation [RAEB-T] by the FAB classification), and AZA was administered at 75 mg/m^2/day as continuous infusion for 7 days every 4 weeks. 49% of patients (21/43 patients) had some type of response; seven in complete response (CR), one in partial response (PR), and 13 with hematological improvement (HI) (responses were redefined using the International Working Group (IWG) criteria [19], which was different from the original criteria used in the trial) [18]. In the next phase II study (CALGB 8921), 70 patients with MDS were enrolled; refractory anemia (RA), 10%; RA with ring sideroblasts (RARS), 6%; RAEB, 27%; RAEB-T, 23%;

Table 19.1 Analysis of response to CALGB9221 study [22]

	Aza C			Supportive care			Crossover		
	No. of patients		%	No. of patients		%	No. of patients		%
No. evaluated		99			92			49	
CR	7		7*	0		0	5		10
PR	16		16*	0		0	2		4
Improved	37		37*	5		5	16		33
Total	60		60*	5		5	23		47

*Significant differences between the arms in CR rate ($P = .01$), CR + PR rate ($P < 0.0001$), and CR + PR + improvement rate ($P < 0.0001$) were observed

chronic myelomonocytic leukemia (CMML), 19%; and AML, 19%. Patients received AZA through s.c. at 75 mg/m^2/day every 4 weeks. Although this study included CMML and AML sharing more than 1/3 of participants, AZA showed a similar response rate as CALGB 8421; 17% of CR, 0% PR, and 23% HI, resulting to 40% of overall response rate [20, 21]. Since there was no standard treatment for MDS patients at that time, these results led CALGB to conduct a randomized, open-label, phase III, multicenter trial (CALGB 9221) to compare the survival benefit of AZA with best supportive care (BSC) [22]. In this study, 191 MDS patients were randomized to AZA group (99 patients) or BSC group (92 patients). There were 36 patients with RA, 13 with RARS, 70 with RAEB, 33 with RAEB-T, 20 with CMML, and 19 with AML, which means that more than 70% of patients were high-risk MDS or AML. AZA was administered 75 mg/m^2 s.c. for 7 days in a 28-day cycle. Criteria to permit crossover from the BSC arm to the AZA arm were established. Treatment response was observed in the 60 cases (60%) including seven cases of CR (7%),16 (16%) PR, and 37 (37%) HI in the AZA arm. Alternatively, only five patients (5%) showed improvement in the BSC arm, but no patient obtained CR or PR. Thus significantly higher-treatment response was found in the AZA arm ($P < 0.0001$). The median time to leukemic transformation or death was 21 months in patients treated with AZA compared with 12 months with BSC, which again showed statistically significant improvement by AZA treatment ($P = 0.007$). The median time of overall survival was 20 months in the AZA arm compared with 14 months in the BSC arm without significant difference. Because 49 patients had crossed over to azacitidine treatment in the BSC arm, a landmark analysis was performed for overall survival, and it showed a significant survival advantage for patients initially treated with AZA or who had crossed over to AZA within 6 months after the inclusion on this study ($P = 0.03$) (Table 19.1). Among CALGB studies, the most frequent adverse events (AEs) were cytopenias induced by AZA. This is also related to infection and febrile neutropenia until HI was obtained. Gastrointestinal events such as nausea, vomiting, and diarrhea were also observed. Those AEs were tolerable, and cytopenias and infections were also critical issues even for those in the BSC arm because of the natural history of MDS.

In response to the results of CALGB9221 study, a multicenter, international, randomized phase III study (AZA-001) was designed to compare the overall survival benefit of AZA treatment with that of the conventional care regimens (CCR) for high-risk MDS [23]. In this study, BSC, low-dose cytarabine (Ara-C) (Ara-C: 20 mg/m^2 s.c. for 14 days), and intensive chemotherapy (ICT) (Ara-C: 100–200 mg/m^2 + daunorubicin: 45–60 mg/m^2 for 3 days or idarubicin: 9–12 mg/m^2 for 3 days or mitoxantrone: 8–12 mg/m^2 for 3 days) were included in CCR arm. Before randomization, the patient and doctor were asked to select one treatment from CCR to be administered if assigned to the CCR arm, and then a randomization was done between AZA and the CCR treatment selected. This trial enrolled 358 patients with high-risk MDS, assessed by an independent review committee for FAB subtypes and International Prognostic Scoring System (IPSS) risk category [24]. One hundred seventy-nine patients were randomized to AZA arm (75 mg/m^2 s.c. for 7 days in a 28-day cycle) and 179 patients were randomized to CCR arm. The patients allocated for CCR arm received either BCS alone (n = 105), low-dose Ara-C (n = 49), or ICT (n = 25). Median age of patients was 69 years old. Median overall survival was 24.5 months for patients in the AZA arm compared with 15 months in CCR arm, and a statistically significant difference was observed (P = 0.0001). Time to progression to AML was also significantly prolonged in AZA arm. The survival benefit with AZA was unconcerned with age, percentage of marrow blasts, or chromosomal karyotype (Table 19.2). This study for the first time demonstrated that AZA prolonged overall survival of high-risk MDS patients over other available treatment regimens at that time. By now, AZA is the only one agent to be proven for survival benefit other than allogeneic transplantation. Since allogeneic hematopoietic stem cell transplantation is not indicated for most of MSD patients with various reasons, such as high age, comorbidities, etc., AZA is the first choice for high-risk MDS that lack the indication of transplant.

Additional analyses of AZA-001 trial revealed interesting features of AZA in the treatment of high-risk MDS. In the induction therapy for AML, hematologists expect to achieve CR after one course of treatment, and patients that entered CR after one course of induction regimen usually show better survival (or longer CR duration) than those obtained CR after two or more courses of induction therapy, showing the importance of prompt reduction of leukemia cells by chemotherapy. However, in terms of AZA for MDS, almost 40% of responders show HI or other responses after four courses of AZA treatment (usually more than 4 months after the initial injection). Time to response did not have strong impact on survival as for MDS as AML. Interestingly, survival benefit among patients with stable disease was also suggested after AZA treatment. Not only pharmacologically but also clinically, AZA shows different features than classical chemotherapeutic agents including Ara-C. Considering no other standard therapy is available for high-risk MDS, it makes physicians continue AZA treatment until progression or intolerable situation.

Table 19.2 Analysis of response to AZA-001 study [21]

	BSC only ($n = 222$)				Low-dose cytarabine ($n = 94$)				Intensive chemotherapy ($n = 42$)			
	Azacitidine ($n = 117$)	BSC ($n = 105$)	HR (95% CI)	*p* value	Azacitidine ($n = 45$)	Low-dose cytarabine ($n = 49$)	HR (95% CI)	*p* value	Azacitidine ($n = 17$)	Intensive chemotherapy ($n = 25$)	HR (95% CI)	*p* value
Overall survival (months)	21.1 (10.5-NR)	11.5 (5.7-NR)	0.58 (0.40–0.85)	0.0045	24.5 (8.4–34.7)	15.3 (4.9–25.8)	0.36 (0.20–0.65)	0.0006	25.1 (10.0-NR)	15.7 (8.2–24.1)	0.76 (0.33–1.74)	0.51
Time to transformationto AML (months)	15.0 (8.8–27.6)	10.1(3.9–19.8)	0.41 (0.27–0.63)	<0.0001	15.0 (7.3–25.5)	14.5 (4.9–19.2)	0.55 (0.28–1.11)	0.097	23.1 (6.4–25.4)	10.7 (4.6–15.4)	0.48 (0.16–1.45)	0.19

Data are median (IQR). Hazard ratios calculated with stratified Cox proportional hazards model adjusted for treatment, subgroup, Eastern Cooperative Oncology Group performance status, lactate dehydrogenase, hemoglobin, number of previous red blood cell transfusions, and presence or absence of cytogenetic −7/del (7q) abnormality. No subgroup-by-treatment interactions were significant ($p > 0.20$)

BCS best supportive care, *NR* not reached, *HR* hazard ratio, *AML* acute myeloid leukemia

19.2.2 Clinical Studies of Decitabine in MDS

Decitabine (DAC) is another nucleoside analog with the capacity to induce DNA hypomethylation through the inhibition of DNMT. The mechanism of hypomethylation of DNA is the same as seen in AZA. Since AZA but no other treatment including chemotherapy with anthracyclins and Ara-C showed clinical efficacy for MDS, DNA hypomethylation was thought to be very important for the treatment of MDS. Considering the mode of action of DAC in which 100% of DAC theoretically works as DNMT inhibitor, DAC was expected to show higher efficacy than AZA of which about 20% would be incorporated into DNA to inhibit DNMT. The clinical trials with the middle or the high dose of DAC were conducted initially. However, there was no preeminence with many adverse events as compared with other drug, and then clinic development was discontinued. After, the demethylation activity of DAC drew attention, and clinical trials with low-dose DAC were conducted. Wijermans et al. conducted a phase II clinical study with decitabine for 66 patients of MDS to test the efficacy and toxicity of DAC [25]. DAC was administered at a dose of 15 mg/m^2 infusion over a 4 h period every 8 h (45 mg/m^2/day) for 3 consecutive days. DAC treatment courses were repeated every 6 weeks up to six courses. Primary endpoint was response rate. There were eight cases of RA or RARS, 29 of RAEB, 20 of RAEB-T, and nine CMML cases, and most of them (76%, 50 out of 66 cases) were included in the higher-risk group of IPSS category. Among them, 32 patients (49%) showed clinical response, including CR (n = 13, 19.7%), PR (n = 3, 4.5%), and improvement (n = 16, 24.2%) of cytopenia as defined by the protocol (reduction of at least 50% of transfusion requirements, etc.). Response rates by the risk category of IPSS were as follows: 25% in the intermediate (Int)-1 category, 48% in Int-2, and 64% in high-risk category. The median time of response duration was 31 weeks. These suggested the clinical efficacy of DAC over the risk of MDS predicted by IPSS. The treatment-related mortality (toxic death) was 7.6% (n = 5), and non-hematological toxicity of grade 3–4 was observed at only 13.6% (n = 9). There were 17 cases (26%) of disease progression. These results were comparable or even better than those of AZA trials mainly conducted by CALGB (mentioned above).

Based on these, a randomized trial was performed in which response rate and time to AML or death were compared between DAC with BSC and BSC alone in MDS at 18 years or older [26]. In this study, the dose of decitabine was 15 mg/m^2 and administered intravenously over 3 h every 8 h for 3 days (at a dose of 45 mg/m^2/day and 135 mg/m^2 per course) and which repeated every 6 weeks depending on the recovery from myelosuppression, almost the same schedule as in the previous phase II study. Response was assessed according to the International IWG criteria [19]. A total of 170 patients with MDS (median age was 70 years old) were randomized to receive either DAC or BSC. Fifty-two patients (31%) were categorized into Int-1 risk group of IPSS, 74 patients (44%) into Int-2 risk group of IPSS, and 43 (25%) in high-risk group of IPSS. Overall response rate was 17% (9% with CR and 8% with PR) in DAC and 0% in BSC, and clinical improvement that included CR, PR, and HI was obtained in 30% of cases in DAC arm and 7% in BSC arm. There were statistically significant differences both in overall response rate and clinical improvement rate

Table 19.3 Analysis of response to decitabine [26]

	Decitabine (n = 89) (%)	Supportive care (n = 81) (%)	P value*
Clinical response			
Overall response (CR + PR)	15(17)	0	<0.001
CR	8(9)	0	
PR	7(8)	0	
Clinical improvement			
Overall improvement (CR + PR + HI)	27(30)	6(7)	<0.001
HI	12(13)	6(7)	
Major	12(13)[a]	5(6)[b]	
Minor	0(0)	1(1)	
Response by subgroup (CR + PR)			

CR complete response, *PR* partial response, *HI* hematologic improvement
*Determined using the Fisher 2-sided exact test
[a]Includes 2 major erythroid hematologic improvements, 4 major platelet hematologic improvements, 1 major neutrophil hematologic improvement, 3 major erythroid plus platelet hematologic improvements, and 2 major neutrophil plus erythroid hematologic improvements
[b]Includes 3 major neutrophil hematologic improvements, 1 major platelet hematologic improvement, and 1 major both hematologic improvement; 1 minor platelet hematologic improvement

(both $P < 0.001$). Although DAC group showed a trend toward a longer median time to AML or death than BSC group, there was no significant difference between the two groups (12.1 months for DAC and 7.8 months for BSC, respectively, $P = 0.16$) (Table 19.3). These results led to the approval of DAC for MDS in the USA.

A similar phase III clinical study of DAC for MDS was conducted among European countries by European Organization for Research and Treatment of Cancer Leukemia Group (EORTC) [27]. The administration method of DAC was similar to the prior phase III study, and the primary endpoint was set as overall survival (OS). Two-hundred thirty-three patients were enrolled; 92% of patients had high-risk diseases (IPSS Int-2 and high) with 32% of AML by WHO criteria, and 53% had poor-risk cytogenetics. These patients were randomly assigned to decitabine arm (n = 119) and the BSC arm (n = 114), with a balanced distribution for age, sex, performance status, and risk profile (IPSS subgroup and FAB subtype). DAC (15 mg/m^2) was given intravenously over 4 h three times a day for 3 days in 6-week cycles. The maximum number of treatment cycle was limited to eight (or ten in case CR was achieved after eight courses). As the primary endpoint, OS prolongation in DAC arm was not shown over BSC with statistical significance (median OS, 10.1, and 8.5 months, respectively, $P = 0.38$). Progression-free survival (PFS), defined as time from randomization to progression, relapse after CR or PR or death, prolonged significantly by DAC (1-year PFS rate 27% and 15%, in the DAC and BSC arm, respectively, $P = 0.004$). There was no statistical difference in AML-free survival (AMLFS, defined as time from randomization to AML transformation or death) between the DAC and BSC arms (median AMLFS, 8.8 versus 6.1 months, respectively, $P = 0.24$), although AML transformation was significantly ($P = 0.036$)

reduced at 1 year (from 33% with BSC to 22% with DAC). There was no difference in cumulative incidence of death without AML, either between two arms ($P = 0.17$). Additional analyses suggested the advantage of DAC over BSC in PFS among several subgroups. In terms of toxicity, grade 3 or 4 infections were most frequent AEs followed by gastrointestinal events. Neutropenia and fatigue were also frequently observed, as seen in other DAC studies.

These two phase III clinical trials failed to demonstrate the significant efficacy of DAC on OS for MDS patients. Because two big trials did not meet the overall survival endpoint, it had a big impact for the role of DAC for not only MDS but also for other hematological malignancies, especially for elderly patients. Some investigators considered that the limitation of treatment cycle of DAC (up to eight courses in both studies) or the administration schedule (3-day administration during 6 weeks) might affect these negative results.

Aiming to improve these problems and to find a better administration way of DAC, the new clinical trials were conducted. Among those trials, one of them tried a low-dose prolonged exposure schedule of DAC in a phase I style. A total of 48 patients (35 patients with AML, seven with MDS, one with acute lymphoblastic leukemia, and five with chronic myelogenous leukemia) were entered in this study at the MD Anderson Cancer Center in the USA (two patients were treated twice at two different dose levels) [28]. The initial plan was to treat patient cohorts (six to eight patients) with DAC at 5, 10, or 20 mg/m^2 daily intravenously over 1 h for 10 days (5 days on, 2 days off, 5 days on), approximately every 6 weeks. After the first two cohorts were accrued and clinical activity was confirmed, a cohort with an intermediate dose of 15 mg/m^2 was added. With 15 mg/m^2 of DAC, three administration plans were tested: 10-, 15-, and 20-day schedule (six, eight, and three patients, respectively). Then, 11 patients were added to a 10-day schedule at 15 mg/m^2 daily to examine the efficacy of DAC. Responses were seen at all dose levels. Interestingly, a dose of 15 mg/m^2 for 10-day schedule showed the highest response rate (11 out of 17 patients in total, 65%), with fewer responses seen with prolonged treatment (15- and 20-day schedules, one response among 11 patients, 9%) or treatment with escalated dose (one responder in eight patients in a 20 mg/m^2 for a 10-day schedule, 9%).

In the following study at MD Anderson Cancer Center which focused on the lower dose (at 100 mg/m^2 in one course) DAC and searched for a better administration schedule, a randomized phase II trial was conducted for MDS (Int or high risk of IPSS) and CMML patients. [29]. In this study, patients were randomized to receive DAC in one of three schedules: (1) 20 mg/m^2 intravenously over 1 h daily for 5 days; (2) 20 mg/m^2 daily for 5 days, given in two subcutaneous doses daily for 5 days; or (3) 10 mg/m^2 intravenously over 1 h daily for 10 days. Decitabine was administered in each arm repeatedly more than three courses every 4 weeks. A total of 95 patients were enrolled, and 77 and 18 patients had MDS and CMML, respectively. Median age of participants was 65 years old. Overall, 32 patients (34%) achieved CR; one had PR, 23 with marrow CR, and 13 with HI. In total, 69 (73%) had an objective response by the newly modified International Working Group criteria. The CR rate in patients receiving 20 mg/m^2 intravenously for 5 days, 20 mg/m^2 subcutaneously for 5 days, and 10 mg/m^2 intravenously for 10 days was 39%,

21%, and 24%, respectively, ($P < 0.05$). The patients who administered decitabine with 20 mg/m^2 intravenously for 5 days showed the superior effect compared with other arms. The methylation status of clinical samples (peripheral blood) was also assessed in this trial. LINE-1 assay to see the methylation of LINE-1 in genome was examined as a marker of genome methylation level, and it was shown that the level of LINE-1 methylation dropped about 10 days after the first administration of DAC to −10% to 20% compared with the initial level. The methylation level recovered after that but not to the initial level. This clearly showed the clinically meaningful hypomethylating activity of DAC in human hematopoietic cells.

The result of this study led to a multicenter phase II trial with decitabine 20 mg/m^2 by intravenous infusion daily for 5 consecutive days every 4 weeks (Alternative Dosing for Outpatient Treatment [ADOPT]) by Steensma D et al. to confirm these results [30]. This study assessed the overall response (CR, marrow CR, and PR) rate as a primary endpoint and also the safety of an alternative dosing regimen administered on an outpatient basis in academic and community-based practices. Ninety-nine patients were enrolled with median age of 72 years old. There were 37 patients with RA or RARS, 51 with RAEB or RAEB-T, and 11 with CMML. All except one patients were Int-1 or higher risk in IPSS [52 cases (53%) with Int-1, 23 (23%) with Int-2, and 23 (23%) with High]. The median number of courses administered was five. Overall response rate, the primary endpoint, was 32%; CR, 17%; marrow CR, 15%; and PR, 0%. There is no patient-achieved PR, but HI was observed in 18% of patients. The 1-year survival rate of all patients was 66%, and median survival time was 19.4 months. Cytopenias were the most frequent complication with grade 3 or higher neutropenia, thrombocytopenia, febrile neutropenia, and anemia. Among non-hematologic AEs, pneumonia, and fatigue were found at 11% and 5%, respectively. This study demonstrated that DAC with the alternative schedule would provide clinical benefit to a certain number of MDS patients in the outpatient setting (Table 19.4).

As described above, DAC provided CR, marrow CR, and PR to patients with MDS, probably with higher response rate by the alternative administration schedule. However, so far, overall survival benefit has not been shown in any treatment schedule.

19.2.3 Clinical Studies of Oral Azacitidine

AZA and DAC are extremely potent in inhibiting DNA methylation, but their short half-lives in aqueous solutions and low oral bioavailability complicate their delivery. To solve this problem, Amy Z et al. had synthesized an acetylated derivative of AZA, 2′,3′,5′-triacetyl-5-azacitidine (TAC) to evaluate its possibility as an oral prodrug. The prodrug demonstrated significant pharmacokinetic improvements in bioavailability, solubility, and stability over the parent compound [31]. In the pilot study with the oral administration, four patients with solid malignant tumors, AML, or MDS received single oral doses of 60 or 80 mg, and pharmacokinetics and safety were evaluated. Patients safely tolerated 80 mg of TAC, and the mean bioavailability was 17.4% of subcutaneous administrations. Severe drug-related

Table 19.4 Analysis of responses to ADOPT trial [30]

	ITT ($N = 99$)	
Response by 2006 IWG criteria	No. of patients	%
Overall complete response rate, CR + mCR	32	32
Overall response rate, CR + mCR + PR	32	32
Overall improvement rate, CR + mCR + PR + HI	50	51
Rate of stable disease or better, CR + mCR + PR + HI + SD	74	75
CR	17	17
mCR	15	15
PR	0	0
HI	18	18
SD	24	24
PD	10	10
Not assessable*	15	15

IWG International Working Group, *ITT* intent to treat, *CR* complete response, *mCR* marrow CR, *PR* partial response, *HI* hematologic improvement, *SD* stable disease, *PD* progressive disease

*A total of 15 patients were not assessable for a response assessment because post-therapy bone marrow and/or CBC values were not available. Specifically, five patients were entered onto the study with comorbid conditions (including metastatic lung cancer, preexisting acute respiratory distress syndrome, pulmonary fibrosis, and cardiomyopathy) that resulted in early withdrawal from the study and precluded an opportunity for a response assessment, five patients were withdrawn from the study early for administrative reasons (ie, patient or family decision) without documentation of a study-related adverse event, and five patients had adverse events before the first post-therapy bone marrow evaluation and were withdrawn based on the clinical judgment of the investigator

toxicity was not observed, and these data suggested that oral AZA is bioavailable [32]. Following this pilot study, an open-label, phase I, dose-escalation trial was conducted to identify the maximum tolerated dose (MTD), dose-limiting toxicities (DLTs), safety, pharmacokinetic and pharmacodynamics profiles, and clinical activity of oral AZA in 41 patients with MDS, CMML, and AML [33]. AZA was injected at 75 mg/m^2 daily s.c. for 7 days of a 28-day cycle in cycle one with a standard AZA administration schedule as control, and then they received oral AZA during cycle two and beyond. Oral AZA was given on the same 7-day schedule as s.c. injection. The starting dose of oral AZA was 120 mg, and doses were escalated in 60 mg increments up to a dose of 360 mg, followed by 120 mg increments until the MTD was reached. Because DLT (grade 3/4 diarrhea) developed in a 600 mg cohort, 480 mg was determined to be the MTD. The adverse events of grade 3/4 included febrile neutropenia (19.5%), diarrhea (12.2%), fatigue (9.8%), nausea (7.3%), and vomiting (7.3%). In terms of pharmacokinetics, plasma concentration of AZA after oral administration of 480 mg was less in both peak concentration and the area under the curve than those of s.c. injection of 75 mg/m^2. Along with lower plasma concentration, the number of hypermethylated loci assessed using the array-based genome methylation analysis methods was larger after oral AZA treatment

Table 19.5 Responses in MDS and CMML patients [33]

Response	Previously treated patients[a]			First-line treatment			Duration of response: range
	Responders	Evaluable patients	%	Responders	Evaluable patients	%	(days)
Overall response[b]	6	17	35	11	15	73	30–483[C]
CR[d]	0	17	0	6	15	40	30–152
Any HI[e]	6	16	38	5	9	56	56–483[c]
HI-E	3	10	30	2	4	50	56–483[c]
HI-N	0	10	0	2	7	29	82–321[c]
HI-P	5	14	36	2	6	33	58–351[c]
TI	0	5	0	1	3	33	76
Red blood cell	0	3	0	1	3	33	76
Platelet	0	4	0	0			NA
mCR[e, f]	6	9	67	2	6	33	63–422[g]

Note: At any cycle of azacitidine, International Working Group 2006 criteria were used with modifications

CR complete remission, *E* erythroid, *HI* hematologic improvement, *mCR* bone marrow complete remission, *N* neutrophil, *NA* not applicable, *P* platelet, *TI* transfusion independence

[a]Includes erythropoiesis-stimulating agents, chemotherapy, hypomethylating agents, and investigational and/or other agents

[b]Overall response rate does not include patients achieving mCR only

[c]One or more responses, including that at upper limit of range, are ongoing. Data were censored as of last visit entered into the clinical database

[d]Patients achieving CR were not included in any other categories

[e]One patient with mCR in the previously treated group also achieved HI (both HI-E and HI-P). Two patients with mCR in the first-line treatment group also achieved HI (one patient with HI-P and one patient with both HI-E and HI-N). These patients have been included in both the mCR and HI categories

[f]In the eight patients who achieved mCR, the response began in cycle 1 of subcutaneous (SC) dosing (n 4) or very early in cycle 2 of oral dosing (n 4). Therefore, the contribution of a single SC azacitidine cycle to the induction of these responses is likely relevant

[g]Bone marrow aspirates were not required after 6 cycles of oral azacitidine treatment, therefore follow-up data were not available to confirm upper limit of duration

Data were censored as of last visit entered into the clinical database

compared to s.c. AZA, though the reduction of the number was substantial after either administration way. The median number of oral AZA cycles administered for MDS, CMML, and AML was 6, 12.5, and 4.5, respectively. Among 17 patients that had previous treatment history, oral AZA provided 35% of overall response rate (HI in 6 out of 17 patients). For those whom oral AZA was given as first-line treatment, 11 out of 15 patients (73%) became responders; the number of patients with CR or PR is six (40%) and HI is five (56%). These showed that oral AZA was a candidate new drug especially for MDS and CMML with biologic and clinical activities (Table 19.5).

Since there are many new drugs for MDS/CMML under developmental trials, it is also expected to combine oral AZA and other agents to enhance the efficacy of treatments.

19.3 Conclusion

Hypomethylating agents (AZA and ADC) as epigenetic regulators are unique for the treatment of hematological malignancies, especially for MDS and AML in the elderly. Considering the mechanism of action and the pattern to see the clinical effects on MDS, these are quite different from classical anticancer drugs including cytarabine. So far, there are no other tumors that clinically respond to AZA or DAC than myeloid neoplasms. However, these two drugs clearly demonstrated that epigenetic regulators would be new targets to treat malignancies and that a new strategy for the combination treatments need to be studied to improve the treatment results of hematological neoplasms, in particular, MDS.

References

1. Esterller M. Epigenetics in cancer. N Engl J Med. 2008;358(11):1148–59.
2. Herman JG, Baylin SB. Gene silencing in cancer in association with promoter hypermethylation. N Engl J Med. 2003;349(21):2042–54.
3. Mardis ER, Ding L, Dooling DJ, et al. Recurring mutations found by sequencing an acute myeloid leukemia genome. N Engl J Med. 2009;361(11):1058–66.
4. Ko M, Huang Y, Jankowska AM, et al. Impaired hydroxylation of 5-methylcytosine in myeloid cancers with mutant TET2. Nature. 2010;468(7325):839–43.
5. Ley TJ, Ding L, Walter MJ, et al. DNMT3A mutations in acute myeloid leukemia. N Engl J Med. 2010;363(25):2424–33.
6. Karon M, Sieger L, Leimbrock S, et al. 5-Azacytidine: a new active agent for the treatment of acute leukemia. Blood. 1973;42(3):359–65.
7. McCredie KB, Bodey GP, Burgess MA, et al. Treatment of acute leukemia with 5-azacytidine (NSC-102816). Cancer Chemother Rep. 1973;57(3):319–23.
8. Israili AH, Vogler WR, Mingioli ES, et al. The disposition and pharmacokinetics in humans of 5-azacytidine administered intravenously as a bolus or by continuous infusion. Cancer Res. 1976;36(4):1453–61.
9. Beller RE, Mastrangelo MJ, Engstrom PF, et al. Clinical trial with subcutaneously administered 5-azacytidine (NSC-102816). Cancer Chemother Rep. 1974;58(2):217–22.
10. Armitage JO, Burns CP. Treatment of refractory adult acute nonlymphoblastic leukemia with subcutaneous 5-azacytidine. Cancer Treat Rep. 1977;61(9):1721–3.
11. Ley TJ, DeSimone J, Noguchi CT, et al. 5-Azacytidine increases gamma-globin synthesis and reduces the proportion of dense cells in patients with sickle cell anemia. Blood. 1983;62(2):370–80.
12. Li LH, Olin EJ, Buskirk HH. Cytotoxicity and mode of action of 5-azacytidine on L1210 leukemia. Cancer Res. 1970;30(11):2760–9.
13. Glover AB, Leyland-Jonecs B. Biochemistry of azacitidine: a review. Cancer Treat Rep. 1987;71(10):959–64.
14. Cihák A, Weiss JW, Pitot HC. Characterization of polyribosomes and maturation of ribosomal RNA in hepatoma cells treated with 5-azacytidine. Cancer Res. 1974;34(11):3003–9.
15. Reichaman M, Penman S. The mechanism of inhibition of protein synthesis by 5-azacytidine in HeLa cells. Biochim Biophys Acta. 1973;324(2):282–9.

16. Cihák A. Biological effects of 5-azacytidine in eukaryotes. Oncolgy. 1974;30(5):405–22.
17. Lu LJ, Randerath K. Mechanism of 5-azacytidine-induced transfer RNA cytosine-5-methyltransferase deficiency. Cancer Res. 1980;40(8 Pt 1):2701–5.
18. Stresemann C, Lyko F. Modes of action of the DNA methyltransferase inhibitors azacytidine and decitabine. Int J Cancer. 2008;123(19):8–13.
19. Cheson BD, Bennett JM, Kantarjian H, et al. Report of an International Working Group to standardize response criteria for myelodysplastic syndromes. Blood. 2000;96(12):3671–4.
20. Silverman LR, McKenzie DR, Peterson BL, et al. Further analysis of trials with azacitidine in patients with myelodysplastic syndrome: studies 8421, 8921, and 9221 by the Cancer and Leukemia Group B. J Clin Oncol. 2006;24(24):3895–903.
21. Silverman LR, Holland JF, Weinberg RS, et al. Effects of treatment with 5-azacytidine on the in vivo and in vitro hematopoiesis in patients with myelodysplastic syndromes. Leukemia. 1993;7(Suppl 1):21–9.
22. Silverman LR, Demakos EP, Peterson BL, et al. Randomized controlled trial of azacitidine in patients with the myelodysplastic syndrome: a study of the cancer and leukemia group B. J Clin Oncol. 2002;20(10):2429–40.
23. Fenaux P, Mufi GJ, Hellstrom-Lindberg E, et al. Efficacy of azacitidine compared with that of conventional care regimens in the treatment of higher-risk myelodysplastic syndromes: a randomised, open-label, phase III study. Lancet Oncol. 2009;10(3):223–32.
24. Greenberg P, Cox C, LeBeau MM, et al. International scoring system for evaluating prognosis in myelodysplastic syndromes. Blood. 1997;89(6):2079–88.
25. Wijermans P, Lübbert M, Verhoef G, et al. Low-dose 5-aza-2′-deoxycytidine, a DNA hypomethylating agent, for the treatment of high-risk myelodysplastic syndrome: a multicenter phase II study in elderly patients. J Clin Oncol. 2000;18(5):956–62.
26. Kantarjian H, Issa JP, Rosenfeld CS, et al. Decitabine improves patient outcomes in myelodysplastic syndromes: results of a phase III randomized study. Cancer. 2006;106(8):1794–803.
27. Lubbert M, Suciu S, Baila L, et al. Low-dose decitabine versus best supportive care in elderly patients with intermediate- or high-risk myelodysplastic syndrome (MDS) ineligible for intensive chemotherapy: final results of the randomized phase III study of the European Organisation for Research and Treatment of Cancer Leukemia Group and the German MDS Study Group. J Clin Oncol. 2011;29(15):1987–96.
28. Issa JP, Garcia-Manero G, Giles FJ, et al. Phase 1 study of low-dose prolonged exposure schedules of the hypomethylating agent 5-aza-2′-deoxycytidine (decitabine) in hematopoietic malignancies. Blood. 2004;103(5):1635–40.
29. Kantarjian H, Oki Y, Garcia-Manero G, et al. Results of a randomized study of 3 schedules of low-dose decitabine in higher-risk myelodysplastic syndrome and chronic myelomonocytic leukemia. Blood. 2007;109(1):52–7.
30. Steensma DP, Baer MR, Slack JL, et al. Multicenter study of decitabine administered daily for 5 days every 4 weeks to adults with myelodysplastic syndromes: the alternative dosing for outpatient treatment (ADOPT) trial. J Clin Oncol. 2009;27(23):3842–8.
31. Ziemba A, Hayes E, Freeman 3rd BB, et al. Development of an oral form of azacytidine: 2′3′5′ triacetyl-5-azacytidine. Chemother Res Pract. 2011;2011:965826.
32. Garcia-Manero G, Stoltz ML, Ward MR, et al. A pilot pharmacokinetic study of oral azacitidine. Leukemia. 2008;22(9):1680–4.
33. Garcia-Manero G, Gore SD, Cogle C, et al. Phase I study of oral azacitidine in myelodysplastic syndromes, chronic myelomonocytic leukemia, and acute myeloid leukemia. J Clin Oncol. 2011;29(18):2521–7.
34. O'Dwyer K, Maslak P. Azacitidine and the beginnings of therapeutic epigenetic modulation. Expert Opin Pharmacother. 2008;9(11):1981–6.
35. Cashen AF, Shah AK, Todt L, et al. Pharmacokinetics of decitabine administered as a 3-h infusion to patients with acute myeloid leukemia (AML) or myelodysplastic syndrome (MDS). Cancer Chemother Pharmacol. 2008;61(5):759–66.

Part VI

Therapy Targeting Leukemic Stem Cells

Therapies Targeting Leukemic Stem Cells 20

Taira Maekawa

Abstract

Despite improvements in the treatment of leukemia, relapse remains a substantial problem. Relapse often results from the persistence of leukemic stem cells (LSCs) that are difficult to eradicate with conventional therapies; therefore, novel therapeutic strategies with the ability to target LSCs are required. In principle, differentiated progenitor cells have no self-renewal ability. However, there is a possibility that LSCs originate from these differentiated progenies when they acquire self-renewal ability. To become LSCs, differentiated leukemic progenitors must have self-renewal ability. Molecules that control self-renewal and proliferation, molecules that regulate the cell cycle and differentiation, molecules that enhance cell survival, molecules constituting the hematopoietic (leukemic) niche that exists in hypoxic environments, and cell surface molecules specific for leukemia are candidates for eradicating LSCs. However, to specifically eliminate LSCs while sparing normal hematopoietic stem cells, the detailed molecular mechanisms and pathophysiology of LSCs need to be clarified by sophisticated gene sequencing technologies and disease models. Many patients with incurable leukemias are eagerly awaiting the benefits of new targeted therapeutics.

Keywords

Cancer stem cells • Leukemic stem cells • Self-renewal capacity • Molecular targeted therapy

T. Maekawa (✉)
Department of Transfusion Medicine & Cell Therapy, Center for Cell and Molecular Therapy, Kyoto University Hospital, 54 Kawahara-cho, Shogoin, Sakyo-ku, Kyoto 606-8507, Japan
e-mail: maekawa@kuhp.kyoto-u.ac.jp

T. Ueda (ed.), *Chemotherapy for Leukemia*, DOI 10.1007/978-981-10-3332-2_20

20.1 Introduction

In recent years, the rapid progress in molecular biology and the remarkable advancement of genetic engineering technology have led to the extraordinary development of novel molecular targeted therapeutics for cancer. In addition, the comprehensive and genome-wide development of gene expression analysis technology using next-generation sequencers and developments such as xenotransplantation techniques using highly immunodeficient humanized mice enable detailed studies in which patient cancer specimens can be repopulated. These technologies accelerate the possibilities of translational research, i.e., the clinical development of novel therapies from the bench to the bedside.

Recent evidence suggests that cancer stem cells (CSCs) are critical for the maintenance and development of cancer. CSCs are a unique population of cells within malignant tumors with stemlike properties that are supposedly mandatory drivers of cancer initiation and progression [1]. CSCs are functionally characterized by their ability to undergo unlimited self-renewal and to form tumors in vivo. The concept of hierarchical organization of a tumor cell population, with CSCs positioned at the apex of the cell hierarchy, can explain at least most of the important aspects of the biological and clinical behavior of cancer, such as relapse and the development of therapeutic resistance [2]. This hierarchy, where quiescent and slow-cycling stem cells self-renew and replenish an active cycling population, is well defined in the hematopoietic system.

In the bone marrow (BM), there is a cell population termed hematopoietic stem cells (HSCs), which are characterized by their self-renewal capacity and multilineage differentiation over the lifetime of an individual [3]. Both murine and human studies have attempted to characterize and purify HSCs based on surface markers, as well as in vitro clonogenic and in vivo repopulation assays. Similar to many human cancers, human acute myeloid leukemia (AML) reveals evidence of a hierarchy. The earliest concept of hierarchy in leukemia can be traced to the identification of clonogenic AML progenitors [4]. Recent advances in gene profiling technologies have begun to unravel the regulatory mechanism of HSCs by novel genes, and the stem cell model of hematopoiesis has also led to the concept of leukemic stem cells (LSCs), which involves the presence of a rare population of cells that possess the essential HSC characteristics of a self-renewal capacity, replication, and differentiation into progenies [5]. Despite remarkable improvements in the treatment of leukemia, a considerable number of patients still suffer from relapse. Relapse most often results from a small number of LSCs, which reestablish the full tumor. Evidence for the existence of LSCs was first derived from the study of AML [6]. AML develops from self-renewing LSCs, which should be an ultimate therapeutic target for a complete cure [7]. Currently, many molecular targeted drugs for leukemia and hematological malignancies are clinically used, and some stemness inhibitors are also in various phases of preclinical development, with some used in clinically relevant settings.

Difficulties in eliminating LSCs with conventional chemotherapies seem to be the primary cause of relapse in patients with AML. Therefore, novel therapeutic strategies with the ability to target LSCs are required to improve the prognosis of patients. An essential step toward this goal is the identification of common phenotypic surface markers and biological characteristics that distinguish between LSCs and normal HSCs/progenitor cells across leukemia patients. This work has developed a considerable number of potential therapies specifically targeting LSCs such as those aimed at cell surface molecules, cell signaling transductions, and BM microenvironments. This chapter briefly reviews the basic biology, signal transduction, and immunophenotype of LSCs. The clinical relevance of LSCs and the emerging therapeutic strategies using biological materials and small molecules that directly target LSCs and modulate their microenvironments to eliminate LSCs will also be discussed.

20.2 Identification and Diversity of LSCs

Hematopoiesis proceeds through an organized developmental hierarchy initiated by HSCs that give rise to progressively more committed progenitors and then terminally differentiated blood cells. Murine hematopoiesis is initiated by long-term HSCs that differentiate into a series of multipotent progenitors that exhibit a progressively diminished self-renewal capacity. In human hematopoiesis, populations enriched for HSC activity are the upstream lineage-committed progenitors. Advances in multicolor flow cytometry were used to show that normal HSCs can be highly purified in the $Lin^-CD34^+CD38^-CD90^+CD45RA^-$ fraction. Downstream of this fraction is the $Lin^-CD34^+CD38^-CD90^-CD45RA^+$ fraction containing multipotent progenitors. Cells of this fraction differentiate into the $CD34^+CD38^+$ fraction. Common myeloid progenitor cells (CMPs), granulocyte lineage-monocyte progenitor cells (GMPs), and erythroid-megakaryocyte progenitor cells are present in the $CD34^+CD38^+$ fraction, and they are fractionated according to the CD123 (IL3RA) and CD45RA expression levels.

In 1997, Dick et al. established an experimental model to repopulate human AML in nonobese diabetic mice with severe combined immunodeficiency disease (NOD/SCID mice) [6]. Regardless of the heterogeneity in the maturation characteristics of leukemic blasts, investigators used flow cytometry to demonstrate that LSCs of AML (AML-LSCs) are exclusively $CD34^{++}CD38^-$, suggesting that normal primitive cells, rather than committed progenitor cells ($CD34^+CD38^+$), are the target for leukemic transformation. AML-LSCs could be differentiated into leukemic blasts and then into leukemic progenitors in vivo, i.e., the leukemic clone constitutes a hierarchy.

In AML, LSC activity was shown to be enriched in the same as the surface antigen is $CD34^+CD38^-$ cell fraction of normal HSCs. In recent years, however, LSCs in some AML patients were not necessarily restricted to the $CD34^+CD38^-$ cell fraction, and it is clear that LSCs are also present in the $CD34^+CD38^+$ cell fraction. Although LSCs are concentrated in the $CD34^+CD38^-$ cell fraction, it is suggested that LSC activity varies according to the individual case, indicating there is more heterogeneity in the LSC compartment than was previously recognized [8, 9].

Indeed, Goardon et al. revealed that, in most primary human $CD34^+$ AMLs, two expanded populations coexist [10]. One is the mature LSC population that is mostly similar to normal GMPs, and the other is the immature LSC population that is functionally similar to lymphoid-primed multipotent progenitors. Both populations demonstrate the self-renewal ability of LSCs and are hierarchically organized. The former LSC population gives rise to the latter population and vice versa. The extensive gene expression profile shows that LSCs are molecularly different and mirror normal progenitors but not stem cells. This suggests that, in most cases, primary $CD34^+$ AML is a progenitor disease in which an abnormal self-renewal potential is acquired. These reports suggest that other biological markers or pathways that are truly specific to LSCs, and are not shared with normal HSCs, need to be identified.

20.3 The Origin of LSCs

Genetic abnormalities of LSCs have been discussed, namely, class I mutations, which lead to acquirement of a growth advantage, and class II mutations, which impair differentiation [11]. As class I mutations, gain-of-function mutations involved in the cell proliferation signal (KIT, FLT3, JAK2, Ras, etc.) are frequently reported. On the other hand, class II mutations of transcription factors that control cell differentiation (RUNX1, PML-RARα, C/EBPα, GATA, etc.) have also been reported. A group of genes involved in epigenetic abnormalities such as DNA methylation and histone modifications (TET2, IDH1/2, DNMT3a, EZH2, and ASXL1) have been reported in relation to AML and myeloproliferative neoplasm. In addition, a group of mutated genes involved in RNA splicing (U2AF35, SF3B1, and SRSF2) has been reported in relation to myelodysplastic syndrome. Furthermore, mutations have also been reported of tumor suppressor genes that control the cell cycle and apoptosis (such as CDKN2A/B and TP53). Such gene mutations, splicing anomalies, and epigenetic alterations are candidates for targeting LSCs (Fig. 20.1).

In recent years, new techniques have begun to revolutionize the diagnosis, prognosis, and classification of leukemia. More recently, the introduction of high-speed analysis of whole-genome sequencing has made it possible to find multiple gene

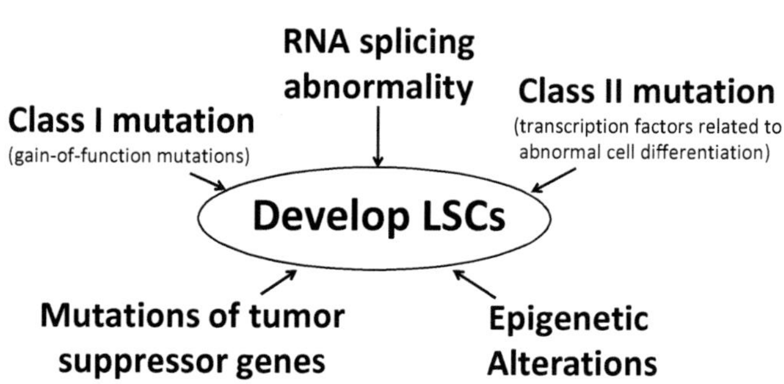

Fig. 20.1 Various causes of LSC development

mutations that are involved in leukemogenesis. During the process by which genetic variation accumulates in HSCs, the fraction termed pre-LSCs gradually expands, and then LSCs are fully established when additional gene mutations are acquired. This final trigger is considered to occur in LSCs in some cases and in progenitor cells differentiated from LSCs in other cases.

As mentioned above, AML-LSCs are present in the $CD34^{+}CD38^{-}$ fraction, which is a phenotype shared with normal HSCs. Thus, leukemia originates from normal HSCs. HSCs have a long lifetime and can undergo a considerable number of divisions; therefore, genetic and epigenetic alterations tend to accumulate in these cells. In addition, because HSCs have molecular mechanisms for self-replication, they fulfill the requirements of LSCs when genes that contribute to a growth advantage and a differentiation block are obtained. In principle, differentiated progenitor cells have no self-renewal ability. However, there is a possibility that LSCs originate from these differentiated progenies after they acquire self-renewal ability. To become LSCs, differentiated leukemic progenitors must have self-renewal ability.

The mixed lineage leukemia (*MLL*) gene present in chromosome 11q23 leads to the development of a variety of diseases by forming various fusion genes such as the *MLL/GAS* fusion gene formed by the 11;17 chromosomal translocation, the *MLL/ENL* rearranged gene formed by the 11;19 translocation, and the *MLL/AF9* formed by the 9;11 translocation [12, 13, 14]. A study examined whether these fusion genes can lead to the development of leukemia upon their introduction into murine HSCs or progenitor cells. The *MLL/GAS7* fusion gene causes leukemia only when introduced into HSCs, while *MLL/ENL* and *MLL/AF9* cause leukemia when introduced not only into HSCs with self-renewal ability but also into GMPs. Similarly, leukemia can develop when the *MOZ/TIF2* fusion gene, which is formed by the inversion of chromosome 8, is introduced into GMPs [15]. These findings indicate that it is possible to develop LSCs from precursor cells, although it is dependent on the type of genetic abnormality.

20.4 Candidate Therapeutic Molecules for Targeting LSCs

20.4.1 Signal Transduction and Metabolic Pathways

The therapeutic strategies for eradicating LSCs are summarized in Table 20.1. Molecules that control self-renewal and proliferation, molecules that regulate the cell cycle and differentiation, molecules that enhance cell survival, molecules constituting the hematopoietic (leukemic) niche that exists in hypoxic environments, and cell surface molecules specific for leukemia are candidates for eradicating LSCs. However, many of these molecules are present even in normal HSCs. To specifically eradicate LSCs while sparing normal HSCs, the specific molecular mechanisms in LSCs need to be clarified.

The canonical Wnt/β-catenin signal is constitutively active in both AML and chronic myeloid leukemia (CML), in addition to many human cancers [16]. Analysis of patient samples demonstrated that LSCs in the chronic phase of CML develop

Table 20.1 Therapeutic strategies targeting LSCs

1. Antibodies specific for LSCs
2. Inhibitors of signal transduction and metabolic pathways
3. Induction of apoptosis
4. Suppression of the self-renewal capacity of LSCs
5. Transition into the cell-cycling state from the quiescent state and differentiation induction
6. Detachment of LSCs from the hypoxic niche
7. Targeting the hematopoietic niche or microenvironment

from HSCs, while those in the accelerated and blastic phases of CML develop by transformation of CMPs or GMPs through activation of the Wnt/β-catenin pathway. β- and γ-catenin are not essential at least for the maintenance of murine normal HSCs, and they are therefore potential therapeutic targets in LSCs [17].

The hedgehog (Hh) pathway is abnormally activated in various types of cancer [18]. During embryonic pattern formation, the Hh signaling pathway regulates proliferation and differentiation. In cancer, the pathway increases tumor invasiveness and regular CSC proliferation. In some preclinical models, aberrant activation of the Hh pathway is necessary for the maintenance of some $CD34^+$ LSCs. PF-04449913 is a novel oral small molecule inhibitor that binds to smoothened (SMO), a membrane protein in the Hh pathway [19]. In AML cell lines and human primary AML cells, PF-04449913 appears to improve sensitivity to cytarabine in dormant LSCs. Multiple phase 1 studies are ongoing with PF-04449913 as a monotherapy or in combination with low-dose cytarabine or hypomethylating agents to treat AML [20]. Vismodegib, a SMO antagonist approved for the treatment of basal-cell carcinoma, in combination with ribavirin with or without decitabine, is also under investigation in relapsed/refractory AML (NCT02073838) [20].

20.4.2 Cell Surface Antigens

Identifying cell surface antigens that are differentially upregulated on LSCs but not on normal HSCs has been a major focus. However, it is difficult to identify such antigens, and thus far no unique antigen has been found that is specifically expressed on $CD34^+CD38^-$ LSCs but not on normal HSCs. Despite these difficulties, many cell surface antigens have been identified that are preferentially expressed on $CD34^+CD38^-$ LSCs compared with normal human HSCs. These include CD25 [21], CD32 [21], CD33 [22], CD44 [23], CD47 [24, 25], CD96 [26], CD123

Table 20.2 Possible target candidates of surface antigens expressed on LSCs

Surface antigen	Characteristics	Expressed on		References
		Normal HSCs	LSCs	
CD25	IL-2Rα chain, expressed on activated T cells	±	+	[21]
CD32	FcγRIIA, expressed on monocytes and neutrophils	±	+	[21]
CD33	Pan-myeloid antigen, clinically used as the antibody gemtuzumab ozogamicin	++	++	[22]
CD44	Adhesion molecule, hyaluronic acid receptor	+	++	[23]
CD47	The ligand for signal regulatory protein alpha (SIRPα), anti-CD47 antibodies induce apoptosis of AML-LSCs	+	++	[24, 25]
CD96	Member of the Ig gene superfamily, expressed in T and NK cells, but not in B cells, granulocytes, monocytes, or red blood cells	+	++	[26]
CD123	IL-3R α chain, expressed on total and $CD34^+CD38^-$ fractions of AML and normal myeloid cells	+	++	[27–29]
TIM-3	T-cell immunoglobulin mucin-3, expressed in $CD4^+$ Th1 lymphocytes and is an important regulator of Th1 cell immunity and tolerance induction	+	++	[30, 31]
IL1RAP	IL1 receptor accessory protein (IL1RAP, IL1R3), expressed on candidate LSCs in the majority of AML patients but not on normal HSCs	−~ ±?	+	[37]
CLL-1	C-type lectin-like molecule-1, expressed on monocytes, neutrophils, and the majority of AML blasts	±	+	[38]

[27–29], TIM-3 [30–32], interleukin (IL)-1 receptor accessory protein (IL1RAP) [37], and C-type lectin-like molecule-1 (CLL-1) [38)], as summarized in Table 20.2.

In normal human BM, CD25 is expressed in a portion of $CD4^+$ T cells (regulatory T cells), and CD32 (Fc gamma receptor II) is expressed in B cells, T cells, and monocytes; however, neither antigen is expressed in $CD34^+CD38^-CD133^+$ HSCs. By demonstrating the functional significance of distinctly expressed genes using analyses including xenotransplantation, it was reported that CD25 and CD32 were most frequently expressed on LSCs of AML patients, 85% of whom were poor risk, and it was suggested that therapeutic strategies targeting these molecules may be effective and improve patient prognosis [21].

CD44 is a cell adhesion molecule whose ligand is hyaluronic acid and which contributes to construction of the LSC niche. The engraftment of human AML into immunodeficient mice is completely inhibited by administration of an anti-CD44 antibody (H90), while that of normal HSCs is only minimally affected [23]. In this paper, Jin et al. reported that CD44 is a key regulator of AML-LSC function and is required for proper homing of AML-LSCs to microenvironments and to maintain

AML-LSCs in a leukemic niche. The finding that AML-LSCs require interactions with a niche to maintain their stem cell properties provides a therapeutic strategy to eliminate dormant AML-LSCs and may be applicable to other types of CSCs.

CD47 belongs to the immunoglobulin (Ig) superfamily and is a ligand of SIRPα (signal regulatory protein alpha) expressed on macrophages. When the IgV region of SIRPα expressed on macrophages combines with CD47 on LSCs, a tyrosine residue of SIRPα is phosphorylated, and the inhibitory signals of phagocytosis ("don't eat me" signal) are transmitted, resulting in the inhibition of phagocytosis by macrophages. On the other hand, when the target cell does not express CD47 or the binding of SIRPα and CD47 is inhibited, the signal of the inhibition is not transmitted, and consequently the target cells are phagocytosed by macrophages. When an anti-CD47 antibody blocks the binding of SIRPα and CD47 expressed on LSCs, the "don't eat me" signal to macrophages is blocked, and LSCs are phagocytosed. Increased phagocytic action by macrophages is a mechanism of action of anti-CD47 antibodies. CD47 is strongly expressed on AML-LSCs compared with normal HSCs. CD47 binds to the ligands thrombospondin-1 and SIRPα, which are involved in apoptosis, proliferation, adhesion, and migration of myeloma cells [24]. In clinical settings, increased expression of CD47 is a poor prognostic factor in AML. Treatment of human AML-engrafted mice with an anti-CD47 antibody could target AML-LSCs [25].

CD96 belongs to the Ig superfamily. Hosen et al. revealed that CD96 is a promising candidate as a specific antigen for LSCs [26]. Applying a signal sequence trap strategy to identify cell surface molecules expressed on human AML-LSCs and fluorescence-activated cell sorting (FACS) analysis demonstrated that CD96 is expressed on $CD34^+CD38^-$ AML cells in the majority of patients. Transplantation of AML cells into immunodeficient mice demonstrated that only $CD96^+$ fractions showed significant levels of engraftment. These results demonstrate that CD96 is a cell surface marker present on AML-LSCs and may be a LSC-specific therapeutic target. Furthermore, FACS analysis demonstrates that CD96 is expressed on the majority of $CD34^+CD38^-$ LSCs of AML, whereas only a few normal HSCs weakly express CD96. Therefore, the authors mentioned that this molecule may be a candidate LSC-specific therapeutic target.

CD123 is an IL-3 receptor α chain, is highly expressed on AML-LSCs compared with their normal counterparts, and is being used to develop an antibody therapy. An anti-CD123-neutralizing antibody (7G3) targeted AML-LSCs, impairing homing to BM and activating innate immunity in NOD/SCID mice. 7G3 treatment profoundly reduced AML-LSC engraftment and improved mouse survival [27]. Targeting LSCs using the 7G3 antibody against CD123 seems to be an attractive approach. A phase 1 clinical study was conducted of relapsed or refractory high-risk AML using CSL360, a chimeric variant of 7G3; however, the remission rate was quite low [28]. One reason for this was the high tumor load, and strategies such as enhancing the ADCC (antibody-dependent cellular cytotoxicity) activity of anti-CD123 antibodies have been investigated. Moreover, it is an immune cell therapy, and preclinical work with a dual-affinity retargeting molecule generated from antibodies against

CD3 and CD123, which is designed to redirect T cells against AML-LSCs, has been reported [29].

T-cell immunoglobulin mucin (TIM)-3 is highly expressed in AML-LSCs, except the FAB classification M3, but is not expressed at all in normal HSCs. While TIM-3-positive AML cells can repopulate AML in mice with high efficiency, TIM-3-negative AML cells do not reconstitute leukemia at all. In immunodeficient mice engrafted with AML cells and treated with an anti-TIM-3 antibody (ATIK2a), AML cells were significantly reduced, and those remaining after treatment with ATIK2a could not succeed in serial passage transplantation in mice, indicating that this antibody can target AML-LSCs [30]. TIM-3 protein is not detectable in normal HSCs or in other myeloerythroid or lymphoid progenitors, although monocyte lineage-committed progenitors begin to upregulate TIM-3. Therefore, expression of TIM-3 is highly specific to human AML-LSCs [31]. TIM-3 was originally identified as being selectively expressed on IFN-γ-secreting Th1 and Tc1 cells [32]. Interaction of TIM-3 with its ligand, galectin-9, triggers cell death in TIM-3$^+$ T cells [33]. Both TIM-3 and PD-1 can function as negative regulators of T-cell responses [34, 35, 36]. Like PD-1, TIM-3 is also an immune checkpoint-associated surface molecule involved in the exhaustion of T cells. Inhibition of TIM-3 functions with an anti-TIM-3 antibody should be an effective treatment strategy. From the perspective of the abovementioned immune checkpoint inhibition, TIM-3 is expressed in some types of hematopoietic cells and seems to have lineage- or cellular context-dependent signal transduction pathways or functions. The role of TIM-3 in AML-LSCs is quite intriguing, and inhibition of this molecule is a promising clinical strategy. Further studies, however, are needed to clarify the specific function of TIM-3 before performing clinical trials to eradicate AML-LSCs.

IL1RAP is a co-receptor of the type 1 IL-1 receptor. IL1RAP is expressed on the cell surface in the majority of AML patients. IL1RAP is upregulated on immature cells in high-risk AML patients with chromosome 7 abnormalities, and AML patients with high IL1RAP expression have a poor prognosis. Ågerstam et al. reported that IL1RAP may become a therapeutic target in AML and that rapid clinical development of an antibody-based IL1RAP therapy for AML is promising [37].

CLL-1 is highly expressed on the blast compartment in the majority of AML cases, while it is completely absent on CD34$^+$CD38$^-$ resting BM cells. CD34$^+$CLL-1$^+$ cells repopulate in sublethally irradiated immunodeficient NOD/SCID mice, indicating that they contain leukemia-initiating cells. Furthermore, culture of normal CD34$^+$ cells in a long-term culture system in the presence of an anti-CLL-1 antibody has no effect on CFU-E and CFU-GM colony formation, suggesting that CLL-1 is a possible target for therapy [38].

20.4.3 Novel Strategy to Exhaust LSCs

The role of CCAAT/enhancer-binding protein β (C/EBPβ), a regulator of emergency granulopoiesis, in the pathogenesis of the chronic phase of CML was examined, and it has been suggested that C/EBPβ is involved in BCR-ABL-mediated myeloid expansion. We found that enforced expression of C/EBPβ in CML-LSCs might induce exhaustion of LSCs, leading to a complete cure of this disease [39]. C/EBPβ-mediated LSC loss might reveal a unique therapeutic strategy to eradicate CML stem cells. Agents that upregulate expression of C/EBPβ in LSCs should be promising (Yokota A, Hirai H, Maekawa T, et al., unpublished observation).

20.4.4 Targeting LSCs Using Small Molecules

In addition to therapies using the antibodies mentioned above, therapies based on small molecules can target intracellular proteins and pathways. Nuclear factor-kappa B (NF-κB) stimulates the transcription of genes encoding Ig of the κ class in B lymphocytes. NF-κB, a dimeric transcription factor complex that controls various aspects of cellular responses to stimuli, is now recognized as a pivotal regulator of cell survival, proliferation, and differentiation. When unstimulated, the complex is sequestered in the cytoplasm by a family of inhibitors of NF-κB (IκBs). NF-κB is constitutively active in AML enriched with LSCs, while its activity was not detectable in unstimulated normal HSCs/progenitor cells. Proteasome inhibitor such as MG-132, which inhibits NF-κB activity by inhibiting IκB degradation, induces the rapid apoptosis of AML-LSCs but not of normal HSCs. Therefore, inhibition of NF-κB signaling may provide a novel therapeutic strategy specific to LSCs [40]. Another molecule with inhibitory activity against NF-κB, parthenolide (PTL), targets primitive AML cells. Agents such as PTL, which is a sesquiterpene lactone that is the major active component in feverfew (*Tanacetum parthenium*), a herbal medicine that has been used to treat migraines and rheumatoid arthritis for a long time, inhibit the ability of LSCs to respond to oxidative stress and make LSCs sensitive to cell death stimuli, while normal stem cells remain relatively unharmed by these agents. The main mechanism of action of these molecules appears to revolve around the altered glutathione metabolism pathway found in leukemia cells [41]. Niclosamide also inhibits the transcription and DNA binding of NF-κB. It blocked tumor necrosis factor-induced IκBα phosphorylation, translocation of p65, and expression of NF-κB-regulated genes [42].

20.4.5 Targeting Antiapoptotic Molecules

A body of investigations has established that AML cells are dependent on antiapoptotic molecules for survival such as the B-cell CLL/lymphoma 2 (Bcl-2) family, which suppresses the intrinsic or mitochondrial apoptotic pathway and plays an important role in AML pathogenesis, prognosis, and responsiveness to chemotherapeutic agents [43]. In addition, the antiapoptotic Bcl-2 family protein myeloid cell leukemia sequence 1 (Mcl-1) is essential for cell survival during the development and maintenance of AML [44, 45].

Normally, the antiapoptotic proteins Bcl-2, Bcl-X_L, and Mcl-1 suppress apoptosis effector molecules such as Bak as well as the proapoptotic BH3-only protein

Bim, thereby preventing apoptosis. The BH3-only proteins Bad and Noxa, as well as BH3-mimetic drugs such as navitoclax and obatoclax, untether the apoptosis effectors and Bim from the antiapoptotic proteins, leading to apoptosis [46]. Apoptosis is initiated when members of the third subfamily, the BH3-only proteins (e.g., Bim, Bad, and Noxa), are activated by various cytotoxic stimuli.

20.5 Gene Abnormalities Involved in Epigenetic Modifications

Gene mutation analyses of leukemia cells using next-generation sequencing greatly assist studies of individual genetic abnormalities in leukemia cells. In addition, the importance of methylation of DNA and histones for epigenetic regulation of gene expression by modulation of the chromatin structure was recently clarified. Abnormalities of genes related to epigenetic modifications are frequently found in many cancers, including AML. There are roughly two types of epigenetic modifications; one is histone modifications including the polycomb group complex-associated gene *ASXL1*, and the other is DNA methylation modifications including the DNA methyltransferase 3A (*DNMT3A*), 10–11 translocation 2 (*TET2*), isocitrate dehydrogenase 1 (*IDH1*), and *IDH2* genes [47, 48]. Gene expression can be controlled by these chemical modifications without changing the genome sequence.

Somatic mutations in genes that encode proteins related to epigenetic alterations play a pivotal role in leukemogenesis. Shlush et al. recently reported that mutations of the *DNMT3A*, *TET2*, and *IDH1/2* genes, which control DNA methylation, and the polycomb group complex-associated gene *ASXL1*, which is involved in histone modifications, are involved in the initiation of pre-LSCs as driver mutations. Such mutations facilitate the self-renewal capacity of pre-LSCs and block the differentiation of hematopoietic stem/progenitor cells. The emergence of these mutations in HSCs can induce their clonal expansion, resulting in a pre-LSC population. Furthermore, HSCs with this *DNMT3A* gene mutation were demonstrated to have a growth advantage in a patient's BM using a xenograft model. Similar findings were observed in HSCs with *ISH2* gene mutation; therefore, *DNMT3A* and *IDH2* gene mutations have a critical role in the preleukemic state [49]. Hemopoietic cells with these gene mutations can remain after a long period of remission achieved by chemotherapy or molecular targeted therapy, and these cells may cause leukemia relapse [50]. The development of a histone deacetylase inhibitor is underway in clinical settings to target such abnormal molecules. AR-42 (OSU-HDAC42) induces NF-κB inhibition, disrupts the ability of heat shock protein 90 to stabilize its oncogenic clients, and causes potent and specific apoptosis of LSCs but not of normal hematopoietic stem and progenitor cells. AR-42 has already been tested in early clinical settings [51].

DNA is methylated at the 5-position carbon in CpG sequences. Methylated cytosine-binding proteins bind to the methylated cytosine, and gene transcription is suppressed together with recruited histone deacetylase and transcriptional repressor. Regions where CpG sequences are condensed are called CpG islands. CpG islands are quite abundant in the promoter region of a gene. CpG islands are usually maintained in a low methylated condition, and gene transcription is activated. In cancer, genome-wide hypomethylation is frequently found, and a specific promoter region is hypermethylated. Genome-wide hypomethylation results in chromosomal instability, along with reactivation of the transposon, which is thought to be the cause of genetic abnormalities. On the other hand, hypermethylation of DNA in CpG islands suppresses the expression of CDK inhibitors, which are negative regulators of the cell cycle and inhibit the expression of tumor suppressor genes and DNA repair genes. Such an altered methylated status has become a therapeutic target, and the development of DNA methylation inhibitors and histone deacetylase inhibitors is under investigation. The detailed mechanism of action in hyper- and hypomethylation will be discussed elsewhere in this book.

20.6 Targeting the Hypoxic Niche of LSCs and Their Interactions

To maintain their undifferentiated state, LSCs, similar to HSCs, adhere to the stem cell niche of the BM microenvironment, which is composed of a variety of cell types, including mesenchymal stem/stromal cells, bone cells, immune cells, neuronal cells, and vascular cells [52]. It is possible that LSCs obtain anticancer drug resistance by lodging in the niche and that the interactions that maintain LSCs are the major cause of leukemia relapse. Angiopoietin-1, Flt3 ligand, thrombopoietin, Wnt/β-catenin [16], CXCL12/SDF-1α [53], CD44, addition of osteopontin, basic fibroblast growth factor, insulin-like growth factor, IL-6, vascular endothelial growth factor, and many other molecules are involved in stem cell maintenance in the niche. By blocking the interaction between LSCs and niches, it is possible to induce quiescent LSCs in the niche to enter the cell cycle, and then these quiescent LSCs could become a target of therapeutic molecules such as chemotherapeutic agents and various inhibitors. HSCs utilize the system of chemokine receptor-4 (CXCR4) and CXCL12/SDF-1α binding [54]. When AML cells were implanted into mice, more engraftment was observed in cases highly expressing CXCR4, and CXCR4/SDF-1α signaling promotes the survival of leukemia cells by inhibiting their differentiation. An anti-CXCR4 agent inhibits the binding of AML-LSCs in the niche, mobilizing AML-LSCs from the niche to the periphery, which is expected to increase sensitivity to chemotherapy [55, 56].

A hallmark of the hematopoietic niche is considered to be low oxygen partial pressure. Hypoxia is necessary for long-term maintenance of hematopoietic stem/progenitor cells. Hypoxia is thought to be a common characteristic of the niche that maintains the quiescence of HSCs and LSCs. In particular, there is an oxygen gradient in BM that ranges from <6% oxygen close to vessels to anoxia in regions that are most distant from blood vessels [57]. However, the O_2 level differs according to the nature of the hematopoietic niche; the partial pressure of oxygen in the sinusoidal niche is around 10 mmHg (equivalent to 1.3% O_2). LSCs share specific niches with normal HSCs. AML is initiated within the BM under local hypoxic conditions

[58]. Bonnet et al. reported that shRNA-based downregulation of mediators of cellular responses to hypoxia, such as hypoxia-inducible factor (HIF)-1α or HIF-2α, induces apoptosis and prevents leukemic engraftment upon transplantation into mice [59]. This observation suggested that HIF-1α or HIF-2α is required for the maintenance of LSCs and may be a potential therapeutic target for AML. However, the first genetic evidence indicates that HIF-2α acts as a tumor suppressor in AML development but is dispensable for LSC-based disease maintenance [60]. Accordingly, this study questions the usefulness of targeting HIFs in AML after critical events in leukemia initiation have occurred.

Overall, these data argue that hypoxia and HIF-mediated signaling play a crucial role in leukemia and leukemogenic processes. However, they provide conflicting results regarding whether HIFs act as oncogenes or tumor suppressors, which is due to the use of different leukemia models, study designs, oxygen levels, and durations of hypoxia. Therefore, therapies targeting hypoxia and HIFs have proven their efficacy in treating mouse models, and detailed studies investigating whether these strategies would truly benefit leukemia patients are required. Representative small molecules in clinical trials or preclinical settings are shown in Table 20.3.

20.7 Conclusions

There are a number of novel approaches to selectively target LSCs, including targeting stem cell properties, such as self-renewal, inducing cycling of quiescent LSCs to sensitize them to conventional agents, employing or inducing immune-based mechanisms, and targeting tumor-specific physiology. We could be at the frontier of a promising new era of novel targeted therapies to specifically eliminate LSCs if these strategies can be performed without adversely affecting normal HSCs/progenitor cells. Therapeutics targeting the pathways that sustain LSCs proliferation and self-renewal might prove to be more effective treatment strategies to eradicate LSCs; however, a number of questions need to be addressed in future studies. A main task for the future is to identify common LSC-specific markers or alterations in a restricted subpopulation of leukemia patients. If every LSC of leukemia patients shows a different and unique fingerprint of markers or genetic alterations, targeting LSCs could be an arduous task. Undoubtedly, however, the remarkably fast-moving advancement of genome-wide analysis of gene expression will resolve these problems, and then many new agents under development will realize a new era in LSC-targeted therapy.

20.8 Future Prospects

Progress toward an ultimate cure for leukemia seems to be made with novel therapeutics directed at specific molecular targets. The approach to achieving this goal may be promoted by modern genomic approaches such as high-speed analysis of whole-genome sequencing and DNA microarray and proteomic strategies to find

Table 20.3 Some possible candidates of small molecules targeting LSCs in clinical trials/ preclinical settings

Target	Agent	Possible mechanism of action	References
Hh pathway			
Hh pathway inhibitor	PF-04449913	Inhibits the binding SMO protein	[20]
	Vismodegib	Binds to and inhibits SMO	[20]
NF-κB pathway			
NF-κB, Hsp90	AR-42	Inhibits NF-κB activity, increases degradation of Hsp90 client proteins	[51]
Multiple targets	Parthenolide	Inhibits NF-κB activity	[41]
	Niclosamide	Inhibits NF-κB activity, increases reactive oxygen species levels	[42]
Anti-apoptosis			
Bcl-2	ABT-263, navitoclax	Inhibits Bcl-2 and Bcl-X_L, suppresses oxidative phosphorylation	[61]
	GX15–070, obatoclax	Inhibits Bcl-2, Bcl-X_L, Mcl-1, and Bcl-w	[62]
Mcl-1, PI3K	PIK-75	Suppresses Mcl-1 through inhibition of CDK7/9, inhibits PI3K signaling	[63]
Epigenetic alterations			
Histone deacetylase inhibitor	Entinostat	Induces expression of Nur77, Nor1, c-Jun, Jun B, TRAIL, Bim, and Noxa	[64]
BRD4	JQ-1	Displaces BRD4 proteins from acetylated histones	[65]
Histone demethylase (KDM1A/LSD1)	Analog of tranylcypromine	Suppresses the oncogenic program in MLL leukemia	[66, 67]
		Enzyme responsible for demethylation of histone H3	
		Sensitizes AML to ATRA in combination use	
G9a histone methyltransferase	UNC0638	Suppresses HoxA9-dependent gene expression	[68] (preclinical)

(continued)

Table 20.3 (continued)

Target	Agent	Possible mechanism of action	References
Others			
HIF-1α	Echinomycin	Inhibits DNA binding and transcriptional activity of HIF-1α	[69] (preclinical)
Telomerase	Imetelstat	Antisense oligonucleotide (13-mer) targeting the RNA component of the telomerase complex	[70] (preclinical)
DNA cross-linking	Evofosfamide	Hypoxia-activated prodrug	[71]
WNT/β-catenin	BC2059	Attenuates β-catenin levels by proteasome-mediated degradation	[72]

novel targets of LSCs and leukemic progenitors with a self-renewal capacity and to identify prognostic indicators. For these developing molecular targeted therapies to provide an ultimate cure, various resistance mechanisms must be clarified, and the aforementioned formidable problems need to be resolved. Although the function and characteristics of LSCs have been considerably unraveled in recent years by the improvement of assays, the self-replicating mechanism of LSCs remains unclear. Solutions to these challenges will require close and continued collaboration between basic researchers and clinical investigators because a considerable number of patients with incurable leukemias are eagerly awaiting the benefits of new targeted therapeutics through the evaluation of well-designed clinical trials.

Acknowledgments This work was supported partly by a Grant-in-Aid for Scientific Research from the Ministry of Education, Culture, Sports, Science and Technology of Japan and nonrestricted Grants from Bristol-Myers Squibb, Astellas, and Novartis Pharmaceuticals Co., Ltd.

References

1. Cabrera MC, Hollingsworth RE, Hurt EM. Cancer stem cell plasticity and tumor hierarchy. World J Stem Cells. 2015;26(7):27–36.
2. Yang M, Lie P, Huang P. Cancer stem cells, metabolism, and therapeutic significance. Tumour Biol. 2016;37:5735–42.
3. Cheung AM, Kwong YL, Liang R, Leung AY. Stem cell model of hematopoiesis. Curr Stem Cell Res Ther. 2006;1:305–15.
4. Moore MA, Williams N, Metcalf D. In vitro colony formation by normal and leukemic hematopoietic cells: characterization of the colony-forming cells. J Natl Cancer Inst. 1973;50:603–23.
5. Warner JK, Wang JC, Hope KJ, Jin L, Dick JE. Concepts of human leukemic development. Oncogene. 2004;23:7164–77.

6. Bonnet D, Dick JE. Human acute myeloid leukemia is organized as a hierarchy that originates from a primitive hematopoietic cell. Nat Med. 1997;3:730–7.
7. Dick JE. Acute myeloid leukemia stem cells. Ann N Y Acad Sci. 2005;1044:1–5.
8. Taussig DC, Miraki-Moud F, Anjos-Afonso F, Pearce DJ, Allen K, Ridler C, et al. Anti-CD38 antibody-mediated clearance of human repopulating cells masks the heterogeneity of leukemia-initiating cells. Blood. 2008;112:568–75.
9. Krivtsov AV, Twomey D, Feng Z, Stubbs MC, Wang Y, et al. Transformation from committed progenitor to leukaemia stem cell initiated by MLL-AF9. Nature. 2006;442:818–22.
10. Goardon N, Marchi E, Atzberger A, Quek L, Schuh A, Soneji S, et al. Coexistence of LMPP-like and GMP-like leukemia stem cells in acute myeloid leukemia. Cancer Cell. 2011;19:138–52.
11. Gilliland DG, Tallman MS. Focus on acute leukemias. Cancer Cell. 2002;1:417–20.
12. Panagopoulos I, Lilljebjörn H, Strömbeck B, Hjorth L, Olofsson T, Johansson B. MLL/GAS7 fusion in a pediatric case of t(11;17) (q23;p13)-positive precursor B-cell acute lymphoblastic leukemia. Haematologica. 2006;91:1287–8.
13. Schwieger M, Schüler A, Forster M, Engelmann A, Arnold MA, Delwel R, et al. Homing and invasiveness of MLL/ENL leukemic cells is regulated by MEF2C. Blood. 2009;114:2476–88.
14. Cavazzini F, Bardi A, Tammiso E, Ciccone M, Russo-Rossi A, Divona D, et al. Validation of an interphase fluorescence in situ hybridization approach for the detection of MLL gene rearrangements and of the MLL/AF9 fusion in acute myeloid leukemia. Haematologica. 2006;91:381–5.
15. Ye M, Zhang H, Yang H, Koche R, Staber PB, Cusan M, et al. Hematopoietic differentiation is required for initiation of acute myeloid leukemia. Cell Stem Cell. 2015;17:611–23.
16. Yao H, Ashihara E, Maekawa T. Targeting the Wnt/β catenin signaling pathway in human cancers. Expert Opin Ther Targets. 2011;15:873–87.
17. Jamieson CH, Ailles LE, Dylla SJ, Muijtjens M, Jones C, Zehnder JL, et al. Granulocyte-macrophage progenitors as candidate leukemic stem cells in blast-crisis CML. N Engl J Med. 2004;351:657–67.
18. Rubin LL, de Sauvage FJ. Targeting the Hedgehog pathway in cancer. Nat Rev Drug Discov. 2006;5:1026–33.
19. Martinelli G, Oehler VG, Papayannidis C, Courtney R, Shaik MN, Zhang X, et al. Treatment with PF-04449913, an oral smoothened antagonist, in patients with myeloid malignancies: a phase 1 safety and pharmacokinetics study. Lancet Haematol. 2015;2:e339–46.
20. Brechbiel J, Miller-Moslin K, Adjei AA. Crosstalk between hedgehog and other signaling pathways as a basis for combination therapies in cancer. Cancer Treat Rev. 2014;40:750–9.
21. Saito Y, Kitamura H, Hijikata A, Tomizawa-Murasawa M, Tanaka S, Takagi S, et al. Identification of therapeutic targets for quiescent, chemotherapy-resistant human leukemia stem cells. Sci Transl Med. 2010;2:17ra9.
22. Taussig DC, Pearce DJ, Simpson C, Rohatiner AZ, Lister TA, Kelly G, et al. Hematopoietic stem cells express multiple myeloid markers: implications for the origin and targeted therapy of acute myeloid leukemia. Blood. 2005;106:4086–92.
23. Jin L, Hope KJ, Zhai Q, Smadja-Joffe F, Dick JE. Targeting of CD44 eradicates human acute myeloid leukemic stem cells. Nat Med. 2006;12:1167–74.
24. Rendtlew Danielsen JM, Knudsen LM, Dahl IM, Lodahl M, Rasmussen T. Dysregulation of CD47 and the ligands thrombospondin 1 and 2 in multiple myeloma. Brit J Haematol. 2007;138:756–60.
25. Majeti R, Chao MP, Alizadeh AA, Pang WW, Jaiswal S, Gibbs Jr KD, et al. CD47 is an adverse prognostic factor and therapeutic antibody target on human acute myeloid leukemia stem cells. Cell. 2009;138:286–99.
26. Hosen N, Park CY, Tatsumi N, Oji Y, Sugiyama H, Gramatzki M, et al. CD96 is a leukemic stem cell-specific marker in human acute myeloid leukemia. Proc Natl Acad Sci U S A. 2007;104:11008–13.

27. Jin L, Lee EM, Ramshaw HS, Busfield SJ, Peoppl AG, Wilkinson L, et al. Monoclonal antibody-mediated targeting of CD123, IL-3 receptor alpha chain, eliminates human acute myeloid leukemic stem cells. Cell Stem Cell. 2009;5:31–42.
28. He SZ, Busfield S, Ritchie DS, Hertzberg MS, Durrant S, Lewis ID, et al. A Phase 1 study of the safety, pharmacokinetics and anti-leukemic activity of the anti-CD123 monoclonal antibody CSL360 in relapsed, refractory or high-risk acute myeloid leukemia. Leuk Lymphoma. 2015;56:1406–15.
29. Al-Hussaini M, Rettig MP, Ritchey JK, Karpova D, Uy GL, Eissenberg LG, et al. Targeting CD123 in acute myeloid leukemia using a T-cell-directed dual-affinity retargeting platform. Blood. 2016;127:122–31.
30. Kikushige Y, Akashi K. TIM-3 as a therapeutic target for malignant stem cells in acute myelogenous leukemia. Ann N Y Acad Sci. 2012;1266:118–23.
31. Kikushige Y, Shima T, Takayanagi S, Urata S, Miyamoto T, Iwasaki H, et al. TIM-3 is a promising target to selectively kill acute myeloid leukemia stem cells. Cell Stem Cell. 2010;7:708–17.
32. Monney L, Sabatos CA, Gaglia J, Ryu A, Waldner H, Chernova T, Manning S, Greenfield EA, Coyle AJ, Sobel RA, et al. Th1-specific cell surface protein Tim-3 regulates macrophage activation and severity of an autoimmune disease. Nature. 2002;415:536–41.
33. Kikushige Y, Miyamoto T, Yuda J, Jabbarzadeh-Tabrizi S, Shima T, Takayanagi S, et al. A TIM-3/Gal-9 autocrine stimulatory loop drives self-renewal of human myeloid leukemia stem cells and leukemic progression. Cell Stem Cell. 2015;17:341–52.
34. Sakuishi K, Apetoh L, Sullivan JM, Blazar BR, Kuchroo VK, Anderson AC, et al. Targeting Tim-3 and PD-1 pathways to reverse T cell exhaustion and restore antitumor immunity. J Exp Med. 2010;207:2187–94.
35. Sakuishi K, Jayaraman P, Behar SM, Anderson AC, Kuchroo VK. Emerging Tim-3 functions in antimicrobial and tumor immunity. Trends Immunol. 2011;32:345–9.
36. Sakuishi K, Ngiow SF, Sullivan JM, Teng MW, Kuchroo VK, Smyth MJ, et al. TIM3 + FOXP3+ regulatory T cells are tissue-specific promoters of T-cell dysfunction in cancer. OncoImmunology. 2013;2:e23849.
37. Ågerstam H, Karlsson C, Hansen N, Sandén C, Askmyr M, von Palffy S, et al. Antibodies targeting human IL1RAP (IL1R3) show therapeutic effects in xenograft models of acute myeloid leukemia. Proc Natl Acad Sci U S A. 2015;112:10786–91.
38. van Rhenen A, van Dongen GA, Kelder A, Rombouts EJ, Feller N, Moshaver B, et al. The novel AML stem cell-associated antigen CLL-1 aids in discrimination between normal and leukemic stem cells. Blood. 2007;110:2659–66.
39. Hayashi Y, Hirai H, Kamio N, Yao H, Yoshioka S, Miura Y, et al. C/EBPβ promotes BCR-ABL-mediated myeloid expansion and leukemic stem cell exhaustion. Leukemia. 2013;27:619–28.
40. Guzman ML, Neering SJ, Upchurch D, Grimes B, Howard DS, Rizzieri DA, et al. Nuclear factor-kappa B is constitutively activated in primitive human acute myelogenous leukemia cells. Blood. 2001;98:2301–7.
41. Guzman ML, Rossi RM, Karnischky L, Li X, Peterson DR, Howard DS, Jordan CT. The sesquiterpene lactone parthenolide induces apoptosis of human acute myelogenous leukemia stem and progenitor cells. Blood. 2005;105:4163–9.
42. Jin Y, Lu Z, Ding K, Li J, Du X, Chen C, et al. Antineoplastic mechanisms of niclosamide in acute myelogenous leukemia stem cells: inactivation of the NF-kappa B pathway and generation of reactive oxygen species. Cancer Res. 2010;70:2516–27.
43. Lagadinou ED, Sach A, Callahan K, Rossi RM, Neering SJ, Minhajuddin M, et al. BCL-2 inhibition targets oxidative phosphorylation and selectively eradicates quiescent human leukemia stem cells. Cell Stem Cell. 2013;12(3):329–41.
44. Glaser SP, Lee EF, Trounson E, Bouillet P, Wei A, Fairlie WD, et al. Anti-apoptotic Mcl-1 is essential for the development and sustained growth of acute myeloid leukemia. Genes Dev. 2012;26:120–5.

45. Okamoto T, Coultas L, Metcalf D, van Delft MF, Glaser SP, Takiguchi M, et al. Enhanced stability of Mcl1, a prosurvival Bcl2 relative, blunts stress-induced apoptosis, causes male sterility, and promotes tumorigenesis. Proc Natl Acad Sci U S A. 2014;111:261–6.
46. Vela L, Marzo I. Bcl-2 family of proteins as drug targets for cancer chemotherapy: the long way of BH3 mimetics from bench to bedside. Curr Opin Pharmacol. 2015;23:74–81.
47. Tefferi A. Novel mutations and their functional and clinical relevance in myeloproliferative neoplasms: JAK2, MPL, TET2, ASXL1, CBL, IDH and IKZF1. Leukemia. 2010;24:1128–38.
48. Chan SM, Majeti R. Role of DNMT3A, TET2, and IDH1/2 mutations in pre-leukemic stem cells in acute myeloid leukemia. Int J Hematol. 2013;98:648–57.
49. Shlush LI, Zandi S, Mitchell A, Chen WC, Brandwein JM, Gupta V, et al. Identification of preleukemic hematopoietic stem cells in acute leukaemia. Nature. 2014;506:328–33.
50. Corces-Zimmerman MR, Hong WJ, Weissman IL, Medeiros BC, Majeti R. Preleukemic mutations in human acute myeloid leukemia affect epigenetic regulators and persist in remission. Proc Natl Acad Sci U S A. 2014;111:2548–53.
51. Guzman ML, Yang N, Sharma KK, Balys M, Corbett CA, Jordan CT, et al. Selective activity of the histone deacetylase inhibitor AR-42 against leukemia stem cells: a novel potential strategy in acute myelogenous leukemia. Mol Cancer Ther. 2014;13:1979–90.
52. Ho AD, Wagner W. Bone marrow niche and leukemia. Ernst Schering Found Symp Proc. 2006;5:125–39.
53. Nagasawa T. CXCL12/SDF-1 and CXCR4. Front Immunol. 2015;6:301.
54. Peled A, Tavor S. Role of CXCR4 in the pathogenesis of acute myeloid leukemia. Theranostics. 2013;3:34–9.
55. Tavor S, Petit I. Can inhibition of the SDF-1/CXCR4 axis eradicate acute leukemia? Semin Cancer Biol. 2010;20:178–85.
56. Konopleva M, Benton CB, Thall PF, Zeng Z, Shpall E, Ciurea S, et al. Leukemia cell mobilization with G-CSF plus plerixafor during busulfan-fludarabine conditioning for allogeneic stem cell transplantation. Bone Marrow Transplant. 2015;50:939–46.
57. Spencer JA, Ferraro F, Roussakis E, Klein A, Wu J, Runnels JM, et al. Direct measurement of local oxygen concentration in the bone marrow of live animals. Nature. 2014;508(7495):269–73.
58. Hoggatt J, Kfoury Y, Scadden DT. Hematopoietic stem cell niche in health and disease. Annu Rev Pathol. 2016;11:555–81.
59. Rouault-Pierre K, Hamilton A, Bonnet D. Effect of hypoxia-inducible factors in normal and leukemic stem cell regulation and their potential therapeutic impact. Expert Opin Biol Ther. 2016;16:463–76.
60. Vukovic M, Guitart AV, Sepulveda C, Villacreces A, O'Duibhir E, Panagopoulou TI, et al. Hif-1α and Hif-2α synergize to suppress AML development but are dispensable for disease maintenance. J Exp Med. 2015;212:2223–34.
61. Kipps TJ, Eradat H, Grosicki S, Catalano J, Cosolo W, Dyagil IS, et al. A phase 2 study of the BH3 mimetic BCL2 inhibitor navitoclax (ABT-263) with or without rituximab, in previously untreated B-cell chronic lymphocytic leukemia. Leuk Lymphoma. 2015;56:2826–33.
62. Brown JR, Tesar B, Yu L, Werner L, Takebe N, Mikler E, et al. Obatoclax in combination with fludarabine and rituximab is well-tolerated and shows promising clinical activity in relapsed chronic lymphocytic leukemia. Leuk Lymphoma. 2015;56:3336–42.
63. Thomas D, Powell JA, Vergez F, Segal DH, Nguyen NY, Baker A, et al. Targeting acute myeloid leukemia by dual inhibition of PI3K signaling and Cdk9-mediated Mcl-1 transcription. Blood. 2013;122:738–48.
64. Batlevi CL, Kasamon Y, Bociek RG, Lee P, Gore L, Copeland A, et al. ENGAGE- 501: phase 2 study of entinostat (SNDX-275) in relapsed and refractory Hodgkin lymphoma. Haematologica. 2016;101(8):968–75.
65. Zuber J, Shi J, Wang E, Rappaport AR, Herrmann H, Sison EA, et al. RNAi screen identifies Brd4 as a therapeutic target in acute myeloid leukaemia. Nature. 2011;478:524–8.

66. McGrath JP, Williamson KE, Balasubramanian S, Odate S, Arora S, Hatton C, et al. Pharmacological inhibition of the histone lysine demethylase KDM1A suppresses the growth of multiple acute myeloid leukemia subtypes. Cancer Res. 2016;76:1975–88.
67. Przespolewski A, Wang ES. Inhibitors of LSD1 as a potential therapy for acute myeloid leukemia. Expert Opin Investig Drugs; 2016, Apr 21:1–10. [Epub ahead of print]
68. Lehnertz B, Pabst C, Su L, Miller M, Liu F, Yi L, et al. The methyltransferase G9a regulates HoxA9-dependent transcription in AML. Genes Dev. 2014;28:317–27.
69. Wang Y, Liu Y, Tang F, Bernot KM, Schore R, Marcucci G, et al. Echinomycin protects mice against relapsed acute myeloid leukemia without adverse effect on hematopoietic stem cells. Blood. 2014;124(7):1127–35.
70. Bruedigam C, Bagger FO, Heidel FH, Paine Kuhn C, Guignes S, Song A, et al. Telomerase inhibition effectively targets mouse and human AML stem cells and delays relapse following chemotherapy. Cell Stem Cell. 2014;15:775–90.
71. Badar T, Handisides DR, Benito JM, Richie MA, Borthakur G, Jabbour E, et al. A phase I study of evofosfamide, an investigational hypoxia-activated prodrug, in patients with advanced leukemia. Am J Hematol. 2016;91:800–5.
72. Fiskus W, Sharma S, Saha S, Shah B, Devaraj SG, Sun B, et al. Pre-clinical efficacy of combined therapy with novel β-catenin antagonist BC2059 and histone deacetylase inhibitor against AML cells. Leukemia. 2015;29:1267–78.

CPI Antony Rowe
Chippenham, UK
2017-04-28 21:23